3D Printing and Bioprinting for Pharmaceutical and Medical Applications

The increasing availability and decreasing costs of 3D printing and bioprinting technologies are expanding opportunities to meet medical needs. *3D Printing and Bioprinting for Pharmaceutical and Medical Applications* discusses emerging approaches related to these game-changer technologies in such areas as drug development, medical devices, and bioreactors.

Key Features

- Offers an overview of applications, the market, and regulatory analysis.
- Analyzes market research of 3D printing and bioprinting technologies.
- Reviews 3D printing of novel pharmaceutical dosage forms for personalized therapies and for medical devices, as well as the benefits of 3D printing for training purposes.
- Covers 3D bioprinting technology, including the design of polymers and decellularized matrices for bio-inks development, elaboration of 3D models for drug evaluation, and 3D bioprinting for musculoskeletal, cardiovascular, central nervous system, ocular, and skin applications.
- Provides risk-benefit analysis of each application.
- Highlights bioreactors, regulatory aspects, frontiers, and challenges.

This book serves as an ideal reference for students, researchers, and professionals in materials science, bioengineering, the medical industry, and healthcare.

Emerging Materials and Technologies

Series Editor:
Boris I. Kharissov

The *Emerging Materials and Technologies* series is devoted to highlighting publications centered on emerging advanced materials and novel technologies. Attention is paid to those newly discovered or applied materials with potential to solve pressing societal problems and improve quality of life, corresponding to environmental protection, medicine, communications, energy, transportation, advanced manufacturing, and related areas.

The series takes into account that, under present strong demands for energy, material, and cost savings, as well as heavy contamination problems and worldwide pandemic conditions, the area of emerging materials and related scalable technologies is a highly interdisciplinary field, with the need for researchers, professionals, and academics across the spectrum of engineering and technological disciplines. The main objective of this book series is to attract more attention to these materials and technologies and invite conversation among the international R&D community.

Nanomaterials for Sustainable Energy Applications
Edited by Piyush Kumar Sonkar and Vellaichamy Ganesan

Materials Science to Combat COVID-19
Edited by Neeraj Dwivedi and Avanish Kumar Srivastava

Two-Dimensional Nanomaterials for Fire-Safe Polymers
Yuan Hu and Xin Wang

3D Printing and Bioprinting for Pharmaceutical and Medical Applications
Edited by Jose Luis Pedraz Muñoz, Laura Saenz del Burgo Martínez, Gustavo Puras Ochoa, and Jon Zarate Sesma

For more information about this series, please visit:
www.routledge.com/Emerging-Materials-and-Technologies/book-series/CRCEMT

3D Printing and Bioprinting for Pharmaceutical and Medical Applications

Edited by
Jose Luis Pedraz Muñoz,
Laura Saenz del Burgo Martínez,
Gustavo Puras Ochoa, and Jon Zarate Sesma

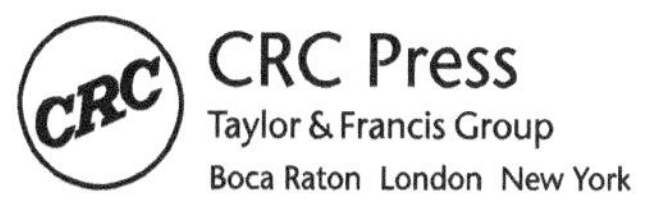

CRC Press is an imprint of the
Taylor & Francis Group, an **informa** business

Designed cover image: Shutterstock

First edition published 2024
by CRC Press
6000 Broken Sound Parkway NW, Suite 300, Boca Raton, FL 33487-2742

and by CRC Press
4 Park Square, Milton Park, Abingdon, Oxon, OX14 4RN

CRC Press is an imprint of Taylor & Francis Group, LLC

ISBN: 978-1-032-22866-2 (hbk)
ISBN: 978-1-032-22867-9 (pbk)
ISBN: 978-1-003-27456-8 (ebk)

DOI: 10.1201/9781003274568

Typeset in Times
by codeMantra

Contents

Editors

Jose Luis Pedraz Muñoz is a Professor and principal researcher in the NanoBioCel group at the University of the Basque Country (UPV/EHU). The research group belongs to the CIBER-BBN of the Carlos III Health Institute, where he serves as the head and director of the medicine formulation laboratory (ICTS) Nanbiosis. Dr. Pedraz is also founder and director of the Pharmaceutical Development Unit of the Basque Country, currently TECNALIA Pharma Labs integrated in the TECNALIA Corporation within a joint project with the UPV/EHU, of which he is scientific director. He had a PhD in Pharmacy from the University of Salamanca.

Laura Saenz del Burgo Martínez is a Professor at the University School of Nursing in Vitoria-Gasteiz and an Associate Professor at the University of the Basque Country (UPV/EHU) in the Department of Pharmacy and Food Sciences. She is a member of the NanoBioCel research group at UPV/EHU and part of the CIBER-BBN and gives technical assistance to the Nanbiosis platform (Drug Formulation). She received a PhD in Pharmacy from UPV/EHU and has worked as a postdoctoral researcher at the Institute of Molecular, Cell and Systems Biology, University of Glasgow.

Gustavo Puras Ochoa is a Professor at the University of the Basque Country (UPV/EHU), Department of Pharmacy and Food Sciences. He is a member of the NanoBioCel research group at UPV/EHU and the National System of Researchers of Mexico (SNI). He is a Professor in the Master's Program of Pharmacology, Development, Evaluation and Rational Use of Medicines at UPV/EHU. He received a PhD in Pharmacy from UPV/EHU.

Jon Zarate Sesma is an Associate Professor in the Department of Pharmacy and Food Sciences, Professor of the Doctoral Program in Drug Research and Evaluation, Application of Pharmaceutical Technology to the Development of Advanced Therapies, and Professor in the Master's Program in Pharmacology, Development, Evaluation and Rational Use of Medicines at the University of the Basque Country (UPV/EHU). He is a member of the NanoBioCel research group at the same institution. He received a PhD in Pharmacy from UPV/EHU.

Contributors

Mohamed Abbas
Electrical Engineering Department, College of Engineering
King Khalid University
Abha, Saudi Arabia
and
Computers and Communications Department, College of Engineering
Delta University for Science and Technology
Gamasa, Egypt

Rouhollah Mehdinavaz Aghdam
School of Metallurgy and Materials Engineering, College of Engineering
University of Tehran
Tehran, Iran

Fouad Alhakim-Khalak
NanoBioCel Research Group, Laboratory of Pharmacy and Pharmaceutical Technology, Department of Pharmacy and Food Science, Faculty of Pharmacy
University of the Basque Country (UPV/EHU)
Vitoria-Gasteiz, Spain
and
Networking Research Centre of Bioengineering, Biomaterials and Nanomedicine (CIBER-BBN)
Institute of Health Carlos III
Madrid, Spain
and
Bioaraba
NanoBioCel Research Group
Vitoria-Gasteiz, Spain

Mohammed Alqahtani
Radiological Sciences Department, College of Applied Medical Sciences
King Khalid University
Abha, Saudi Arabia
and
BioImaging Unit, Space Research Centre, Department of Physics and Astronomy
University of Leicester
Leicester, United Kingdom

Qonita Kurnia Anjan
School of Pharmacy
Queen's University Belfast, Medical Biology Centre
Belfast, United Kingdom

Lijia Cheng
School of Basic Medical Sciences, Clinical Medical College & Affiliated Hospital
Chengdu University
Chengdu, China

Khandmaa Dashnyam
Institute of Tissue Regeneration Engineering
Dankook University
Cheonan, South Korea

Luis Diaz-Gomez
Departamento de Farmacología, Farmacia y Tecnología Farmacéutica, I+D Farma (GI-1645), Facultad de Farmacia, Instituto de Materiais (iMATUS) and Health Research Institute of Santiago de Compostela (IDIS)
Universidad de Santiago de Compostela
Santiago de Compostela, Spain

Patricia Diaz-Rodriguez
Departamento de Farmacología, Farmacia y Tecnología Farmacéutica, I+D Farma (GI-1645), Facultad de Farmacia, Instituto de Materiais (iMATUS) and Health Research Institute of Santiago de Compostela (IDIS)
Universidad de Santiago de Compostela
Santiago de Compostela, Spain

Garry Duffy
CÚRAM, Science Foundation Ireland Research Centre for Medical Devices
University of Galway
Galway, Ireland
and
Discipline of Anatomy and Regenerative Medicine Institute (REMEDI), School of Medicine, College of Medicine, Nursing and Health Sciences
University of Galway
Galway, Ireland
and
Science Foundation Ireland Advanced Materials and BioEngineering Research Centre (AMBER)
Trinity College Dublin & University of Galway
Galway, Ireland

Barkan Kagan Durukan
Department of Metallurgical and Materials Engineering
Atilim University
Ankara, Turkey

Lucía Enriquez-Rodríguez
NanoBioCel Research Group, Laboratory of Pharmacy and Pharmaceutical Technology, Department of Pharmacy and Food Science, Faculty of Pharmacy
University of the Basque Country (UPV/EHU)
Vitoria-Gasteiz, Spain
and
Networking Research Centre of Bioengineering, Biomaterials and Nanomedicine (CIBER-BBN)
Institute of Health Carlos III
Madrid, Spain
and
Bioaraba
NanoBioCel Research Group
Vitoria-Gasteiz, Spain

Jasper Foolen
Orthopaedic Biomechanics, Department of Biomedical Engineering
Eindhoven University of Technology
Eindhoven, the Netherlands
and
Institute of Complex Molecular Systems
Eindhoven University of Technology
Eindhoven, the Netherlands

Idoia Gallego
Laboratory of Pharmaceutics, NanoBioCel Group, Faculty of Pharmacy
University of the Basque Country UPV/EHU
Vitoria-Gasteiz, Spain
and
Biomedical Research Networking Centre in Bioengineering, Biomaterials and Nanomedicine (CIBER-BBN)
Institute of Health Carlos III
Vitoria-Gasteiz, Spain
and
Bioaraba
NanoBioCel Research Group
Vitoria-Gasteiz, Spain

Jiaqi Gao
School of Pharmacy
Queen's University Belfast, Medical Biology Centre
Belfast, United Kingdom

Rossana García-Castro
Gradocell
Parque Científico de Madrid
Tres Cantos, Madrid, Spain

Fátima García-Villén
NanoBioCel Research Group, Laboratory of Pharmacy and Pharmaceutical Technology, Department of Pharmacy and Food Science, Faculty of Pharmacy
University of the Basque Country (UPV/EHU)
Vitoria-Gasteiz, Spain
and
Networking Research Centre of Bioengineering, Biomaterials and Nanomedicine (CIBER-BBN)
Institute of Health Carlos III
Madrid, Spain
and
Bioaraba
NanoBioCel Research Group
Vitoria-Gasteiz, Spain

Luca Gasperini
3B's Research Group, I3Bs - Research Institute on Biomaterials, Biodegradables and Biomimetics
University of Minho, Headquarters of the European Institute of Excellence on Tissue Engineering and Regenerative Medicine, AvePark, Parque de Ciência e Tecnologia, Zona Industrial da Gandra
Barco, Guimarães, Portugal
and
ICVS/3B's–PT Government Associate Laboratory
Braga/Guimarães, Portugal

Carmine Gentile
University of Technology Sydney
Ultimo, NSW, Australia

Rand Ghanma
School of Pharmacy
Queen's University Belfast, Medical Biology Centre
Belfast, United Kingdom

Hodei Gómez-Fernández
Laboratory of Pharmaceutics, NanoBioCel Group, Faculty of Pharmacy
University of the Basque Country UPV/EHU
Vitoria-Gasteiz, Spain
and
AJL Ophthalmic S.A.
Miñano, Spain

Álvaro Goyanes
Department of Pharmaceutics, UCL School of Pharmacy
University College London
London, United Kingdom
and
FabRx Ltd.
Henwood House, Henwood
Ashford, United Kingdom
and
Departamento de Farmacología, Farmacia y Tecnología Farmacéutica, I+D Farma Group (GI-1645), Facultad de Farmacia, iMATUS and Health Research Institute of Santiago de Compostela (IDIS)
Universidade de Santiago de Compostela (USC)
Santiago de Compostela, Spain

Achmad Himawan
School of Pharmacy
Queen's University Belfast, Medical Biology Centre
Belfast, United Kingdom

Qingxi Hu
Rapid Manufacturing Engineering Center, School of Mechatronic Engineering and Automation
Shanghai University
Shanghai, China
and
Shanghai Key Laboratory of Intelligent Manufacturing and Robotics, School of Mechatronic Engineering and Automation
Shanghai University
Shanghai, China
and
National Demonstration Center for Experimental Engineering Training Education
Shanghai University
Shanghai, China

Alireza Jenabi
School of Metallurgy and Materials Engineering, College of Engineering
University of Tehran
Tehran, Iran

Hirokazu Kaji
Department of Biomechanics, Institute of Biomaterials and Bioengineering
Tokyo Medical and Dental University
Tokyo, Japan

Hae-Won Kim
Institute of Tissue Regeneration Engineering
Dankook University
Cheonan, South Korea
and
Department of Nanobiomedical Science, BK21 NBM Global Research Center for Regenerative Medicine
Dankook University
Cheonan, South Korea
and
Mechanobiology Dental Medicine Research Center
Dankook University
Cheonan, South Korea

Marcelo Javier Kogan
Departamento de Química Farmacológica y Toxicológica, Facultad de Ciencias Químicas y Farmacéuticas
Universidad de Chile, Santos Dumont, Independencia
Santiago, Chile

Anna Korelidou
School of Pharmacy, Queen's University Belfast
Medical Biology Centre
Belfast, United Kingdom

Markel Lafuente-Merchan
Laboratory of Pharmaceutics, NanoBioCel Group, Faculty of Pharmacy
University of the Basque Country UPV/EHU
Vitoria-Gasteiz, Spain
and
Biomedical Research Networking Centre in Bioengineering, Biomaterials and Nanomedicine (CIBER-BBN)
Institute of Health Carlos III
Vitoria-Gasteiz, Spain
and
Bioaraba
NanoBioCel Research Group
Vitoria-Gasteiz, Spain

Eneko Larrañeta
School of Pharmacy
Queen's University Belfast, Medical Biology Centre
Belfast, United Kingdom

Jung-Hwan Lee
Institute of Tissue Regeneration Engineering
Dankook University
Cheonan, South Korea
and

Department of Nanobiomedical Science, BK21 NBM Global Research Center for Regenerative Medicine
Dankook University
Cheonan, South Korea
and
Mechanobiology Dental Medicine Research Center
Dankook University
Cheonan, South Korea

Linlin Li
School of Pharmacy
Queen's University Belfast, Medical Biology Centre
Belfast, United Kingdom

Suihong Liu
Centre for Translational Bone, Joint and Soft Tissue Research, Faculty of Medicine and University Hospital Carl Gustav Carus
Technische Universität Dresden
Dresden, Germany
and
Rapid Manufacturing Engineering Center, School of Mechatronic Engineering and Automation
Shanghai University
Shanghai, China
and
Shanghai Key Laboratory of Intelligent Manufacturing and Robotics, School of Mechatronic Engineering and Automation
Shanghai University
Shanghai, China

Yakui Liu
Rapid Manufacturing Engineering Center, School of Mechatronic Engineering and Automation
Shanghai University
Shanghai, China

Stephanie Ly
University of Technology Sydney
Ultimo, NSW, Australia

Iván Maldonado
Laboratory of Pharmaceutics, NanoBioCel Group, Faculty of Pharmacy
University of the Basque Country UPV/EHU
Vitoria-Gasteiz, Spain
and
Biomedical Research Networking Centre in Bioengineering, Biomaterials and Nanomedicine (CIBER-BBN)
Institute of Health Carlos III
Vitoria-Gasteiz, Spain
and
Bioaraba
NanoBioCel Research Group
Vitoria-Gasteiz, Spain

Abhik Mallick
CÚRAM, Science Foundation Ireland Research Centre for Medical Devices
University of Galway
Galway, Ireland

Alexandra P. Marques
3B's Research Group, I3Bs - Research Institute on Biomaterials, Biodegradables and Biomimetics
University of Minho, Headquarters of the European Institute of Excellence on Tissue Engineering and Regenerative Medicine, AvePark, Parque de Ciência e Tecnologia, Zona Industrial da Gandra, Barco
Guimarães, Portugal
and
ICVS/3B's–PT Government Associate Laboratory
Braga/Guimarães, Portugal

Eva Martín-Becerra
Gradocell
Parque Científico de Madrid
Tres Cantos, Madrid, Spain

Niina Matthews
University of Technology Sydney
Ultimo, NSW, Australia

Mary B. McGuckin
School of Pharmacy
Queen's University Belfast, Medical Biology Centre
Belfast, United Kingdom

Tapas Mitra
Discipline of Anatomy and Regenerative Medicine Institute (REMEDI), School of Medicine, College of Medicine, Nursing and Health Sciences
University of Galway
Galway, Ireland

Yara Naser
School of Pharmacy
Queen's University Belfast, Medical Biology Centre
Belfast, United Kingdom

Jorge Ordoyo-Pascual
NanoBioCel Research Group, Laboratory of Pharmacy and Pharmaceutical Technology, Department of Pharmacy and Food Science, Faculty of Pharmacy
University of the Basque Country (UPV/EHU), Paseo de la Universidad 7
Vitoria-Gasteiz, Spain
and
Networking Research Centre of Bioengineering, Biomaterials and Nanomedicine (CIBER-BBN)
Institute of Health Carlos III
Madrid, Spain
and
Bioaraba
NanoBioCel Research Group
Vitoria-Gasteiz, Spain

Muireann O'Reilly
Discipline of Anatomy and Regenerative Medicine Institute (REMEDI), School of Medicine, College of Medicine, Nursing and Health Sciences
University of Galway
Galway, Ireland
and
CÚRAM, Science Foundation Ireland Research Centre for Medical Devices
University of Galway
Galway, Ireland

Serge Ostrovidov
Department of Biomechanics, Institute of Biomaterials and Bioengineering
Tokyo Medical and Dental University
Tokyo, Japan

Santiago Daniel Palma
Unidad de Investigación y Desarrollo en Tecnología Farmacéutica (UNITEFA), CONICET and Departamento de Farmacia, Facultad de Ciencias Químicas
Universidad Nacional de Córdoba, Ciudad Universitaria
Córdoba, Argentina

Jeong-Hui Park
Institute of Tissue Regeneration Engineering
Dankook University
Cheonan, South Korea
and
Department of Nanobiomedical Science, BK21 NBM Global Research Center for Regenerative Medicine
Dankook University
Cheonan, South Korea
and

Mechanobiology Dental Medicine Research Center
Dankook University
Cheonan, South Korea

Jose Luis Pedraz Muñoz
NanoBioCel Research Group, Laboratory of Pharmacy and Pharmaceutical Technology, Faculty of Pharmacy
University of the Basque Country (UPV/EHU)
Vitoria-Gasteiz, Spain
and
Networking Research Centre of Bioengineering, Biomaterials and Nanomedicine
Institute of Health Carlos III
Madrid, Spain

Ke Peng
School of Pharmacy
Queen's University Belfast, Medical Biology Centre
Belfast, United Kingdom

Camila Picco
School of Pharmacy
Queen's University Belfast, Medical Biology Centre
Belfast, United Kingdom

Gustavo Puras
NanoBioCel Research Group, Laboratory of Pharmacy and Pharmaceutical Technology, Department of Pharmacy and Food Science, Faculty of Pharmacy
University of the Basque Country (UPV/EHU)
Vitoria-Gasteiz, Spain
and
Networking Research Centre of Bioengineering, Biomaterials and Nanomedicine (CIBER-BBN)
Institute of Health Carlos III
Madrid, Spain
and
Bioaraba
NanoBioCel Research Group
Vitoria-Gasteiz, Spain

Seeram Ramakrishna
Center for Nanofibers and Nanotechnology, Department of Mechanical Engineering
National University Singapore
Singapore, Singapore

Murugan Ramalingam
Institute of Tissue Regeneration Engineering
Dankook University
Cheonan, South Korea
and
Department of Nanobiomedical Science, BK21 NBM Global Research Center for Regenerative Medicine
Dankook University
Cheonan, South Korea
and
Mechanobiology Dental Medicine Research Center
Dankook University
Cheonan, South Korea
and
School of Basic Medical Sciences, Clinical Medical College & Affiliated Hospital
Chengdu University
Chengdu, China
and
Department of Metallurgical and Materials Engineering
Atilim University
Ankara, Turkey

Daniel Andrés Real
Departamento de Química Farmacológica y Toxicológica, Facultad de Ciencias Químicas y Farmacéuticas

Universidad de Chile
Independencia, Santiago, Chile

Juan Pablo Real
Unidad de Investigación y Desarrollo en Tecnología Farmacéutica (UNITEFA), CONICET and Departamento de Farmacia, Facultad de Ciencias Químicas
Universidad Nacional de Córdoba, Ciudad Universitaria
Córdoba, Argentina

Daniel P. Reis
3B's Research Group, I3Bs - Research Institute on Biomaterials, Biodegradables and Biomimetics, University of Minho, Headquarters of the European Institute of Excellence on Tissue Engineering and Regenerative Medicine, AvePark, Parque de Ciência e Tecnologia
Zona Industrial da Gandra, Barco
Guimarães, Portugal
and
ICVS/3B's–PT Government Associate Laboratory
Braga/Guimarães, Portugal

Sandra Ruiz-Alonso
NanoBioCel Research Group, Laboratory of Pharmacy and Pharmaceutical Technology. Department of Pharmacy and Food Science, Faculty of Pharmacy
University of the Basque Country (UPV/EHU), Paseo de la Universidad 7
Vitoria-Gasteiz, Spain
and
Networking Research Centre of Bioengineering, Biomaterials and Nanomedicine (CIBER-BBN)
Institute of Health Carlos III
Madrid, Spain
and
Bioaraba
NanoBioCel Research Group
Vitoria-Gasteiz, Spain

Laura Saenz del Burgo
NanoBioCel Research Group, Laboratory of Pharmacy and Pharmaceutical Technology, Department of Pharmacy and Food Science, Faculty of Pharmacy
University of the Basque Country (UPV/EHU)
Vitoria-Gasteiz, Spain
and
Networking Research Centre of Bioengineering, Biomaterials and Nanomedicine (CIBER-BBN)
Institute of Health Carlos III
Madrid, Spain
and
Bioaraba
NanoBioCel Research Group
Vitoria-Gasteiz, Spain

Myriam Sainz-Ramos
Laboratory of Pharmaceutics, NanoBioCel Group, Faculty of Pharmacy
University of the Basque Country UPV/EHU
Vitoria-Gasteiz, Spain
and
Biomedical Research Networking Centre in Bioengineering, Biomaterials and Nanomedicine (CIBER-BBN)
Institute of Health Carlos III
Vitoria-Gasteiz, Spain
and
Bioaraba
NanoBioCel Research Group
Vitoria-Gasteiz, Spain

Hilal Turkoglu Sasmazel
Department of Metallurgical and Materials Engineering
Atilim University
Ankara, Turkey

Denis Scaini
International School for Advanced Studies (SISSA/ISAS)
Trieste, Italy
and
Basque Foundation for Science Ikerbasque
Bilbao, Spain
and
Faculty of Pharmacy
University of Basque Country
Vitoria-Gasteiz, Spain

Iria Seoane-Viaño
Department of Pharmaceutics, UCL School of Pharmacy
University College London
London, United Kingdom
and
Department of Pharmacology, Pharmacy and Pharmaceutical Technology, Paraquasil Group (GI-2109), Faculty of Pharmacy
University of Santiago de Compostela (USC), and Health Research Institute of Santiago de Compostela (IDIS)
Santiago de Compostela, Spain

Zheng Shi
School of Basic Medical Sciences, Clinical Medical College & Affiliated Hospital
Chengdu University
Chengdu, China

Janne Spierings
Orthopaedic Biomechanics, Department of Biomedical Engineering
Eindhoven University of Technology
Eindhoven, the Netherlands
and
Institute of Complex Molecular Systems
Eindhoven University of Technology
Eindhoven, The Netherlands

Ana Torres-García
Gradocell
Parque Científico de Madrid, Tres Cantos
Madrid, Spain

Ilia Villate-Beitia
NanoBioCel Research Group, Laboratory of Pharmacy and Pharmaceutical Technology. Department of Pharmacy and Food Science, Faculty of Pharmacy
University of the Basque Country (UPV/EHU), Paseo de la Universidad 7
Vitoria-Gasteiz, Spain
and
Networking Research Centre of Bioengineering, Biomaterials and Nanomedicine (CIBER-BBN)
Institute of Health Carlos III
Madrid, Spain
and
Bioaraba
NanoBioCel Research Group
Vitoria-Gasteiz, Spain

Victoria Ward
Discipline of Anatomy and Regenerative Medicine Institute (REMEDI), School of Medicine, College of Medicine, Nursing and Health Sciences
University of Galway
Galway, Ireland
and
Science Foundation Ireland Advanced Materials and BioEngineering Research Centre (AMBER)
Trinity College Dublin & University of Galway
Galway, Ireland

Jon Zarate
NanoBioCel Research Group, Laboratory of Pharmacy and Pharmaceutical Technology, Department of Pharmacy and Food Science, Faculty of Pharmacy
University of the Basque Country (UPV/EHU)
Vitoria-Gasteiz, Spain
and
Networking Research Centre of Bioengineering, Biomaterials and Nanomedicine (CIBER-BBN)
Institute of Health Carlos III
Madrid, Spain
and
Bioaraba
NanoBioCel Research Group
Vitoria-Gasteiz, Spain

Haiguang Zhang
Rapid Manufacturing Engineering Center, School of Mechatronic Engineering and Automation
Shanghai University
Shanghai, China
and
Shanghai Key Laboratory of Intelligent Manufacturing and Robotics, School of Mechatronic Engineering and Automation
Shanghai University
Shanghai, China
and
National Demonstration Center for Experimental Engineering Training Education
Shanghai University
Shanghai, China

1 3D Printing and Bioprinting Technologies in Pharmaceutics

Commercial Perspectives and Market Analytics

Suihong Liu
Technische Universität Dresden
Shanghai University

Yakui Liu
Shanghai University

Qingxi Hu and Haiguang Zhang
Shanghai University

Jeong-Hui Park
Dankook University

Khandmaa Dashnyam
Dankook University

Jung-Hwan Lee
Dankook University

Lijia Cheng and Zheng Shi
Clinical Medical College & Affiliated
Hospital, Chengdu University

Barkan Kagan Durukan and
Hilal Turkoglu Sasmazel
Atilim University

DOI: 10.1201/9781003274568-1

Serge Ostrovidov and Hirokazu Kaji
Institute of Biomaterials and Bioengineering,
Tokyo Medical and Dental University

Rouhollah Mehdinavaz Aghdam and Alireza Jenabi
College of Engineering, University of Tehran

Mohammed Alqahtani
College of Applied Medical Sciences, King Khalid University
University of Leicester

Mohamed Abbas
College of Engineering, King Khalid University
College of Engineering, Delta University
for Science and Technology

Jose Luis Pedraz Muñoz
University of the Basque Country (UPV/EHU)
Networking Research Centre of Bioengineering,
Biomaterials and Nanomedicine,
Institute of Health Carlos III

Seeram Ramakrishna
National University Singapore

Hae-Won Kim
Dankook University

Murugan Ramalingam
Dankook University
Clinical Medical College & Affiliated
Hospital, Chengdu University
Atilim University

CONTENTS

1.1 INTRODUCTION

Three-dimensional (3D) printing is a fast-emerging applied technology that has had a major impact on healthcare applications, particularly the pharmaceutical field, over the last decades. 3D printing, also known as additive manufacturing (AM), has been used for building a wide range of 3D structures and complex geometries layer by layer through a computer-aided design since the early 1980s [1]. 3D printing widens the manufacturing window, allowing the production of customized medical devices from metals, ceramics, and polymers without the need for molds or machining which was typically used in conventional formative and subtractive manufacturing [1,2]. Since the early 2000s, 3D printing has been successfully applied in pharmaceutics, tissue engineering, and regenerative medicine due to its capability for the fabrication of 3D biological constructs with high shape complexity and fidelity [3,4]. 3D printing involving biological substances is called 3D bioprinting, where bioinks, which comprise a choice of biomaterials, cells, drugs, proteins, or growth factors, play a major role in printing desired constructs or devices [5]. 3D bioprinting could transform the future of medicine, that is, the way drugs and complex living tissues are made.

Along with technological advancement, the commercial market value of 3D bioprinting is growing day by day. For example, the global 3D bioprinting market size reached 1.7 billion USD in 2021 and is expected to expand at a compound annual growth rate of 21% by 2030 [6]. According to the latest market research by Mordor Intelligence, the global bioprinting industry was valued at 586.13 million USD in 2019 and is expected to reach 1,949.94 million USD by 2025 [7]. Meanwhile, numerous new companies have emerged to exploit 3D printing, and most of them are based on their unique value proposition of providing bioprinting services or partnerships for manufacturing medical devices, pills, or tissue constructs. The majority of these bioprinting companies are based in North America, and the rest in Europe and Asia. Statistics shows that almost three-quarters of all bioprinting companies have been established within the last 5–10 years. In fact, 20% of all the companies have been in operation for less than 3 years, and this shows the dynamism of this sector [8]. The development of these companies has also further promoted the expanded applications of 3D bioprinting in drug discovery, development, and delivery with a huge commercial market for the pharmaceutical industry [9–11].

Considering these aspects, this chapter deals with 3D printing and bioprinting technologies in pharmaceuticals and related fields from the commercial perspectives and market analytics.

1.2 IMPACT OF BIOPRINTING ON PHARMACEUTICS

Rapid progress of 3D bioprinting in the recent decade has had a revolutionary impact on tissue engineering and biomedicine, particularly in pharmaceutics. The traditional development process of new drugs was overturned by this novel technique, opening a new era of pharmaceutical industry as various 3D bioprinting technologies developed. Currently, the primary applications of 3D bioprinting focus on pharmaceutics, tissue engineering, and regenerative medicine. With regard to pharmaceutical aspects, the 3D bioprinting technique could be applied in different fields, including printing of personalized medicine (i.e., drug products), drug screening and delivery, and vaccines, as shown in Figure 1.1. With the development of precision medicine, there is increasing interest in customized drugs, and 3D bioprinting plays an immense role in this process due to its unique advantages. Meanwhile, high-throughput screening (HTS) of drugs also has gained benefits. However, the rapid development of 3D bioprinting is inseparable from the development of bioinks. Among the various bioinks, hydrogel as a common biomaterial plays a vital role in the exploration of bioinks because it could mimic ECM microenvironments for cell survival and proliferation; meanwhile, it is also widely applied in biomedical developments, including drug delivery, target discovery, and drug penetration, as shown in Figure 1.2 [12]. Due to the diversity and different requirements of drug discovery and development, different 3D bioprinting technologies are used in different aspects during the development of new drugs to meet the needs. The main applications of different bioprinting techniques are listed in Table 1.1, as well as corresponding principles of each technique, their strengths and limitations, and specific application cases in pharmaceutics of different bioprinting approaches. For example, the inkjet-based bioprinting technique has high printing resolution and good adaptability and formability for rather low-viscosity bioinks (3.5–12 mPa/s), and is thus widely used in drug screening, particularly in high-throughput drug screening, due to its capability of rapid and mass production. This strategy not only could structure

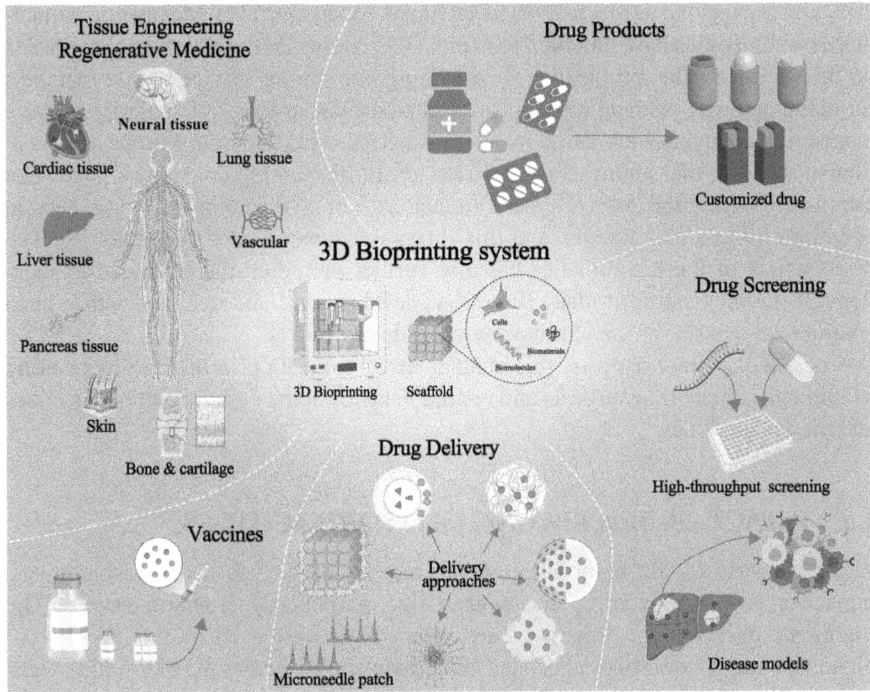

FIGURE 1.1 Schematic showing the 3D bioprinting applications in pharmaceutics and therapeutics.

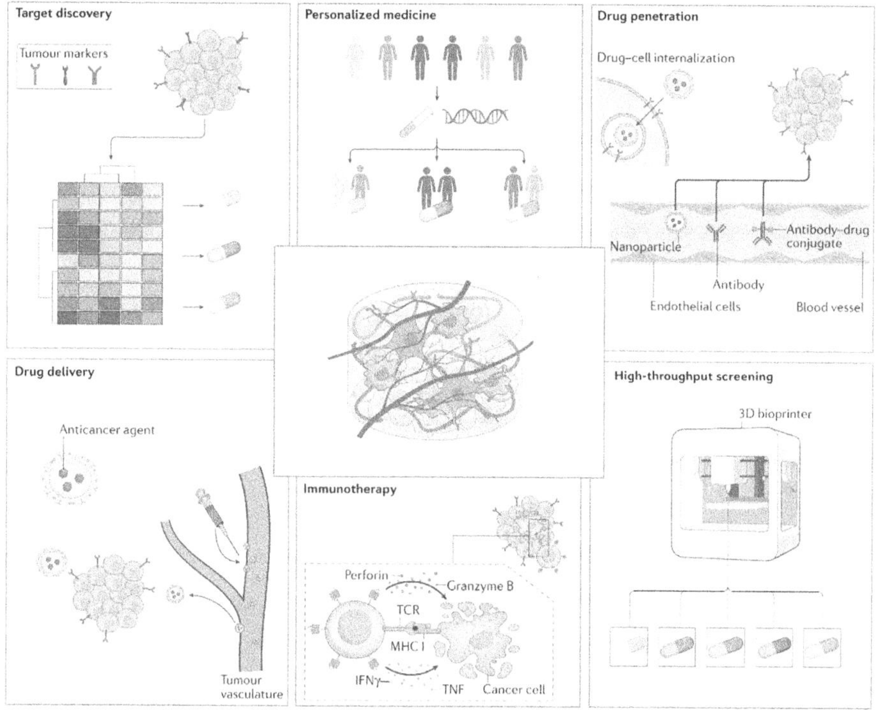

FIGURE 1.2 Applications of 3D-bioprinted constructs for drug developments and efficacy. Source: Neufeld et al. [12] used with permission.

TABLE 1.1
Key Bioprinting Techniques with Their Merits and Demerits in Pharmaceuticals and Tissue Therapeutics

	Principle	Strengths	Limitations	Applications
Extrusion-based bioprinting	Use pneumatic-, piston-, or solenoid-driven actuators to extrude bioinks through a nozzle onto a printing substrate	• Compatibility with viscosities in a wide range • Rapid prototyping	• Substantial cell damage due to shear stress • Not practical for high-throughput bioprinting	Disease model [24] Drug delivery [25] Drug screening [26] Tissue engineering [27–29]
Inkjet-based bioprinting	Use thermal, piezoelectric, or electromagnetic approaches to dispense precise droplets of bioink on printing stage.	• High resolution; • Compatibility with small viscosities in the range of 3.5–12 mPa/s;	• Frequent nozzle clogging; • potential damage to cells; • material restrictions;	Drug delivery [30]; Drug screening [31]; Tissue engineering [32];

(Continued)

TABLE 1.1 (*Continued*)
Key Bioprinting Techniques with Their Merits and Demerits in Pharmaceuticals and Tissue Therapeutics

	Principle	Strengths	Limitations	Applications
DLP-based bioprinting	Use the micro-optoelectromechanical system to monitor the intensity of light for every pixel of the printing area, wherein light polymerizes the polymer materials that are sensitive to light	• Complex designs with high resolution • Compatibility with viscosities in a wide range	• Material restrictions • High equipment costs • Large time expenditure • Potential damage to cells	Disease model [33] Tissue engineering [34]
Laser-based bioprinting	A laser pulse is focused on the donor ribbon and converted into a shockwave to activate the bioink layer underneath. Then, the bioink travels to the recipient slide from the donor slide.	• High feature resolution • Good cell viability	• High equipment costs • Labor-intensive and time-consuming preparation • Material restrictions	Disease model [35] Tissue engineering [36,37]

much more close to the human body 3D microenvironment than to the 2D well plate but also could accelerate the drug development process. Notably, the appropriate or best application of different bioprinting techniques in pharmaceutics could be successfully achieved via the selection and/or combination of the existed bioprinting approach, as well as further developing or upgrading the bioprinting strategy according to the specific requirements of drug development cases [9,11,13]. Thus, we could find that the 3D bioprinting technique has great impact on current drug discovery and development, and the current bioprinting technique performed an opening and multi-possible development trend for future biomedical application.

With regard to the drug product application, the current developments of new drugs mostly focus on customized (i.e., personalized) drugs, toward patient-specific delivery or personalization, to shift the current practice of producing medicines with a 'one-size-fits-all' manner [9,13]. Commonly, the fabrication process of drug does not contain living components (such as cells); thus, there has been a significant development in the 3D bioprinting of drug products in recent years. As shown in Figure 1.3, 3D printing has been applied in different aspects of drug products and also has shown several unique advantages, such as cost-effectiveness, personalized geometrics and regiments, continuous manufacturing, and personalized medicines. Personalized medicine could integrate the pharmacogenetic profiles and pharmacokinetic characteristics of patients individually or in a subgroup with clinical tools and treatments that will consider their genetic variations to develop therapies that are suitable for their conditions, while reducing adverse drug reactions and delivering

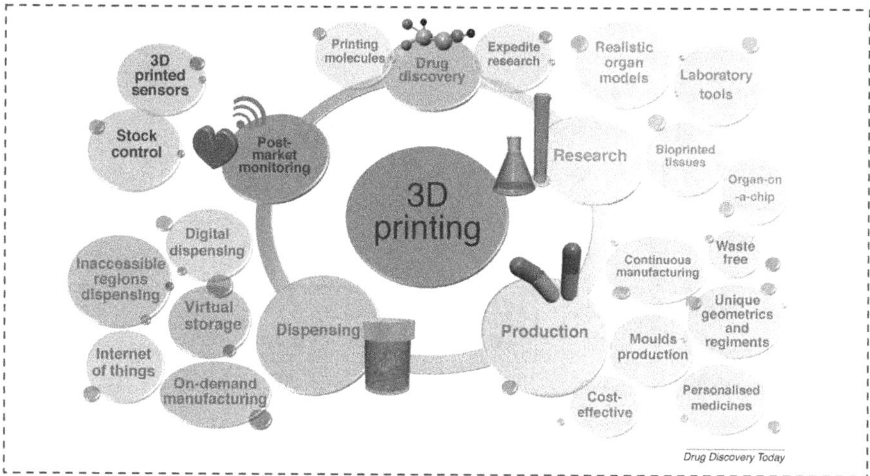

FIGURE 1.3 Graphical representation of potential applications and advantages of 3D printing in pharmaceutics and therapeutics. Source: Awad et al. [9] used with permission.

more efficient treatments [13,14]. In this process, different components of drugs can be formulated and spatially assembled by using the 3D printing technique according to the personalized requirements of patients, and the drugs could also be wrapped by different materials to control and adjust the releasing or working time. Moreover, other different specific functions of personalized medicine (such as drug targeted releasing) could be designed and performed via combining 3D printing with other techniques, such as smart materials. However, the printing resolution of 3D bioprinting influences the efficacy of produced drugs [9,15] and thus needs further improvement for the precision medicine. More details of fabrication strategies, principles, and progress of personalized drugs with different printing technologies can be found in Wallis et al. and Trenfield et al. [13,15].

Drug screening is an extremely important step in drug development, which is used to identify and optimize potential drugs and components that will be evaluated in clinical trials to achieve a good evaluation of drug efficiency and potential toxicity [4,16]. Thus, 3D bioprinting has been widely applied for drug screening aspects, attracting more and more pharmaceutical companies' and researchers' sight. Currently, the main applications of bioprinting techniques include but are not limited to fabrication of 3D drug models (disease models), HTS of drug candidates, and precision medicine [10], as shown in Figures 1.1 and 1.2. Among them, the HTS of drug candidates is the main application aspect of bioprinting [17] because 3D bioprinting can produce uniform 3D drug models in batches within a short duration. For example, the HTS of a tumor drug can be performed by using a 3D-printed hanging drop dripper (3D-phd) for studying tumor spheroid generation, drug-induced cell death, and metastasis in extracellular matrix gel (the schematic diagram is shown in Figure 1.4) [17]. Drug screening is a critical step during the drug development process, which contributes to reduce the unnecessary time and money investments. Importantly, thanks to 3D (bio)printing ineffective drugs or components can be excluded in the

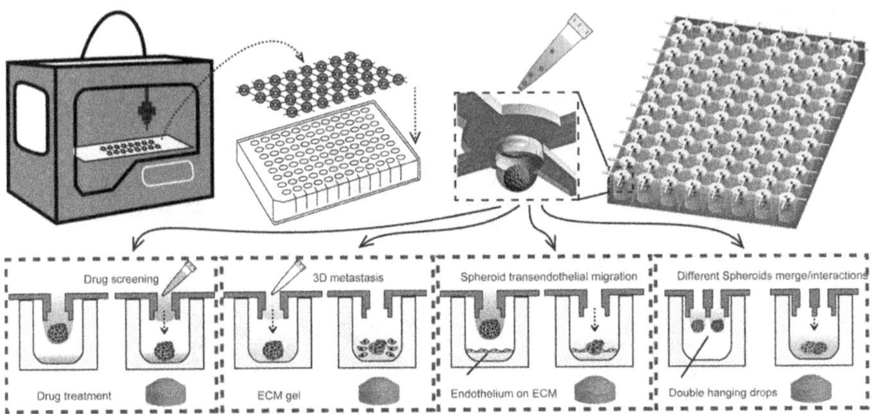

FIGURE 1.4 Graphical representation of high-throughput drug screening using a 3D printed hanging drop dripper (3D-phd) for studying tumor spheroid generation, drug-induced cell death, and metastasis in extracellular matrix gel. Source: Zhao et al. [17] used with permission.

early preclinical phase [18]. In addition, in future, 3D bioprinting could also reduce and replace the costs of drug development in the clinical phase via the fabrication of an *in vitro* bio-functional living system, which will serve not only as a disease model for functional testing of drugs and as a normal native-mimic tissue/organ model system for biosecurity and toxicity of drugs [19,20]. Drug screening research is being carried out in recent years by using the 3D bioprinting technique, and many valuable research works and achievements were proposed [21,22]. Therefore, it is indisputable and predicts the fact that 3D bioprinting will further innovate drug screening and occupy a main position in the drug development as well as commercial market in pharmaceutics.

The 3D bioprinting technology is also rapidly becoming a powerful method in vaccine development and delivery, including directly producing RNA vaccines and therapeutic drugs [23], as shown in Figure 1.5. The current advancement and more details of the application of 3D bioprinting for manufacturing vaccines, therapeutics, and delivery systems can be referred to in Yi et al. [23]. Nevertheless, it can be predicted that there is great potential and commercial market prospect of 3D bioprinting techniques in vaccine development and corresponding delivery system exploration.

1.3 CURRENT ADVANCES OF BIOPRINTING TECHNOLOGIES IN PHARMACEUTICS

Currently, the majority of bioprinting research in pharmaceutical applications focuses on the drug screening at early-phase drug development via the fabrication of physiologically relevant 3D tissue models [10,38,39]. Such screening strategy could exclude the ineffective and/or unacceptable drugs or toxic compounds as early as possible to accelerate drug discovery and reduce the cost burden. In addition, the 3D bioprinting technique contributes to high-throughput sample evaluation

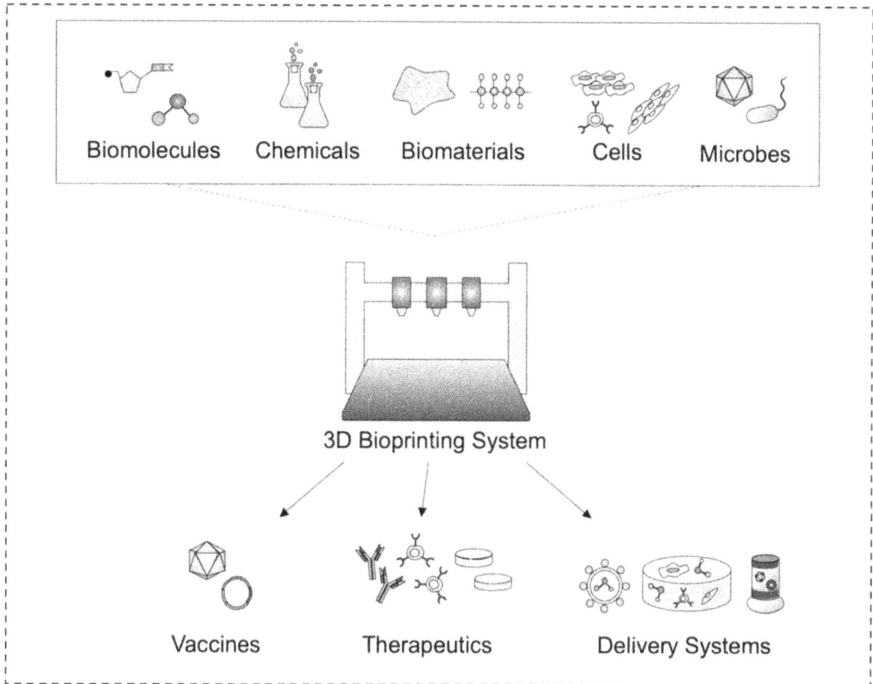

FIGURE 1.5 Applications of 3D bioprinting for manufacturing of vaccines, therapeutics, and delivery systems. Source: Yi et al. [23] used with permission.

with the advantages of high yield, less time consumption, and convenience culture medium replenishment. Thus, numerous same constructs can be bioprinted for drug HTS, which enables parallel investigation of efficacy or toxicity of hundreds of drugs [40]. For instance, Demirci et al. developed an acoustic-based bioprinting method with various cells (including mouse embryonic stem cells (ESCs), fibroblasts, AML-12 hepatocytes, human Raji cells, and HL-1 cardiomyocytes) for HTS applications [41]. Single cells (or a few cells) ejected from an open pool in acoustic picoliter droplets of around 37 μm in diameter at rates varying from 1 to 10,000 droplets per second, while the viability of cells was over 89.8% across various cell types. Then, the group achieved the high-throughput bioprinting of high-viscosity collagen bioink encapsulating rat bladder smooth muscle cells with the use of a mechanical valve ejector [42,43]. Next, using this printing system, constructs were bioprinted with uniform cell seeding, yielding a layer-by-layer 3D cell pattern with controlled spatial resolution and maintaining high viability over long-term cell culture. They also integrated micro-valve bioprinting with hanging drop method to create controllable, uniform-sized embryoid bodies from ESCs, as shown in Figure 1.6a [44]. However, most bioprinting drug screening model studies have evolved around monocellular and single-cell tissue construction [11], yet native tissues or organs are heterocellular in nature with multiple cell types patterned in a

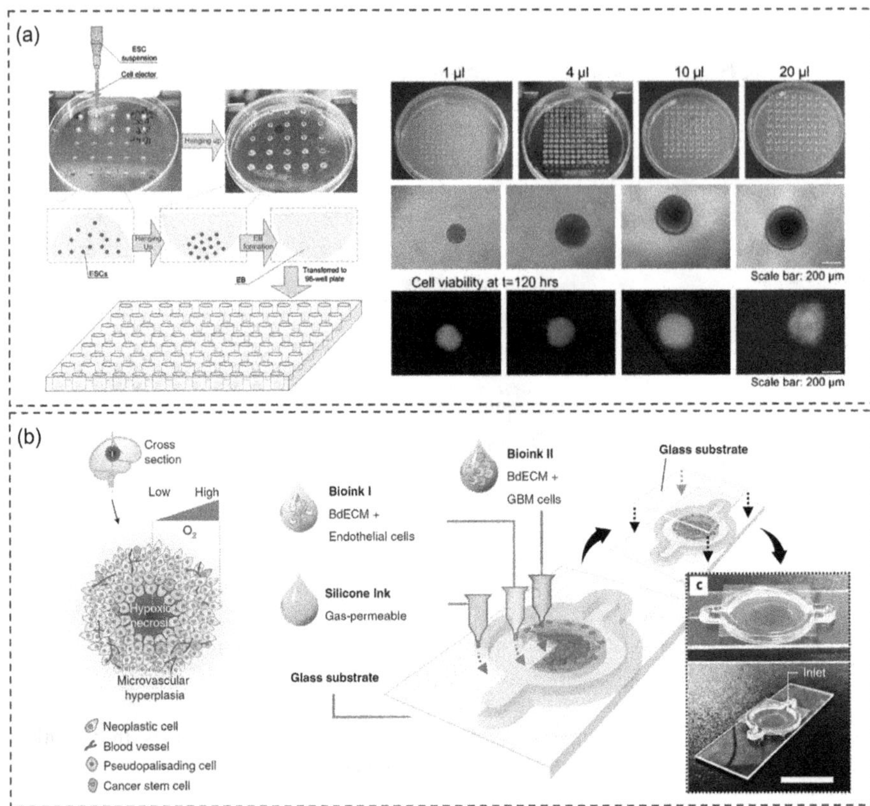

FIGURE 1.6 (a) Schematic of the embryoid body formation process using the 3D bioprinting approach. An array of droplets of cell medium suspension were bioprinted onto the lid of a Petri dish; uniform-sized droplets encapsulating ESCs were bioprinted to form embryoid bodies with droplet sizes of 1, 4, 10, and 20 μL; and the corresponding bright-field morphologies of droplets at $t=72$ hours and fluorescent images of green fluorescent protein (GFP)-positive embryoid bodies at $t=96$ hours stained with ethidium homodimer. Source: Xu et al. [44] used with permission. (b) Schematic representation of a tumor cross-section depicting the hypoxic core and different biological components typically found in a tumor microenvironment, and the schematic illustration of the bioinks and 3D bioprinting multicellular 'glioblastoma-on-a-chip' model, as well as mock representation of bioink compartments of brain dECM laden with HUVECs, and brain dECM with glioblastoma (GBM) cells in a bioprinted model (scale bar, 2 cm). Source: Yi et al. [50] used with permission.

highly complex anatomy [45]. Therefore, the construction of bio-functional tissues/organ models for pharmaceutics, involving appropriate multiple cell types to stimulate cell-to-cell and cell-to-matrix interactions, is necessary [45,46]. Recently, there has been a fast-growing trend toward the bioprinting of heterocellular tissue models, such as the building of complex pancreas, liver, muscle/tendon, kidney, heart, and various tumor models [21,47–49]. For instance, a representative

3D bioprinted multicellular model, 'glioblastoma-on-a-chip', was established using patient-derived glioblastoma cells co-cultured with endothelial cells in the decellularized extracellular matrix environment, as shown in Figure 1.6b [50]. In this study, they developed a cancer stroma concentric ring structure, which maintained the radial oxygen gradient and mimicked the *in vivo* tumor-like microenvironment. Furthermore, the drug-testing experiments with this model exhibited a great clinical significance for drug discovery and development by reproducing patient-specific resistance to concurrent chemoradiation and temozolomide drugs. Such bioprinting modeling was applied to construct various diseases models, which served for the screening of developed new drugs, or effective drugs and treatment modalities for different patients who are resistant to conventional treatments or drugs [21]. In addition, to further duplicate or mimic the native physiological and dynamic microenvironment, bionic engineering integrating the principles of microfluidics and 3D bioprinting with co-culture techniques can improve the effectiveness of *in vitro* models for disease biology and drug testing [51–54]. Thus, we could find that the current advances in 3D bioprinting in pharmaceutics (i.e., drug development) are still in the early stages of research, such as bioprinting of reliable drug or disease models, and long-way needs to go for the construction of human tissue or organ relevantly multicellular model structure. Certainly, its development is limited by various aspects, such as material science for the development of appropriate biomaterials, biomedicine for the understanding of the mechanism of various disease models, and molecular biology for the clarification of cell-to-cell and cell-to-material interactions. However, great potential of 3D bioprinting in drug discovery and screening has been demonstrated, and a series of fruits in pharmaceutical and therapeutic aspects are achieved, and the promising commercial market prospect is bright and worth looking forward in the near future.

1.4 COMMERCIAL PERSPECTIVES AND MARKET ANALYTICS OF BIOPRINTING

The fascination of 3D bioprinting is the capability of construction of anatomically shaped tissue or organ structures as substitutes for injured or damaged tissue or organ, or applied for various biomedical research studies, such as disease mechanism and drug discovery and development. Although this technology in clinical application mostly remains at an early stage and almost applications of bioprinting research is still in the laboratory stage, a certain commercial market share of 3D bioprinting and accessory products has been rapidly occupied in recent years. The novel 3D bioprinting technology could solve several problems in tissue engineering and regenerative medicine, which cannot reached by conventional tissue engineering techniques; thus, 3D bioprinting has become a strongest competitor in commercial market aspect at present. In addition, with the aggravation of population aging, the people's demand for the regenerative substitutes of tissues and organs is more urgent year by year; thus, much investment has been put into this area by governments, industry, and financial market, which attributes to the rapid development of 3D bioprinting in these years. Accordingly, the commercial market analytics of this revolutionary technology is necessary and help us deeply understand and further predict the 3D bioprinting development perspectives, as well as explore the potential commercial market and investment.

As surveyed, the global 3D bioprinting market was valued at 875.33 million (USD) in 2021 and is forecasted to reach a value of 4,815.02 million (USD) by 2030 at a compound annual growth rate of 21% between 2022 and 2030 (Figure 1.7a) [55], similarly to another report mentioned above [7]. Among them, 50.7% of the increase will originate from North America [55], which is closely relevant to the developed commercial 3D printing companies and corresponding advance technologies. There is no doubt that the development of new technology will drive the growth of related commercial market, and 3D bioprinting is no exception and will help in rapid development in next few years (Figure 1.7a). Moreover, business development is inseparable from the establishment of enterprises. Globally, there

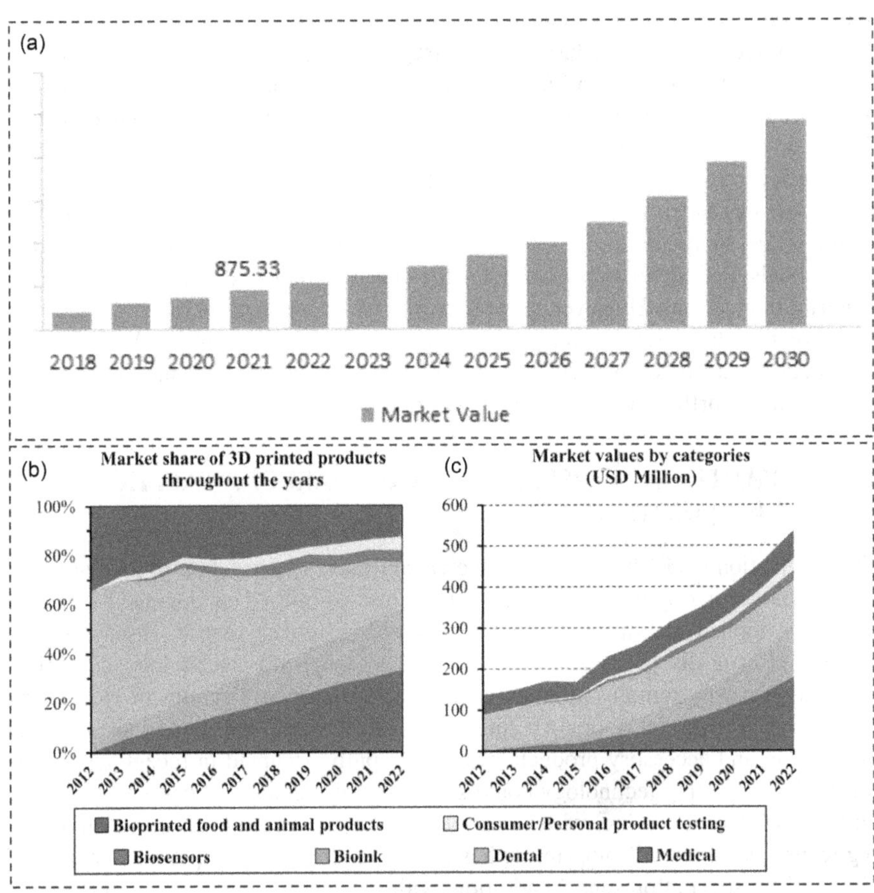

FIGURE 1.7 (a) Global 3D bioprinting market value (USD, million) analysis and forecast, 2017–2030. Source: Coherent Market Insights [55] used with permission. (b) The global market share of 3D printed products (i.e., 3D printing sectors) during 2012–2022 as a percentage of the whole bioprinting market and relative values (c) in absolute dollar amounts. Data reproduced with permission from Grand View Research [56].

are a number of companies and startups contributing to various niches within the bioprinting field (Figure 1.8a [57]), and these companies are spread across different regions of the world and focus on different aspects of 3D bioprinting. Thus, some companies have focused on the printing hardware and/or software (such as 3D bioprinter and corresponding CAD/CAM systems such as RegenHU and GeSiM companies), whereas other companies have focused on the development and printing of bioinks (such as CELLINK). Furthermore, other companies have applied bioprinting technologies and/or strategies to the development of high-throughput assays, commercialized tissue models, and grafting products for trauma repair

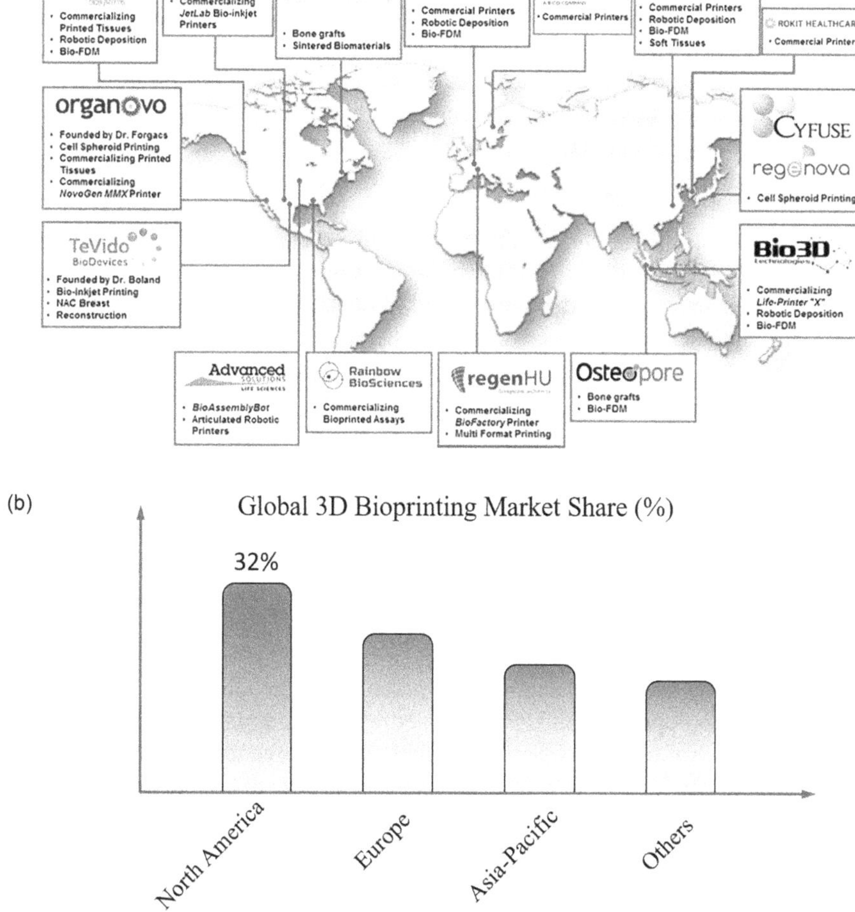

FIGURE 1.8 (a) Representative list of major companies involved in 3D bioprinting. Modified from Source: Jose et al. [57] used with permission. (b) The distribution of 3D bioprinting market share in global percentage (%). Source: Coherent Market Insights [55] used with permission.

such as Organovo. 3D bioprinting, as an independent printing field, does not affect and is limited by polymer or metal printing techniques such as FDM and SLS; thus, many startups have developed from university labs. Meanwhile, some big 3D printing companies (e.g., *Stratasys* and 3D *Systems*) gradually went into the bioprinting market, as well as Hewlett-Packard (HP, Palo Alto, CA) deployed in the biotechnology space and established the bioplotting platform (HP D300e). All these efforts accelerate the development speed of 3D bioprinting and made it rapidly occupied a certain commercial market. In terms of geographical distribution of main bioprinting companies, North America (such as the US and Canada) held a dominant position in the global 3D bioprinting market and has a vast number of companies, which corresponds to the distribution of market shares (Figure 1.8b) in global and produced market values, as mentioned above, followed by Europe (such as Germany, the UK, France, and Sweden) and Asia-Pacific (China, Japan, and South Korea) countries, and others. The rapid development of this bioprinting technology in the North America is inseparable from these objective reasons of business development, technological advancements, increasing research and development activities, and enhancing healthcare infrastructure. Meanwhile, the high healthcare expenditure, growing geriatric population, and increasing prevalence of chronic diseases are supporting the demand for this technology, especially in the pharmaceutical industry. However, geriatric population increase and expensive healthcare expenditure are problems that are faced, which include Europe, Asia-Pacific, and others; thus, these growing basic demands for peoples' health further promote the development of 3D bioprinting globally. Furthermore, the main end-users of 3D bioprinters and derived products can be summarized within five categories at present: pharmaceutical companies, research and academic institutions, medical device manufacturers, food industry, and contract research organizations. Among them, applications in pharmaceutics occupied a main role and achieved rapid development, especially in drug development and discovery, as mentioned above (Sections 9.2 and 9.3).

With such rapid growth of 3D bioprinting in these years, a certain market share and values of the corresponding 3D (bio)printed products, byproducts, and derivatives also have been produced in the last decade (2012–2022). The occupied market share and corresponding market value of each product or applied industry are shown in Figure 1.7b and c [56]. According to the principle and process of 3D bioprinting and tissue regeneration, the engineering tissue or organ substitutes could be bioprinted using appropriate bioink encapsulated with cells, isolated from the patient to decrease the risk of rejection from host tissues, and cultured under certain conditions to mature for repair or replace the damaged tissue or organ. However, during this process, the appropriate ECM-mimicking microenvironments provided by biomaterials are extremely important to ensure the cell survival, attachment, proliferation, differentiation, and maturation. Therefore, majority of research institutes or companies focus on the development of various bioinks for different tissues, and significant progress and rapid development of bioinks has been made in recent years, as shown by the fact that this bioink development holds main market shares and values in the last decade (Figure 1.7b and c) [56]. Furthermore, an interesting tendency could be noted that the global market share of bioink gradually has decreased over year, while increasing yearly in the dental and medical market share, and even the medical market share more than bioink in 2022. We could speculate that it may be because the developed bioinks have been more and more applied in dental and medical fields, leading to the rapid growth of these fields in recent years. Certainly, we can forecast that the rapid development of biomedical applications will continue and expand in the near future. Moreover, the food industry and animal product fields also have a certain market share in 3D bioprinting. 3D printing technology has the advantages of customized foods, contributing to nutritional balance and health. Overall, the market values of all the products are increasing yearly (Figure 1.7c), which means the market requirements of 3D bioprinting are rapidly increasing over the years and further reveals the broad market prospects of 3D bioprinted products.

In addition, two main applications of 3D bioprinting in the biomedical field are tissue engineering and pharmaceutics. The main driver of the rapid development of the 3D bioprinting market relies on the increasing use of this technique in the pharmaceutical industries. Thus, many companies are increasingly adopting 3D bioprinting products and technologies in the drug discovery and development process, and many bioprinters from different companies have been used in drug development (summarized and listed in Table 1.2), such as in drug screening and disease modeling. Furthermore, more and more bioprinting startups for drug development are established and growing in recent years. Compared to the traditional drug-testing method used in the pharmaceutical industry, the novel 3D bioprinting method enables accelerating the drug development and discovery and saves costs, particularly in the safety testing phase. Different types of 3D printing technologies have been utilized in pharmaceutical industries, such as

TABLE 1.2
Examples of Commercial Bioprinters and Their Potential Applications in Pharmaceuticals and Tissue Therapeutics

Company	Relative Printer	Applications
Advanced Solutions	BioAssemblyBot200 BioAssemblyBot400 BioAssemblyBot500	Disease models [58] Tissue engineering [59,60]
BRINTER	BRINTER ONE	Drug products [61]
CELLINK	INKREDIBLE+ BIO X BIO X6	Drug delivery [62–65] Drug products [66,67] Drug screening[68]
GeSiM	BioScaffolder Nano-Plotter Micro-contact Printer	Tissue engineering [69–71] Drug delivery (Microneedle) [72,73]
Inventia	RASTRUM	Drug screening [74]
Organovo	NovoGen MMX	Disease models [75] Tissue engineering [76]
RegenHU	R-GEN 100 R-GEN 200	Disease models [77] Tissue engineering [78] Drug delivery [79] Drug screening [80]

extrusion-based bioprinting, inkjet-based bioprinting, DLP-based bioprinting, and laser-based bioprinting techniques according to their advantages mentioned above (Section 9.2, Table 1.1). Corresponding working mechanisms, strength, and limitations of these techniques are listed in Table 1.1, as well as the relative study cases of 3D bioprinting applied in pharmaceuticals and therapeutics. Thus, 3D bioprinted disease models for drug efficacy tests and normal tissue models for drug safety tests are current main technique strategies in pharmaceutical application. 3D bioprinted tissue models can be applied in the early stages and during preclinical trials of new drug development. Advantages offered by 3D bioprinting include reduced use of animals for drug testing, enhanced productivity, and shortened drug discovery process. However, there are also some limitations. Thus, due to the continuous technological advancements, the field has a growing requirement of highly qualified and skilled professionals who should possess multiple field knowledge (not limited to the 3D bioprinting technique). We can speculate that a large number of 3D bioprinting operator/engineer jobs will emerge in the near future, and this increase in employment will be a key characteristic of the commercialization of the 3D bioprinting technique. Moreover, the consistency in the AM process is altered between machines due to the uncontrolled process variables and material differences. In addition, there are only limited data available on process control, and the capacity to develop detailed and accurate mathematical models through AM has been difficult. These limitations in process control, preproduction, and planning have often resulted in manufacturing failure and expensive errors. At least, the printing process is still slow, and a faster printing and scale-up process is required to become commercially acceptable. Thus, we can see that if the market prospect is broad and bright for 3D bioprinting, there will be several obstacles that need to be overcome to reach the full marketization.

Based on these market analysis and relevant challenges in 3D bioprinting, the prediction of 3D bioprinting development is essential for industrial distribution and investment. Some ongoing and anticipated or potential growth and developing momentum of 3D bioprinting in next years is listed as follows: (i) the adoption of 3D printing will increase and explore and enter into newer markets; (ii) 3D printing workflow automation and collaboration with other techniques, such as robots, will increase; (iii) there will be an increase in the development and qualification of high-performance 3D printing materials and biopolymers (particularly in ECM-mimicking bioinks); (iv) there will be an increase in the development of large-format 3D bioprinting systems; (v) improvement in the reliability and repeatability of bioprinting can be witnessed; (vi) the 3D bioprinting industry standardization and increasing 3D bioprinting technician training will improve; (vii) there will be an increase in the integration of on-demand, just-in-time manufacturing through applying a novel technique, such as Internet of Things, to achieve intelligent bioprinting; and (viii) relative ethics regulation for clinical application will be established. Indeed, real commercialization of a technology and its entry into the market require relevant standards and regulation for evaluation and constraint, which are also suitable for 3D bioprinting and relevant products.

Overall, from the market analytics of 3D bioprinting technology in the total global market share and value, global distribution of market share, 3D bioprinting company development, market share and value of 3D bioprinted products, and biomedical application of 3D bioprinting in tissue engineering and pharmaceutics, we could observe that 3D bioprinting has broad and sight commercial prospects and exhibit an increasing trend. Certainly, the opportunities and challenges coexisted with the rise of new industry, and there are numerous obstacles and long muddy way to reach the real commercialization of 3D bioprinting.

1.5 CONCLUSION AND FUTURE PERSPECTIVES

As discussed in this chapter, 3D printing, in particular 3D bioprinting, is a relatively new yet evolving technique mainly used in pharmaceutics, tissue engineering, and regenerative medicine. It revolutionizes the pharmaceutical formulation toward personalized drugs. There is considerable evidence that supports the development process of new drugs and vaccines in a rapid and cost-effective manner. It will also bring significant changes to pharmaceutical testing due to its unique advantages of precise spatial control, reproducibility, automation, high-throughput, and fabrication of desired structures. The 3D-printed structures, especially tissue-mimicking structures, not only allow tissue repair but could also be applied in the bio-safety and bio-toxicity testing of drugs. In recent days, the advent of commercial bioprinting has revolutionized the field of pharmaceutics and therapeutics. Within a short span, numerous companies working in the bioprinting business and selling their bioprinters and relevant products in the market have developed. This bioprinting industry now has a worldwide reach with companies in almost all major markets. The constant increase in recent years in financial support and investments in 3D bioprinting for pharmaceutics from governments, institutes, and big companies shows a flourishing financial market and an industry that has value. Although the advantages of bioprinting in pharmaceutics have emerged, the commercial level of customized bioprinted products still remains limited, and it is expected to rapidly grow in the near future. This is an exciting time to be involved in the research and development of clinically translatable 3D-printed drugs and biological constructs as a new modality in personalized medicine.

REFERENCES

1. S.C. Ligon, R. Liska, J. Stampfl, M. Gurr, R. Mülhaupt, Polymers for 3D Printing and Customized Additive Manufacturing, *Chemical Reviews* 117(15) (2017) 10212–10290.
2. M.A. Alhnan, T.C. Okwuosa, M. Sadia, K.-W. Wan, W. Ahmed, B. Arafat, Emergence of 3D Printed Dosage Forms: Opportunities and Challenges, *Pharmaceutical Research* 33(8) (2016) 1817–1832.
3. A.C. Fonseca, F.P.W. Melchels, M.J.S. Ferreira, S.R. Moxon, G. Potjewyd, T.R. Dargaville, S.J. Kimber, M. Domingos, Emulating Human Tissues and Organs: A Bioprinting Perspective Toward Personalized Medicine, *Chemical Reviews* 120(19) (2020) 11093–11139.
4. G. Gao, M. Ahn, W.-W. Cho, B.-S. Kim, D.-W. Cho, 3D Printing of Pharmaceutical Application: Drug Screening and Drug Delivery, *Pharmaceutics* 13 (2021) 1373.
5. J. Malda, J. Visser, F.P. Melchels, T. Jüngst, W.E. Hennink, W.J.A. Dhert, J. Groll, D.W. Hutmacher, 25th Anniversary Article: Engineering Hydrogels for Biofabrication, *Advanced Materials* 25(36) (2013) 5011–5028.

6. GVR Report cover3D Bioprinting Market Size, Share & Trends Report 3D Bioprinting Market Size, Share & Trends Analysis Report by Technology (Magnetic Levitation, Inkjet-based), by Application (Medical, Dental, Biosensors, Bioinks), by Region, and Segment Forecasts, 2022–2030.
7. S. Santoni, S.G. Gugliandolo, M. Sponchioni, D. Moscatelli, B.M. Colosimo, 3D Bioprinting: Current Status and Trends—A Guide to the Literature and Industrial Practice, *Bio-Design and Manufacturing* 5(1) (2022) 14–42.
8. D. Choudhury, S. Anand, M.W. Naing, The Arrival of Commercial Bioprinters - Towards 3D Bioprinting Revolution!, *International Journal of Bioprinting* 4(2) (2018) 139.
9. A. Awad, S.J. Trenfield, A. Goyanes, S. Gaisford, A.W. Basit, Reshaping Drug Development Using 3D Printing, *Drug Discovery Today* 23(8) (2018) 1547–1555.
10. W. Peng, P. Datta, B. Ayan, V. Ozbolat, D. Sosnoski, I.T. Ozbolat, 3D Bioprinting for Drug Discovery and Development in Pharmaceutics, *Acta Biomaterialia* 57 (2017) 26–46.
11. W. Peng, D. Unutmaz, I.T. Ozbolat, Bioprinting towards Physiologically Relevant Tissue Models for Pharmaceutics, *Trends in Biotechnology* 34(9) (2016) 722–732.
12. L. Neufeld, E. Yeini, S. Pozzi, R. Satchi-Fainaro, 3D Bioprinted Cancer Models: From Basic Biology to Drug Development, Nature Reviews Cancer 22(12) (2022) 679–692.
13. M. Wallis, Z. Al-Dulimi, D.K. Tan, M. Maniruzzaman, A. Nokhodchi, 3D Printing for Enhanced Drug Delivery: Current State-of-the-Art and Challenges, *Drug Development and Industrial Pharmacy* 46(9) (2020) 1385–1401.
14. A.M. Issa, Personalized Medicine and the Practice of Medicine in the 21st Century, *McGill Journal of Medicine* 10(1) (2020) 56–57.
15. S.J. Trenfield, A. Awad, A. Goyanes, S. Gaisford, A.W. Basit, 3D Printing Pharmaceuticals: Drug Development to Frontline Care, *Trends in Pharmacological Sciences* 39(5) (2018) 440–451.
16. O. Jung, M.J. Song, M. Ferrer, Operationalizing the Use of Biofabricated Tissue Models as Preclinical Screening Platforms for Drug Discovery and Development, *SLAS Discovery* 26(9) (2021) 1164–1176.
17. L. Zhao, J. Xiu, Y. Liu, T. Zhang, W. Pan, X. Zheng, X. Zhang, A 3D Printed Hanging Drop Dripper for Tumor Spheroids Analysis Without Recovery, *Scientific Reports* 9(1) (2019) 19717.
18. M.J. Waring, J. Arrowsmith, A.R. Leach, P.D. Leeson, S. Mandrell, R.M. Owen, G. Pairaudeau, W.D. Pennie, S.D. Pickett, J. Wang, O. Wallace, A. Weir, An Analysis of the Attrition of Drug Candidates from Four Major Pharmaceutical Companies, *Nature Reviews Drug Discovery* 14(7) (2015) 475–486.
19. X. Ma, J. Liu, W. Zhu, M. Tang, N. Lawrence, C. Yu, M. Gou, S. Chen, 3D Bioprinting of Functional Tissue Models for Personalized Drug Screening and In Vitro Disease Modeling, *Advanced Drug Delivery Reviews* 132 (2018) 235–251.
20. I.T. Ozbolat, W. Peng, V. Ozbolat, Application Areas of 3D Bioprinting, *Drug Discovery Today* 21(8) (2016) 1257–1271.
21. P. Datta, M. Dey, Z. Ataie, D. Unutmaz, I.T. Ozbolat, 3D Bioprinting for Reconstituting the Cancer Microenvironment, *NPJ Precision Oncology* 4(1) (2020) 18.
22. A.P. Tiwari, N.D. Thorat, S. Pricl, R.M. Patil, S. Rohiwal, H. Townley, Bioink: A 3D-Bioprinting Tool for Anticancer Drug Discovery and Cancer Management, *Drug Discovery Today* 26(7) (2021) 1574–1590.
23. H.-G. Yi, H. Kim, J. Kwon, Y.-J. Choi, J. Jang, D.-W. Cho, Application of 3D Bioprinting in the Prevention and the Therapy for Human Diseases, *Signal Transduction and Targeted Therapy* 6(1) (2021) 177.
24. R. Chang, K. Emami, H. Wu, W. Sun, Biofabrication of a Three-Dimensional Liver Micro-Organ as an In Vitro Drug Metabolism Model, *Biofabrication* 2(4) (2010) 045004.

25. J.E. Snyder, Q. Hamid, C. Wang, R. Chang, K. Emami, H. Wu, W. Sun, Bioprinting Cell-Laden Matrigel for Radioprotection Study of Liver by Pro-Drug Conversion in a Dual-Tissue Microfluidic Chip, *Biofabrication* 3(3) (2011) 034112.
26. S.M. King, S.C. Presnell, D.G. Nguyen, Abstract 2034: Development of 3D Bioprinted Human Breast Cancer for In Vitro Drug Screening, *Cancer Research* 74(19_Supplement) (2014) 2034–2034.
27. T. Agarwal, M. Costantini, T.K. Maiti, Extrusion 3D Printing with Pectin-Based Ink Formulations: Recent Trends in Tissue Engineering and Food Manufacturing, *Biomedical Engineering Advances* 2 (2021) 100018.
28. S. Pant, S. Subramanian, S. Thomas, S. Loganathan, R.B. Valapa, Tailoring of Mesoporous Bioactive Glass Composite Scaffold Via Thermal Extrusion based 3D Bioprinting and Scrutiny on Bone Tissue Engineering Characteristics, *Microporous and Mesoporous Materials* 341 (2022) 112104.
29. D. Kilian, S. Holtzhausen, W. Groh, P. Sembdner, C. Czichy, A. Lode, R. Stelzer, M. Gelinsky, 3D Extrusion Printing of Density Gradients by Variation of Sinusoidal Printing Paths for Tissue Engineering and Beyond, *Acta Biomaterialia* 158 (2022) 308–323.
30. A.B. Owczarczak, S.O. Shuford, S.T. Wood, S. Deitch, D. Dean, Creating Transient Cell Membrane Pores Using a Standard Inkjet Printer, *Journal of Visualized Experiments: JoVE* (61) (2012): 3681.
31. J.I. Rodríguez-Dévora, B. Zhang, D. Reyna, Z.-D. Shi, T. Xu, High Throughput Miniature Drug-Screening Platform Using Bioprinting Technology, *Biofabrication* 4(3) (2012) 035001.
32. R.E. Saunders, B. Derby, Inkjet Printing Biomaterials for Tissue Engineering: Bioprinting, *International Materials Reviews* 59(8) (2014) 430–448.
33. X. Ma, X. Qu, W. Zhu, Y.-S. Li, S. Yuan, H. Zhang, J. Liu, P. Wang, C.S.E. Lai, F. Zanella, G.-S. Feng, F. Sheikh, S. Chien, S. Chen, Deterministically Patterned Biomimetic Human iPSC-Derived Hepatic Model Via Rapid 3D Bioprinting, *Proceedings of the National Academy of Sciences* 113(8) (2016) 2206–2211.
34. W. Zhu, X. Qu, J. Zhu, X. Ma, S. Patel, J. Liu, P. Wang, C.S.E. Lai, M. Gou, Y. Xu, K. Zhang, S. Chen, Direct 3D Bioprinting of Prevascularized Tissue Constructs with Complex Microarchitecture, *Biomaterials* 124 (2017) 106–115.
35. Z. Ma, S. Koo, M.A. Finnegan, P. Loskill, N. Huebsch, N.C. Marks, B.R. Conklin, C.P. Grigoropoulos, K.E. Healy, Three-Dimensional Filamentous Human Diseased Cardiac Tissue Model, *Biomaterials* 35(5) (2014) 1367–1377.
36. D. Hakobyan, O. Kerouredan, M. Remy, N. Dusserre, C. Medina, R. Devillard, J.-C. Fricain, H. Oliveira, Laser-Assisted Bioprinting for Bone Repair, in: J.M. Crook (Ed.), *3D Bioprinting: Principles and Protocols*, Springer US, New York, NY, 2020, pp. 135–144.
37. R.D. Ventura, An Overview of Laser-assisted Bioprinting (LAB) in Tissue Engineering Applications, *Medical Lasers* 10(2) (2021) 76–81.
38. S. Ostrovidov, S. Salehi, M. Costantini, K. Suthiwanich, M. Ebrahimi, R.B. Sadeghian, T. Fujie, X. Shi, S. Cannata, C. Gargioli, A. Tamayol, M.R. Dokmeci, G. Orive, W. Swieszkowski, A. Khademhosseini, 3D Bioprinting in Skeletal Muscle Tissue Engineering, *Small* 15(24) (2019) 1805530.
39. S. Ostrovidov, M. Ramalingam, H. Bae, G. Orive, T. Fujie, X. Shi, H. Kaji, Latest Developments in Engineered Skeletal Muscle Tissues for Drug Discovery and Development, *Expert Opinion on Drug Discovery* 18(1) (2023) 47–63. doi: 10.1080/17460441.2023.2160438. Epub 2022 Dec 26. PMID: 36535280.
40. D.A. Pereira, J.A. Williams, Origin and Evolution of High Throughput Screening, *British Journal of Pharmacology* 152(1) (2007) 53–61.

41. U. Demirci, G. Montesano, Single Cell Epitaxy by Acoustic Picolitre Droplets, *Lab on a Chip* 7(9) (2007) 1139–1145.
42. F. Xu, S.J. Moon, A.E. Emre, E.S. Turali, Y.S. Song, S.A. Hacking, J. Nagatomi, U. Demirci, A Droplet-Based Building Block Approach for Bladder Smooth Muscle Cell (SMC) Proliferation, *Biofabrication* 2(1) (2010) 014105.
43. S. Moon, S.K. Hasan, Y.S. Song, F. Xu, H.O. Keles, F. Manzur, S. Mikkilineni, J.W. Hong, J. Nagatomi, E. Haeggstrom, A. Khademhosseini, U. Demirci, Layer by Layer Three-dimensional Tissue Epitaxy by Cell-Laden Hydrogel Droplets, *Tissue Engineering Part C: Methods* 16(1) (2009) 157–166.
44. F. Xu, B. Sridharan, S. Wang, U.A. Gurkan, B. Syverud, U. Demirci, Embryonic Stem Cell Bioprinting for Uniform and Controlled Size Embryoid Body Formation, *Biomicrofluidics* 5(2) (2011) 022207.
45. B. Nelson, 3-Dimensional Bioprinting Makes Its Mark: New Tissue and Organ Printing Methods Are Yielding Critical New Tools for the Laboratory and Clinic, *Cancer Cytopathology* 123(4) (2015) 203–204.
46. A.M. Bejoy, K.N. Makkithaya, B.B. Hunakunti, A. Hegde, K. Krishnamurthy, A. Sarkar, C.F. Lobo, D.V.S. Keshav, D. G, D.D. S, S. Mascarenhas, S. Chakrabarti, S.R.R.D. Kalepu, B. Paul, N. Mazumder, An Insight on Advances and Applications of 3d Bioprinting: A Review, *Bioprinting* 24 (2021) e00176.
47. N.S. Bhise, V. Manoharan, S. Massa, A. Tamayol, M. Ghaderi, M. Miscuglio, Q. Lang, Y. Shrike Zhang, S.R. Shin, G. Calzone, N. Annabi, T.D. Shupe, C.E. Bishop, A. Atala, M.R. Dokmeci, A. Khademhosseini, A Liver-on-a-Chip Platform with Bioprinted Hepatic Spheroids, *Biofabrication* 8(1) (2016) 014101.
48. M. Rimann, S. Laternser, H. Keller, O. Leupin, U. Graf-Hausner, 3D Bioprinted Muscle and Tendon Tissues for Drug Development: biotechnet Switzerland, *CHIMIA* 69(1–2) (2015) 65.
49. S. Knowlton, S. Onal, C.H. Yu, J.J. Zhao, S. Tasoglu, Bioprinting for Cancer Research, *Trends in Biotechnology* 33(9) (2015) 504–513.
50. H.-G. Yi, Y.H. Jeong, Y. Kim, Y.-J. Choi, H.E. Moon, S.H. Park, K.S. Kang, M. Bae, J. Jang, H. Youn, S.H. Paek, D.-W. Cho, A Bioprinted Human-Glioblastoma-on-a-Chip for the Identification of Patient-Specific Responses to Chemoradiotherapy, *Nature Biomedical Engineering* 3(7) (2019) 509–519.
51. M. Singh, Y. Tong, K. Webster, E. Cesewski, A.P. Haring, S. Laheri, B. Carswell, T.J. O'Brien, C.H. Aardema, R.S. Senger, J.L. Robertson, B.N. Johnson, 3D Printed Conformal Microfluidics for Isolation and Profiling of Biomarkers from Whole Organs, *Lab on a Chip* 17(15) (2017) 2561–2571.
52. J. Ma, Y. Wang, J. Liu, Bioprinting of 3D Tissues/Organs Combined with Microfluidics, *RSC Advances* 8(39) (2018) 21712–21727.
53. R. Amin, S. Knowlton, A. Hart, B. Yenilmez, F. Ghaderinezhad, S. Katebifar, M. Messina, A. Khademhosseini, S. Tasoglu, 3D-Printed Microfluidic Devices, *Biofabrication* 8(2) (2016) 022001.
54. B. Zhang, A. Korolj, B.F.L. Lai, M. Radisic, Advances in Organ-on-a-Chip Engineering, *Nature Reviews Materials* 3(8) (2018) 257–278.
55. 3d Bioprinting Market Analysis, 3d Bioprinting Market Analysis, Aug 2022. https://www.coherentmarketinsights.com/market-insight/3d-bioprinting-market-5166
56. A. Tong, Q.L. Pham, P. Abatemarco, A. Mathew, D. Gupta, S. Iyer, R. Voronov, Review of Low-Cost 3D Bioprinters: State of the Market and Observed Future Trends, *SLAS Technology* 26(4) (2021) 333–366.
57. R.R. Jose, M.J. Rodriguez, T.A. Dixon, F. Omenetto, D.L. Kaplan, Evolution of Bioinks and Additive Manufacturing Technologies for 3D Bioprinting, *ACS Biomaterials Science & Engineering* 2(10) (2016) 1662–1678.

58. Y. Aghazadeh, F. Poon, F. Sarangi, F.T.M. Wong, S.T. Khan, X. Sun, R. Hatkar, B.J. Cox, S.S. Nunes, M.C. Nostro, Microvessels Support Engraftment and Functionality of Human Islets and hESC-Derived Pancreatic Progenitors in Diabetes Models, *Cell Stem Cell* 28(11) (2021) 1936–1949.e8.
59. T. Später, F.S. Frueh, R.M. Nickels, M.D. Menger, M.W. Laschke, Prevascularization of Collagen-Glycosaminoglycan Scaffolds: Stromal Vascular Fraction versus Adipose Tissue-Derived Microvascular Fragments, *Journal of Biological Engineering* 12 (2018) 24.
60. S.M. Moss, M. Ortiz-Hernandez, D. Levin, C.A. Richburg, T. Gerton, M. Cook, J.J. Houlton, Z.H. Rizvi, P.C. Goodwin, M. Golway, B. Ripley, J.B. Hoying, A Biofabrication Strategy for a Custom-Shaped, Non-Synthetic Bone Graft Precursor with a Prevascularized Tissue Shell, *Frontiers in Bioengineering and Biotechnology* 10 (2022) 838415.
61. E. Sjöholm, R. Mathiyalagan, L. Lindfors, X. Wang, S. Ojala, N. Sandler, Semi-Solid Extrusion 3D Printing of Tailored ChewTs for Veterinary Use - A Focus on Spectrophotometric Quantification of Gabapentin, *European Journal of Pharmaceutical Sciences* 174 (2022) 106190.
62. S. Naeimipour, F. Rasti Boroojeni, R. Selegård, D. Aili, Enzymatically Triggered Deprotection and Cross-Linking of Thiolated Alginate-Based Bioinks, *Chemistry of Materials* 34(21) (2022) 9536–9545.
63. F. Vashahi, M.R. Martinez, E. Dashtimoghadam, F. Fahimipour, A.N. Keith, E.A. Bersenev, D.A. Ivanov, E.B. Zhulina, P. Popryadukhin, K. Matyjaszewski, M. Vatankhah-Varnosfaderani, S.S. Sheiko, Injectable Bottlebrush Hydrogels with Tissue-Mimetic Mechanical Properties, *Science Advances* 8(3) (2022) eabm2469.
64. J. Rahman, J. Quodbach, Versatility on Demand – The Case for Semi-Solid Micro-Extrusion in Pharmaceutics, Advanced Drug Delivery Reviews 172 (2021) 104–126.
65. G. Bovone, E.A. Guzzi, S. Bernhard, T. Weber, D. Dranseikiene, M.W. Tibbitt, Supramolecular Reinforcement of Polymer–Nanoparticle Hydrogels for Modular Materials Design, *Advanced Materials* 34(9) (2022) 2106941.
66. L. Zhang, Y. Xiang, H. Zhang, L. Cheng, X. Mao, N. An, L. Zhang, J. Zhou, L. Deng, Y. Zhang, X. Sun, H.A. Santos, W. Cui, A Biomimetic 3D-Self-Forming Approach for Microvascular Scaffolds, *Advanced Science* 7(9) (2020) 1903553.
67. R. Ajdary, N.Z. Ezazi, A. Correia, M. Kemell, S. Huan, H.J. Ruskoaho, J. Hirvonen, H.A. Santos, O.J. Rojas, Multifunctional 3D-Printed Patches for Long-Term Drug Release Therapies after Myocardial Infarction, *Advanced Functional Materials* 30(34) (2020) 2003440.
68. G. Janani, S. Priya, S. Dey, B.B. Mandal, Mimicking Native Liver Lobule Microarchitecture In Vitro with Parenchymal and Non-Parenchymal Cells Using 3D Bioprinting for Drug Toxicity and Drug Screening Applications, *ACS Applied Materials & Interfaces* 14(8) (2022) 10167–10186.
69. D. Kilian, S. Cometta, A. Bernhardt, R. Taymour, J. Golde, T. Ahlfeld, J. Emmermacher, M. Gelinsky, A. Lode, Core–Shell Bioprinting as a Strategy to Apply Differentiation Factors in a Spatially Defined Manner Inside Osteochondral Tissue Substitutes, *Biofabrication* 14(1) (2022) 014108.
70. A.D. Štiglic, F. Gürer, F. Lackner, D. Bračič, A. Winter, L. Gradišnik, D. Makuc, R. Kargl, I. Duarte, J. Plavec, U. Maver, M. Beaumont, K.S. Kleinschek, T. Mohan, Organic Acid Cross-Linked 3D Printed Cellulose Nanocomposite Bioscaffolds with Controlled Porosity, *Mechanical Strength, and Biocompatibility, iScience* 25(5) (2022) 104263.
71. D. Kilian, M. von Witzleben, M. Lanaro, C.S. Wong, C. Vater, A. Lode, M.C. Allenby, M.A. Woodruff, M. Gelinsky, 3D Plotting of Calcium Phosphate Cement and Melt Electrowriting of Polycaprolactone Microfibers in One Scaffold: A Hybrid Additive Manufacturing Process, *Journal of Functional Biomaterials* 13(2) (2022) 75. doi: 10.3390/jfb13020075. PMID: 35735931; PMCID: PMC9225379.

72. C.P.P. Pere, S.N. Economidou, G. Lall, C. Ziraud, J.S. Boateng, B.D. Alexander, D.A. Lamprou, D. Douroumis, 3D Printed Microneedles for Insulin Skin Delivery, *International Journal of Pharmaceutics* 544(2) (2018) 425–432.
73. T. von Strauwitz Né Ahlfeld, A.R. Akkineni, Y. Förster, T. Köhler, S. Knaack, M. Gelinsky, A. Lode, Design and Fabrication of Complex Scaffolds for Bone Defect Healing: Combined 3D Plotting of a Calcium Phosphate Cement and a Growth Factor-Loaded Hydrogel, *Annals of Biomedical Engineering* 45 (2017) 224–236.
74. R.H. Utama, L. Atapattu, A.P. O'Mahony, C.M. Fife, J. Baek, T. Allard, K.J. O'Mahony, J.C.C. Ribeiro, K. Gaus, M. Kavallaris, J.J. Gooding, A 3D Bioprinter Specifically Designed for the High-Throughput Production of Matrix-Embedded Multicellular Spheroids, *iScience* 23(10) (2020) 101621.
75. E.M. Langer, B.L. Allen-Petersen, S.M. King, N.D. Kendsersky, M.A. Turnidge, G.M. Kuziel, R. Riggers, R. Samatham, T.S. Amery, S.L. Jacques, B.C. Sheppard, J.E. Korkola, J.L. Muschler, G. Thibault, Y.H. Chang, J.W. Gray, S.C. Presnell, D.G. Nguyen, R.C. Sears, Modeling Tumor Phenotypes In Vitro with Three-Dimensional Bioprinting, *Cell Reports* 26(3) (2019) 608–623.e6.
76. C. Norotte, F.S. Marga, L.E. Niklason, G. Forgacs, Scaffold-Free Vascular Tissue Engineering Using Bioprinting, *Biomaterials* 30(30) (2009) 5910–5917.
77. S. D'Agostino, M. Rimann, P. Gamba, G. Perilongo, M. Pozzobon, M. Raghunath, Macromolecular Crowding Tuned Extracellular Matrix Deposition in a Bioprinted Human Rhabdomyosarcoma Model, *Bioprinting* 27 (2022) e00213.
78. J. Kajtez, S. Buchmann, S. Vasudevan, M. Birtele, S. Rocchetti, C.J. Pless, A. Heiskanen, R.A. Barker, A. Martínez-Serrano, M. Parmar, J.U. Lind, J. Emnéus, 3D-Printed Soft Lithography for Complex Compartmentalized Microfluidic Neural Devices, *Advanced Science* 8(12) (2021) 2101787.
79. S. Madiedo-Podvrsan, J.-P. Belaïdi, S. Desbouis, L. Simonetti, Y. Ben-Khalifa, C. Collin-Djangone, J. Soeur, M. Rielland, Utilization of Patterned Bioprinting for Heterogeneous and Physiologically Representative Reconstructed Epidermal Skin Models, *Scientific Reports* 11(1) (2021) 6217.
80. L.C.C. Ferre, Collagen-Tannic Acid Spheroids for b-Cell Encapsulation Fabricated by 3d Bioprinting, *Tissue Engineering Part A* 28 (2022) S616–S617.

2 3D Printing of New Drugs
Pharmaceutical Dosage Forms in Personalised Therapies

Álvaro Goyanes
University College London
FabRx Ltd.
iMATUS and Health Research Institute of Santiago de Compostela (IDIS), Universidade de Santiago de Compostela (USC)

Iria Seoane-Viaño
University College London
University of Santiago de Compostela (USC), and Health Research Institute of Santiago de Compostela (IDIS)

CONTENTS

2.1 INTRODUCTION

Three-dimensional (3D) printing has the potential to revolutionise the manufacturing of pharmaceutical drug products by creating structures with an unprecedented level of complexity and functionality [1,2]. In contrast to conventional mass manufacture, this flexible manufacturing platform uses digital computer-aided design software to design and create dosage forms in a layer-by-layer manner, with personalised

DOI: 10.1201/9781003274568-2

geometries, dosages, drug combinations and specific release characteristics [3,4]. In 2015, the Food and Drug Administration (FDA) approved the commercialisation of the first 3D-printed tablet (Spritam®) for the treatment of epilepsy [5]. The technology used is based on the use of a binder jet printing apparatus adapted for mass manufacturing capable of producing fast-dispersing tablets containing drug loads up to 1,000 mg.

The unique properties of 3D printing make it an ideal candidate to take part in the new digital healthcare era together with non-invasive diagnostics (e.g., medical imaging) and drug monitoring techniques (e.g., biosensors and artificial intelligence tools) [6,7]. The digital information with the specific requirements of each patient provided by diagnostic tools will allow the production of personalised medicines by means of 3D printing adapted to those specific needs [8,9].

From the production of bespoke formulations for preclinical and first-in-human trials, to the production of tailored medications (termed "Printlets™") at the point of care, 3D printing can streamline the entire pharmaceutical manufacturing chain and provide unique advantages over conventional manufacturing processes (Figure 2.1) [1]. Small batches of formulations can be prepared for preclinical studies in animals adapted, for example, to different routes of administration [10,11]. In the clinical arena, the production of medications using 3D printing can enhance patient adherence to medication by the creation of patient-friendly formulations, such as chewable or flavoured dosage forms [12–15]. Drug products could also be designed with different release profiles [16,17], targeted at different sections of the gastrointestinal (GI) tract [18,19], or formulated for different routes of administration other than oral [20,21]. Apart from dosage forms, medical devices such as punctal plugs [22], bladder devices [23], scaffolds [24], microneedles [25] and implants [26] can also be created using this technology.

One of the advantages of 3D printing is its portability and the reduced cost and size of some 3D printers, which makes this technology an ideal candidate for use in remote areas, such as disaster zones or the outer space [27]. More recently, the use of 3D printed has been proposed to the preparation of veterinary medicines as the number of approved veterinary drugs is limited so animals are usually treated with compounded dosage forms or off-label human medications [28].

Five main 3D printed technologies are used for pharmaceutical applications (Figure 2.2). Binder jetting [29,30] and material jetting (in particular, inkjet printing)

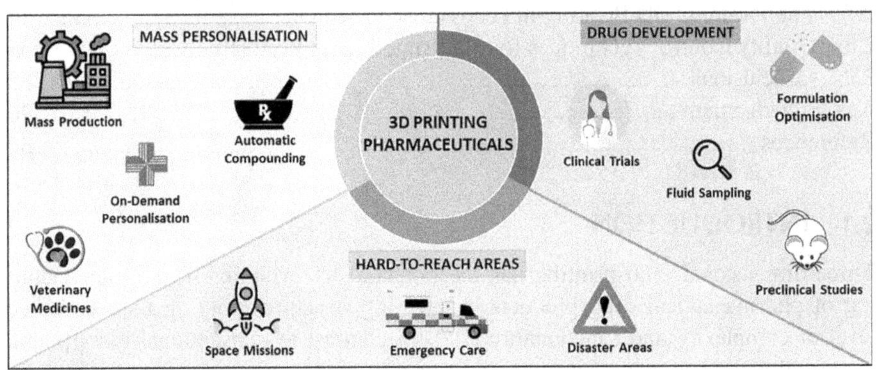

FIGURE 2.1 Some applications of 3D printing in healthcare. Reproduced with permission from Ref. [1].

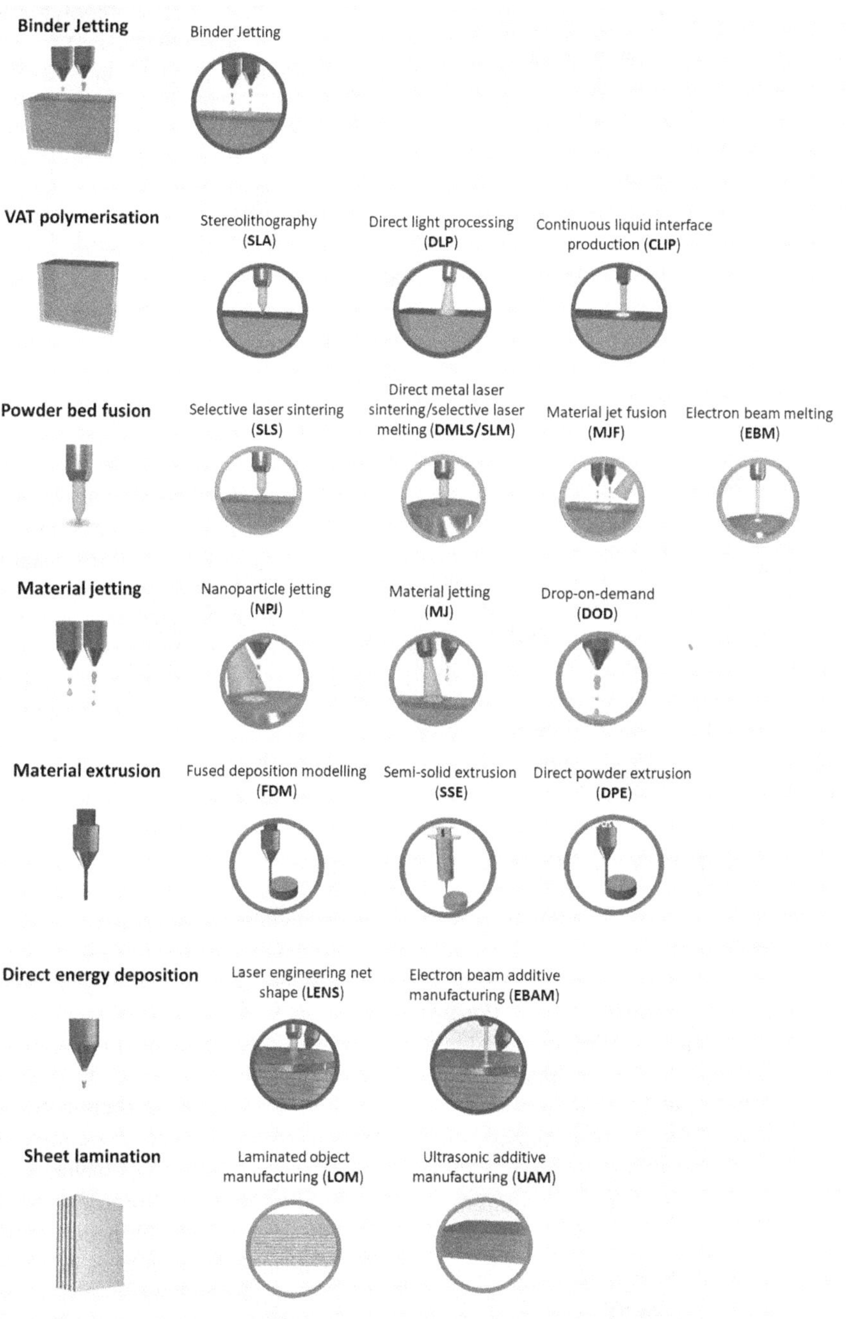

FIGURE 2.2 The seven main 3D printing technologies, only the first five are used for pharmaceutical purposes. Reproduced with permission from Ref. [1].

[31,32], in which droplets of ink are deposited onto a substrate. Vat photopolymerisation [33,34] uses a light source to solidify a liquid resin and powder bed fusion [35,36] uses a laser to melt and fuse powder particles together. And finally, material extrusion, in which the feedstock material could be in the form of filaments [16,37,38], powder [39–41], or semisolid material [42–44].

As these technologies have been extensively reviewed elsewhere [45–47], this chapter will focus on how these 3D printing technologies have been applied in healthcare to develop personalised medical devices and dosage forms in both the preclinical and clinical arena.

2.2 OPPORTUNITIES OF 3D PRINTING IN PRECLINICAL DRUG DEVELOPMENT

In preclinical studies, a drug candidate is administered to animals to test its efficacy, safety and pharmacokinetic behaviour across a wide dose range [48,49]. To save costs and speed up the drug development process, it is crucial to identify and discard the toxic or ineffective molecules as soon as possible [50]. Rodents are commonly used as animal models for these early-stage studies. Drug candidates are usually administered as liquid formulations or included within small capsules [51]. However, these formulation preparation approaches are labour-intensive and essential parameters such as the correct solubilisation of the drug may not be ensured. 3D printing allows the production of small batches of dosage forms adapted to the animal and route of administration. Printlets can be created with a wide variety of doses and sizes combining different excipients so that parameters such as drug stability and interactions can also be tested.

2.3 3D-PRINTED ORAL DOSAGE FORMS

Dosage forms can be designed to release the drug immediately or in a more sustained manner. The pharmacokinetic behaviour of these dosage forms is evaluated *in vitro* and *in vivo* in animals. Some 3D printed oral drug products have already been tested in animals with promising results. For instance, two anti-tuberculosis drugs, isoniazid and rifampicin, were incorporated into a 3D printed dosage form with two compartments to keep the drug separate and prevent interactions between them (Figure 2.3a) [52]. The *in vivo* release profiles showed a more rapid release of rifampicin and a more delayed release of isoniazid from the 3D printed form. Another example of the application of 3D printing in preclinical research is the creation of tablets with different sizes adapted for small animal administration (Figure 2.3b). These small tablets were fabricated with the aim of testing the *in vivo* pharmacokinetics of the drug warfarin administered in solution compared with its administration in a personalised tablet [53]. The *in vivo* results showed more controlled pharmacokinetic profiles with the drug administered as 3D-printed tablets, which is very important in the case of narrow therapeutic index drugs such as warfarin. In another study, 3D printed capsules containing the radiotracer ^{18}F-FDG were employed to assess intestinal behaviour in rats by the use of PET/CT imaging [54]. The capsules were fabricated using pharmaceutical excipients with different solubilities and release

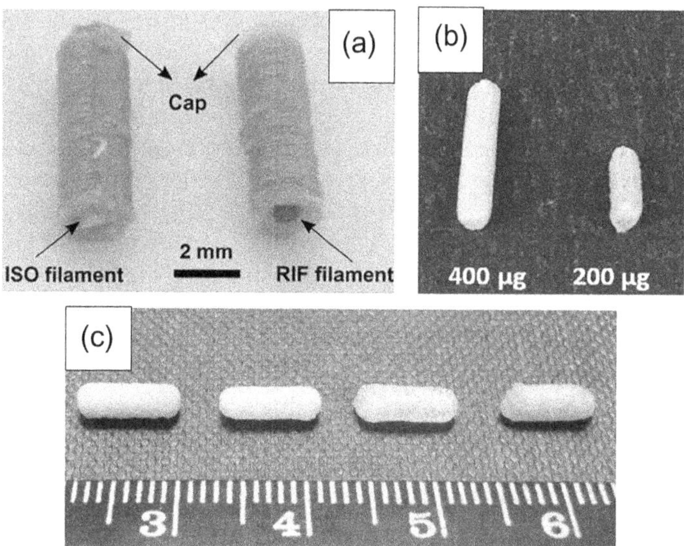

FIGURE 2.3 (a) Picture of the 3D printed dosage forms with two compartments loaded with rifampicin and isoniazid. (b) Photograph of 3D printed tablets adapted in size to be administered by oral gavage to rats. (c) Pictures of 3D printed devices for PET/CT studies in rats fabricated using different materials: Kollicoat IR, Klucel EF, Aqualon N7 and Aquasolve-LG, from left to right. Scale in cm. Reproduced with permission from Refs. [52–54].

characteristics (Kollicoat IR, Klucel EF, Aqualon N7 and Aquasolve-LG) (Figure 2.3c). Surprisingly, the capsules never emptied from the stomach even though they were manufactured in the recommended sizes (9 and 9h) for rodents. This inconsistency was investigated in a subsequent study, in which the use of anaesthetic agents and the size of the capsule were found to greatly influence gastric emptying [51].

2.4 3D PRINTED DEVICES FOR DRUG DELIVERY

Gastroretentive systems have also been fabricated by 3D printing. Gastroretentive formulations represent a useful approach to increase the gastric residence time of the formulation. One approach could be to include a commercial tablet within a floating 3D printed device, as shown in two studies using a sustained-release tablet of acyclovir [55] and an amoxicillin capsule [56]. In both studies, gastric residence time was prolonged as shown by X-ray images of the devices in beagle dogs and rabbits, respectively. Another approach could be to 3D print the floating device using filaments loaded with the drug, in this case domperidone [57]. The residence time was also evaluated using X-ray imaging in rabbits. The images revealed a prolonged drug release from the 3D printed device compared with commercial domperidone tablets.

More complex gastroretentive devices could also be manufactured using 3D printing. An example is found in the manufacturing of long-acting drug delivery devices capable of releasing anti-malarial drugs for at least 1 week [58]. The folded device is administered inside a gelatin capsule that dissolves in the stomach and releases the drug delivery system. The device then unfolds its arms and is able to stay in pigs' stomachs for 10 days. This approach could be especially useful for patients in remote areas with diseases for which obtaining constant drug blood levels over several days is crucial for treatment efficacy.

Biomedical electronics and 3D printing can also be combined to create personalised devices with both diagnostic and therapeutic functions [2]. Electronic devices that can be ingested rather than needing to be implanted represent a feasible approach to deliver drugs while collecting other data from the organism, such as temperature or pH. For instance, the creation of a wireless gastroretentive electronic device able to maintain in vivo wireless communication while releasing drugs was made possible using 3D printing [59]. The device was designed with two arms (Figure 2.4) to achieve a diameter greater than the pylorus so that it can be retained in the stomach for at least 36 days until it disintegrates and is excreted.

Fluid sampling represents another application of orally administered 3D-printed devices. Currently, gut microbiome testing often depends on easily accessible samples, such as faeces, which are not representative of the microbiome that can be found throughout the GI tract. The possibility of sampling gut microbiota from different regions of the GI tract could offer different perspectives on how human health is influenced by changes in the microbiome [60]. In this sense, using 3D printing, it was possible to create a miniaturised pill with microfluidic channels and an osmotic sampler capable of taking samples from different regions of the intestine of non-human primates and pigs [61]. The microbiota populations retrieved from the pill closely resembled the microbiome in the different regions the pill passed through, including the upper parts of the gastrointestinal tract.

In addition to oral dosage forms and devices, 3D printing has also been used to fabricate lipid-based suppositories. Initially, the suppositories were designed in different sizes and loaded with the drug tacrolimus for the treatment of ulcerative colitis

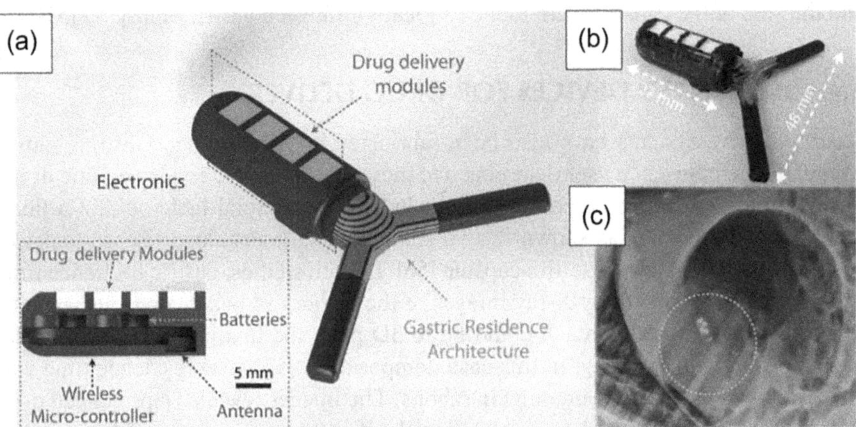

FIGURE 2.4 (a) Computer-aided design model of the gastroretentive electronic device showing its architecture, wireless system for communication and drug delivery compartments. (b) Dimensions of the device. (c) X-ray image of a porcine stomach with the gastroretentive device inside. Reproduced with permission from Ref. [59].

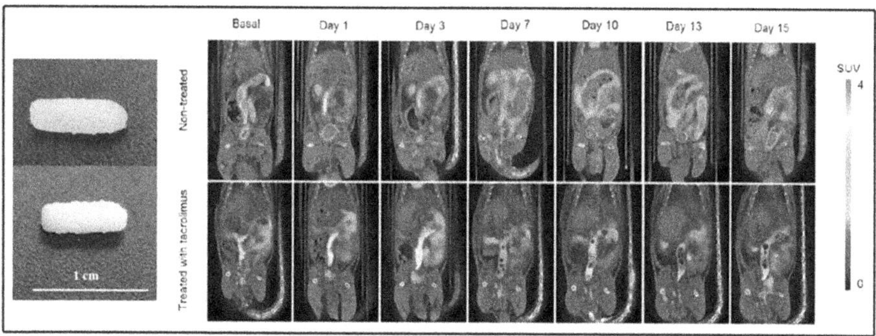

FIGURE 2.5 On the left, picture of the 3D printed rectal devices adapted in dose and size for administration to rats. On the right, PET/CT scan images over 15 days of the control group and the animals treated with the 3D printed tacrolimus rectal devices. A lower radiotracer uptake in the colon can be appreciated from day 7, which indicates that the animal is recovering from the illness. Reproduced with permission from Ref. [11].

in humans [20]. In subsequent work, the formulations were adapted for administration to small animals and tested *in vivo* in a colitis disease model in rats (Figure 2.5) [11]. PET/CT imaging technique was employed to evaluate the progression of the illness after daily administration of the suppositories to the rats, confirming a remission of the disease from day 7 after the beginning of treatment compared with the control group [62].

2.5 CLINICAL OPPORTUNITIES OF 3D PRINTING

The first clinical study in humans that reported the use of 3D printing for the manufacturing of personalised medicines in a hospital pharmacy service was published in 2019 [12]. It involved the preparation of chewable isoleucine printlets to treat children with a rare genetic disorder called maple syrup urine disease. The printlets were fabricated with different flavours and colours to be more attractive to children (Figure 2.6). Plasma drug concentration levels after administration of printlets were closer to the target value than those obtained with the isoleucine prepared trough manual compounding. This study represents an example of how 3D printing can be an alternative to the conventional extemporaneous preparation of medicines. Manual compounding is generally used at hospital pharmacies to prepare patient-specific drugs when they are not commercially available or are not available in the dose that the patient requires. However, it is a labour-intensive and time-consuming task that is not exempt of risks such as weighing errors. In this instance, an automatic technology like 3D printing capable of formulating medicines containing an exact dosage would prevent formulation errors from occurring as well as save time and costs.

Since this first study, several clinical studies have been conducted in humans to assess the use of 3D printing to prepare patient tailored medicines. Tablet splitting is another common practice among patients and caregivers, as most medications are marketed as limited dose strengths [63]. Thus, the dose is usually adjusted manually by

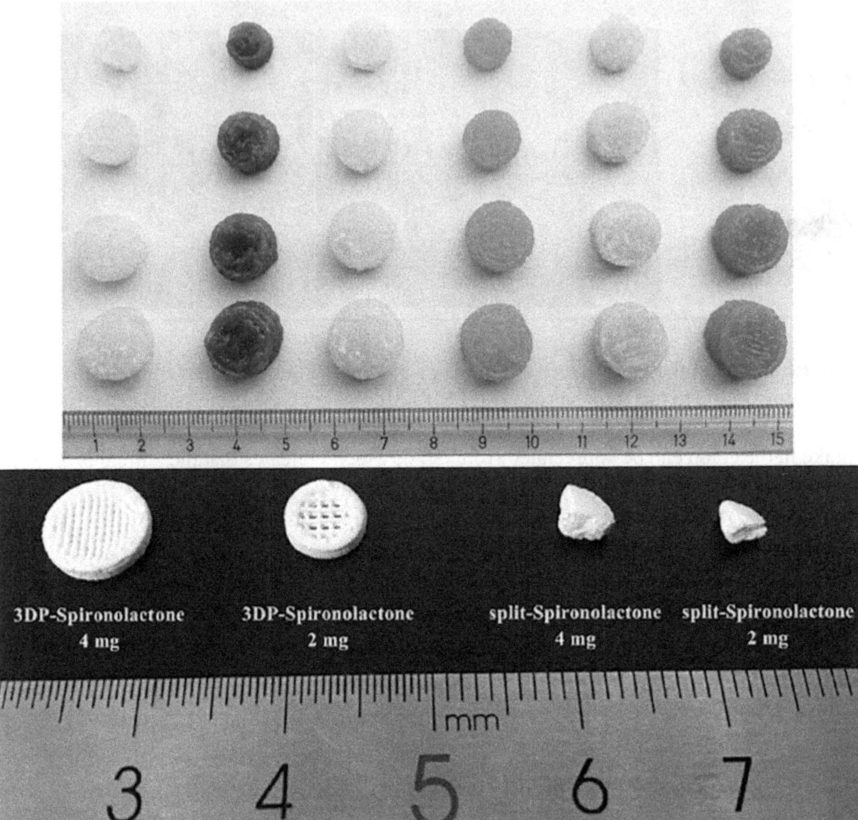

FIGURE 2.6 On top, chewable isoleucine printlets fabricated in different colours and flavours to treat children a genetic disorder called maple syrup urine disease. At the bottom, 3D printed spironolactone tablets compared with the commercial split tablets. Reproduced with permission from Refs. [12,66].

splitting or crushing the tablet to achieve the correct dosage. This practice involves the serious risk of inaccurate dosing as well as formulation failure, for example, if enteric-coated tablets are divided [64,65]. It has been shown in a study how tablets with exact doses of spironolactone and hydrochlorothiazide can be manufactured by 3D printing instead of using subdivided tablets obtained by pharmacists' splitting [66]. In addition to the better appearance of the 3D printed tablets (Figure 2.6), the 3D printed formulations showed better drug content and uniformity compared with the split tablets.

Paediatric and geriatric populations could specially benefit from this approach, as they often have different dosage and formulation requirements compared with the standard adult. For instance, children usually require personalised dosages of medicines based on their weight or body surface area. Also, children's acceptance of medicines is higher if they have particular formulation characteristics, such as being chewable or having a particular flavour or colour. This has been shown in a study [67] among children aged 4–11 years that highlighted children's preference for 3D printed chewable tablets. Taste adversity is another reason of medication refusal in children [68]. As shown in a study [69], 3D printing offers the possibility of preparing tablets with appealing forms also employing taste-masking approaches to improve treatment adherence. Printlets incorporating indomethacin as a model drug and mimicking Starmix® sweets were prepared in different forms (bear, lion, heart) and given to healthy volunteers to assess their taste-masking properties. The volunteers reported no aftertaste or bitterness, which is important for paediatric drug acceptance. Several works have focused on developing medicines especially focused on improving children's acceptance, for example by creating chocolate and gelatin-based dosage forms with attractive forms [43,70].

On the other hand, the needs of the elderly differ slightly from those of children. For example, it is more common among geriatric populations to have swallowing or visual impairments that make it more difficult to properly administer medications [71]. The perceptions and preferences of polypharmacy patients concerning 3D printed drugs were assessed in a study [14]. These patients tended to prefer not only conventional and easy-to-swallow shapes, but also forms that were easy to handle. A previous study in humans has already shown that people prefer printlets with a physical appearance to conventional dosage forms, although in this case the formulation with the highest score was the torus-shaped printlet [72]. Visually impaired patients may also benefit from 3D printed medicines. Printlets with Braille and moon patterns can be created for these patients to identify medications (Figure 2.7) [73,74]. The readability of the formulations was evaluated by blind people, who reported adequate legibility of the texts.

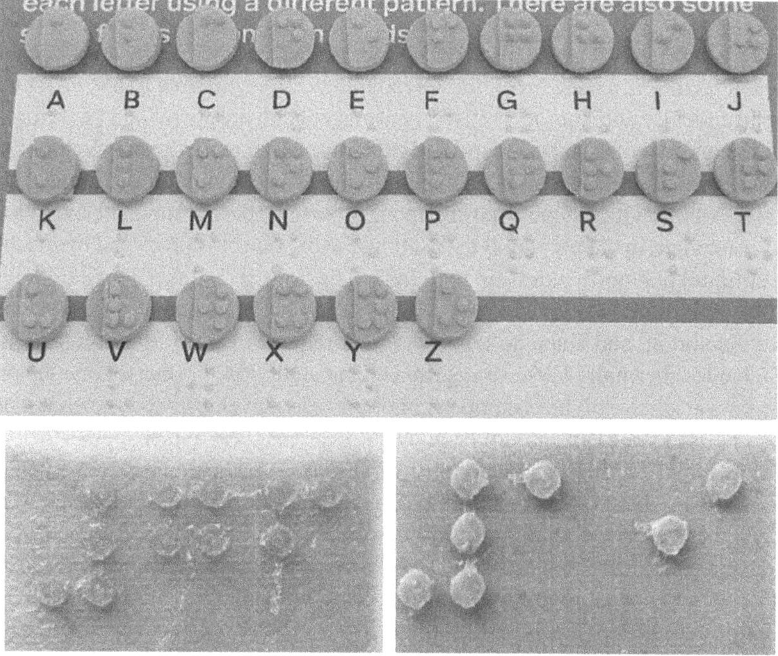

FIGURE 2.7 On top, photograph of printlets containing the 26 Braille alphabets. At the bottom, pictures of Braille dots onto the surface of two 3D printed films. Reproduced with permission from Refs. [73,74].

Another special population is represented by polypharmacy patients. Polypharmacy involves the use of two or more medicines at a time, especially among geriatric patients. People affected by a high tablet burden find it more difficult to follow their treatment regime, since a strong discipline with the therapy is needed [75,76]. The flexibility of 3D printing enables the creation of polypills (also called polyprintlets) to reduce the complexity of multi-drug treatments. Several studies have reported the creation of polyprintlets using 3D printing technologies [77–80]. For example, in one study [81], a polypill containing four different drugs was manufactured by combining 3D printing technology with hot-filling syringes. The drugs used in the treatment of cardiovascular pathologies (indapamide, amlodipine, lisinopril and rosuvastatin) were included in separate modules of the dosage form. In turn, the modular compartments had different spatial distributions and shell thickness to achieve different drug release profiles. Gastroplus® was used for *in silico* simulation of pharmacokinetics to offer an estimate *in vitro* plasma profile that could aid in the creation of a polyprintlet tailored to individual patient requirements. As with polypharmacy patients, another potential application of 3D printing in the clinical practice is the formulation of exact doses of narrow therapeutic index drugs for a specific patient. Achieving an exact dose of a narrow therapeutic index drug (i.e. drugs with small differences between therapeutic and toxic doses) is of the utmost importance to ensure adequate plasma levels of the drug, and thus ensure its efficacy and safety [82].

2.6 POTENTIAL 3D PRINTING TECHNOLOGIES FOR CLINICAL STUDIES

The 3D printing techniques used for these clinical studies were mainly material extrusion techniques, since with these technologies it is possible to use conventional pharmaceutical excipients to prepare pharmaceutical products, and therefore, it is easier to comply with pharmaceutical regulations. More recently, vat photopolymerisation technologies have also been explored for the production of medicines. Unlike material extrusion techniques that create 3D objects by depositing material in a layer-by-layer manner, in vat photopolymerisation, the 3D object is produced by irradiating a vat of liquid photopolymer resin with light. The light activates polymerisation reaction that solidifies the irradiated resin [83]. Structures 3D printed in this way have a higher resolution, and since no temperature is required for printing, the technology is suitable for thermally labile drugs. In a recent study [34], a smartphone 3D printer based on vat photopolymerisation technology was developed for the manufacture of personalised warfarin sodium printlets in different sizes and shapes (Figure 2.8).

The features of this compact smartphone-based 3D printing system make it a good candidate to be incorporated into future digital healthcare for the manufacture of medicines at the point of care, in emergency situations, hard-to-reach areas or low-resource settings. This platform is also an example of how 3D printing can make health technologies more affordable and accessible to all.

Another study [33] took advantage of a recently developed vat polymerisation technology known as volumetric 3D printing. This technology is based on the simultaneous irradiation of an entire volume of a photosensitive resin to create an entire 3D structure simultaneously (Figure 2.9).

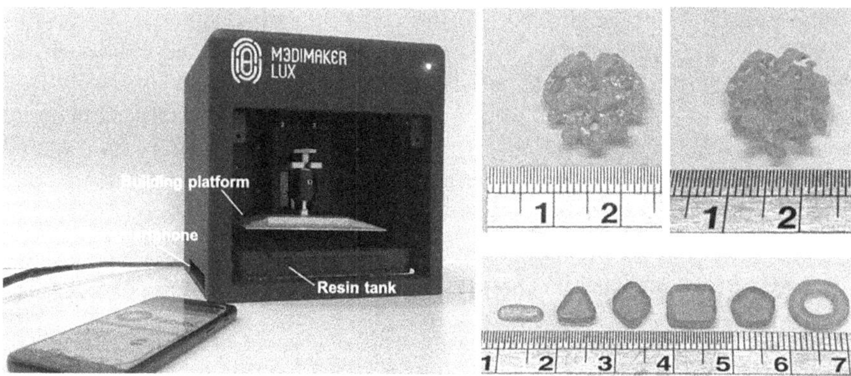

FIGURE 2.8 Photograph of the smartphone-based 3D printer alongside a smartphone. On the right, photograph of printlets in various geometries. Reproduced with permission from Ref. [34].

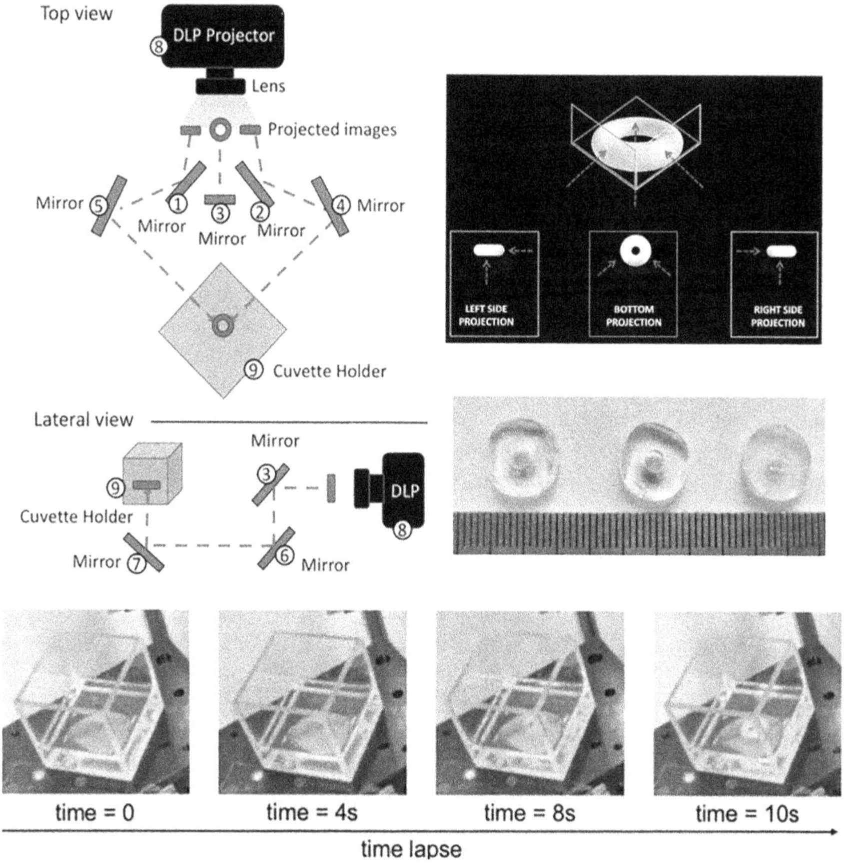

FIGURE 2.9 Schematic showing the volumetric 3D printing apparatus and the irradiance of the photosensitive resin with three orthogonal light beams, and picture of the fabricated printlets (scale in cm). Below, time lapse view of the cuvette during the manufacturing process. Reproduced with permission from Ref. [33].

The results of this study confirm the suitability of volumetric 3D printing technology for the fast and on-demand production of medicines. However, the main drawback of vat photopolymerisation technologies is the biocompatibility of the photosensitive materials used. More research is needed on the toxicological profile of the individual components of the formulation as well as on the products derived from the photopolymerisation reaction before its implementation in the clinic.

2.7 THE FUTURE OF 3D PRINTING IN PERSONALISED MEDICINE

3D printing is a constantly evolving field with new applications constantly being developed. These applications will not only be limited to the preparation of personalised human drugs at the point of care or in a hospital setting. For instance, a natural progression of this technology will take place towards the veterinary medicine sector due to its potential to prepare formulations suitable for animals in a wide range of dosages [15]. Currently, the number of approved veterinary drugs is limited, so it is common to resort to manual compounding and off-label use of human-marketed drugs, with the inherent risk of dosage errors. Recently, a few studies focused on the application of 3D printing to produce veterinary pet-friendly chewable medications [28,84]. With the growing awareness of animal welfare, it is likely that 3D printing will be soon implemented for production of veterinary formulations close to the point of care.

Hard-to-reach areas, disaster zones or even space are other fields that could certainly benefit from 3D printing technologies. The portable and decentralised nature of the technology makes it ideal for use in remote areas, and the low number of materials needed to prepare small batches of medicines makes the technology also suitable for areas where resources are scarce [1]. For example, future deep space missions to Mars or other planets will require technologies that enable on-demand manufacturing of pharmaceuticals, as stored drugs are prone to degradation over time, especially in a harsh environment like outer space [85]. NASA has already begun to include additive manufacturing technologies in missions for on-demand manufacturing of spare parts, logistics and maintenance [86]. For the future of space exploration to be successful, it will be necessary to develop new technologies capable of helping maintain the health of the crew. 3D printing holds that potential, as the small size of the printers would make them easily transportable on board. Medicines could be prepared on-demand using excipients and drugs stored or synthesised on board (Figure 2.10) [27].

However, space medicine is just one of the achievements that may be possible by combining 3D printing with other digital technologies, such as artificial intelligence, robots and biosensors [6,87]. A new and digitalised healthcare model would be based on a decentralised manufacturing platform, where tailored medicines can be produced both at the point of care or in remote areas based on digital prescriptions.

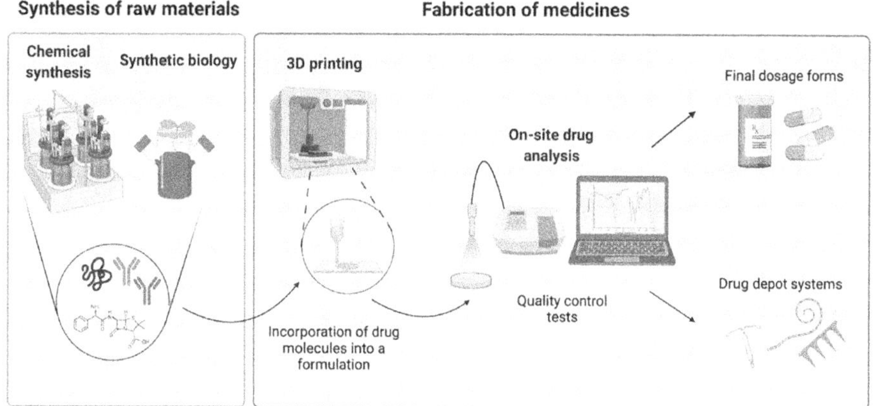

FIGURE 2.10 An example of the possible role of 3D printing in future space travel. Reproduced with permission from Ref. [27].

2.8 QUALITY CONTROL TECHNIQUES FOR 3D PRINTED DRUG PRODUCTS

An important aspect in this future scenario will be the quality control (QC) of processes and final products to guarantee the safety and efficacy of medicines. Traditional QC measures based on laborious and destructive techniques would not be suitable for 3D-printed medicines. These conventional techniques must be replaced by non-destructive analytical methods, such as spectroscopic analytical technologies. Near-infrared (NIR) and Raman spectroscopy have already shown great potential for rapid non-destructive analysis of drug content in 3D printed products [88]. Furthermore, the portability of these analytical sensors makes them ideal to be used in remote areas or clinical settings in conjunction with 3D printers. Final drug products should also comply with regulatory standards for medicines [89] and 3D printers must meet Good Manufacturing Practice (GMP) requirements [90]. But all efforts to move towards digitalisation of health systems are in vain if regulatory agencies do update legislations to ensure that they are up to date with the current technological advances. Regulatory bodies must find a balance between protecting patients and healthcare workers without impeding the advancement of digital technologies such as 3D printing.

2.9 CONCLUSIONS

This chapter briefly reviews the main recent research on the applications of 3D printing technology in the areas of clinical and preclinical research. 3D printing enables the on-demand manufacturing of small batches of dosage forms with different dosages suited for preclinical or clinical studies, which is currently unfeasible with conventional manufacturing techniques. Moreover, the affordability and portability of 3D printers make them well suited to be implemented in clinical settings, at the point of care, or even in remote areas such as the outer space. However, it is still necessary to develop quality control measures adapted to this new technology and review and update the regulations before this new pharmaceutical model becomes a reality.

ACKNOWLEDGEMENT

I.S.-V. acknowledges Consellería de Cultura, Educación e Universidade for her Postdoctoral Fellowship (Xunta de Galicia, Spain; ED481B-2021-019).

REFERENCES

1. Seoane-Viaño I, Trenfield SJ, Basit AW, Goyanes A. Translating 3D printed pharmaceuticals: From hype to real-world clinical applications. *Adv Drug Deliv Rev.* 2021;174:553–75.
2. Ghosh U, Ning S, Wang Y, Kong YL. Addressing unmet clinical needs with 3D printing technologies. *Adv Healthc Mater.* 2018;7(17):e1800417.
3. Goyanes A, Wang J, Buanz A, Martinez-Pacheco R, Telford R, Gaisford S, et al. 3D printing of medicines: Engineering novel oral devices with unique design and drug release characteristics. *Mol Pharm.* 2015;12(11):4077–84.
4. Wang J, Zhang Y, Aghda NH, Pillai AR, Thakkar R, Nokhodchi A, et al. Emerging 3D printing technologies for drug delivery devices: Current status and future perspective. *Adv Drug Deliv Rev.* 2021;174:294–316.
5. Aprecia_Pharmaceuticals. FDA approves the first 3D printed drug product. https://wwwapreciacom/pdf/2015_08_03_Spritam_FDA_Approval_Press_Releasepdf, last accessed 9, 2018. 2015.
6. Ong JJ, Pollard TD, Goyanes A, Gaisford S, Elbadawi M, Basit AW. Optical biosensors - Illuminating the path to personalized drug dosing. *Biosens Bioelectron.* 2021;188:113331.
7. Trenfield SJ, Awad A, McCoubrey LE, Elbadawi M, Goyanes A, Gaisford S, et al. Advancing pharmacy and healthcare with virtual digital technologies. *Adv Drug Deliv Rev.* 2022;182:114098.
8. Awad A, Trenfield SJ, Pollard TD, Ong JJ, Elbadawi M, McCoubrey LE, et al. Connected healthcare: Improving patient care using digital health technologies. *Adv Drug Deliv Rev.* 2021;178:113958.
9. Andreadis, II, Gioumouxouzis CI, Eleftheriadis GK, Fatouros DG. The advent of a new era in digital healthcare: A role for 3D printing technologies in drug manufacturing? *Pharmaceutics.* 2022;14(3):609.
10. Awad A, Fina F, Trenfield SJ, Patel P, Goyanes A, Gaisford S, et al. 3D printed pellets (miniprintlets): A novel, multi-drug, controlled release platform technology. *Pharmaceutics.* 2019;11(4):148.
11. Seoane-Viaño I, Gómez-Lado N, Lázare-Iglesias H, García-Otero X, Antúnez-López JR, Ruibal Á, et al. 3D printed tacrolimus rectal formulations ameliorate colitis in an experimental animal model of inflammatory bowel disease. *Biomedicines.* 2020;8(12):563.
12. Goyanes A, Madla CM, Umerji A, Duran Piñeiro G, Giraldez Montero JM, Lamas Diaz MJ, et al. Automated therapy preparation of isoleucine formulations using 3D printing for the treatment of MSUD: First single-centre, prospective, crossover study in patients. *Int J Pharm.* 2019;567:118497.

13. Lafeber I, Ruijgrok EJ, Guchelaar HJ, Schimmel KJM. 3D printing of pediatric medication: The end of bad tasting oral liquids?-A scoping review. *Pharmaceutics.* 2022;14(2):416.
14. Fastø MM, Genina N, Kaae S, Kälvemark Sporrong S. Perceptions, preferences and acceptability of patient designed 3D printed medicine by polypharmacy patients: A pilot study. *Int J Clin Pharm.* 2019;41(5):1290–8.
15. Rodríguez-Pombo L, Awad A, Basit AW, Alvarez-Lorenzo C, Goyanes A. Innovations in chewable formulations: The novelty and applications of 3D printing in drug product design. *Pharmaceutics.* 2022;14(8):1732.
16. Fanous M, Bitar M, Gold S, Sobczuk A, Hirsch S, Ogorka J, et al. Development of immediate release 3D-printed dosage forms for a poorly water-soluble drug by fused deposition modeling: Study of morphology, solid state and dissolution. *Int J Pharm.* 2021;599:120417.
17. Ghanizadeh Tabriz A, Nandi U, Hurt AP, Hui HW, Karki S, Gong Y, et al. 3D printed bilayer tablet with dual controlled drug release for tuberculosis treatment. *Int J Pharm.* 2021;593:120147.
18. Almeida A, Linares V, Mora-Castaño G, Casas M, Caraballo I, Sarmento B. 3D printed systems for colon-specific delivery of camptothecin-loaded chitosan micelles. *Eur J Pharm Biopharm.* 2021;167:48–56.
19. Saviano M, Bowles BJ, Penny MR, Ishaq A, Muwaffak Z, Falcone G, et al. Development and analysis of a novel loading technique for FDM 3D printed systems: Microwave-assisted impregnation of gastro-retentive PVA capsular devices. *Int J Pharm.* 2022;613:121386.
20. Seoane-Viaño I, Ong JJ, Luzardo-Álvarez A, González-Barcia M, Basit AW, Otero-Espinar FJ, et al. 3D printed tacrolimus suppositories for the treatment of ulcerative colitis. *Asian J Pharm Sci.* 2021;16(1):110–9.
21. Tagami T, Ito E, Hayashi N, Sakai N, Ozeki T. Application of 3D printing technology for generating hollow-type suppository shells. *Int J Pharm.* 2020;589:119825.
22. Xu X, Awwad S, Diaz-Gomez L, Alvarez-Lorenzo C, Brocchini S, Gaisford S, et al. 3D Printed punctal plugs for controlled ocular drug delivery. *Pharmaceutics.* 2021;13(9):1421.
23. Xu X, Goyanes A, Trenfield SJ, Diaz-Gomez L, Alvarez-Lorenzo C, Gaisford S, et al. Stereolithography (SLA) 3D printing of a bladder device for intravesical drug delivery. *Mater Sci Eng C, Mater Biol Appl.* 2021;120: 111773.
24. Koffler J, Zhu W, Qu X, Platoshyn O, Dulin JN, Brock J, et al. Biomimetic 3D-printed scaffolds for spinal cord injury repair. *Nat Med.* 2019;25(2):263–9.
25. Economidou SN, Pere CPP, Reid A, Uddin MJ, Windmill JFC, Lamprou DA, et al. 3D printed microneedle patches using stereolithography (SLA) for intradermal insulin delivery. *Mater Sci Eng C, Mater Biol Appl.* 2019;102:743–55.
26. Liaskoni A, Wildman RD, Roberts CJ. 3D printed polymeric drug-eluting implants. *Int J Pharm.* 2021;597:120330.
27. Seoane-Viaño I, Ong JJ, Basit AW, Goyanes A. To infinity and beyond: Strategies for fabricating medicines in outer space. *Int J Pharm: X.* 2022;4:100121.
28. Sjöholm E, Mathiyalagan R, Lindfors L, Wang X, Ojala S, Sandler N. Semi-solid extrusion 3D printing of tailored ChewTs for veterinary use - A focus on spectrophotometric quantification of gabapentin. *Eur J Pharm Sci.* 2022;174:106190.
29. Kozakiewicz-Latała M, Nartowski KP, Dominik A, Malec K, Gołkowska AM, Złocińska A, et al. Binder jetting 3D printing of challenging medicines: From low dose tablets to hydrophobic molecules. *Eur J Pharm Biopharm.* 2022;170:144–59.
30. Infanger S, Haemmerli A, Iliev S, Baier A, Stoyanov E, Quodbach J. Powder bed 3D-printing of highly loaded drug delivery devices with hydroxypropyl cellulose as solid binder. *Int J Pharm.* 2019;555:198–206.

31. He Y, Foralosso R, Trindade GF, Ilchev A, Ruiz-Cantu L, Clark EA, et al. A reactive prodrug ink formulation strategy for inkjet 3D printing of controlled release dosage forms and implants. *Adv Ther.* 2020;3(6):1900187.
32. Evans SE, Harrington T, Rodriguez Rivero MC, Rognin E, Tuladhar T, Daly R. 2D and 3D inkjet printing of biopharmaceuticals - A review of trends and future perspectives in research and manufacturing. *Int J Pharm.* 2021;599:120443.
33. Rodríguez-Pombo L, Xu X, Seijo-Rabina A, Ong JJ, Alvarez-Lorenzo C, Rial C, et al. Volumetric 3D printing for rapid production of medicines. *Addit Manuf.* 2022;52:102673.
34. Xu X, Seijo-Rabina A, Awad A, Rial C, Gaisford S, Basit AW, et al. Smartphone-enabled 3D printing of medicines. *Int J Pharm.* 2021;609:121199.
35. Awad A, Fina F, Goyanes A, Gaisford S, Basit AW. 3D printing: Principles and pharmaceutical applications of selective laser sintering. *Int J Pharm.* 2020;586:119594.
36. Yang Y, Xu Y, Wei S, Shan W. Oral preparations with tunable dissolution behavior based on selective laser sintering technique. *Int J Pharm.* 2021;593:120127.
37. Awad A, Gaisford S, Basit AW. Fused deposition modelling: Advances in engineering and medicine. In: Basit AW, Gaisford S, editors. *3D Printing of Pharmaceuticals.* Springer International Publishing; 2018. pp. 107–32.
38. Goyanes A, Fina F, Martorana A, Sedough D, Gaisford S, Basit AW. Development of modified release 3D printed tablets (printlets) with pharmaceutical excipients using additive manufacturing. *Int J Pharm.* 2017;527(1–2):21–30.
39. Goyanes A, Allahham N, Trenfield SJ, Stoyanov E, Gaisford S, Basit AW. Direct powder extrusion 3D printing: Fabrication of drug products using a novel single-step process. *Int J Pharm.* 2019;567:118471.
40. Ong JJ, Awad A, Martorana A, Gaisford S, Stoyanov E, Basit AW, et al. 3D printed opioid medicines with alcohol-resistant and abuse-deterrent properties. *Int J Pharm.* 2020;579:119169.
41. Zheng Y, Deng F, Wang B, Wu Y, Luo Q, Zuo X, et al. Melt extrusion deposition (MED™) 3D printing technology - A paradigm shift in design and development of modified release drug products. *Int J Pharm.* 2021;602:120639.
42. Seoane-Viaño I, Januskaite P, Alvarez-Lorenzo C, Basit AW, Goyanes A. Semi-solid extrusion 3D printing in drug delivery and biomedicine: Personalised solutions for healthcare challenges. *J Control Release.* 2021;332:367–89.
43. Karavasili C, Gkaragkounis A, Moschakis T, Ritzoulis C, Fatouros DG. Pediatric-friendly chocolate-based dosage forms for the oral administration of both hydrophilic and lipophilic drugs fabricated with extrusion-based 3D printing. *Eur J Pharm Sci.* 2020;147:105291.
44. Chatzitaki A-T, Tsongas K, Tzimtzimis EK, Tzetzis D, Bouropoulos N, Barmpalexis P, et al. 3D printing of patient-tailored SNEDDS-based suppositories of lidocaine. *J Drug Deliv Sci Tec.* 2021;61:102292.
45. Seoane-Viaño I, Otero-Espinar FJ, Goyanes Á. Chapter 18-3D printing of pharmaceutical products. In: Pou J, Riveiro A, Davim JP, editors. *Additive Manufacturing.* Elsevier; 2021. pp. 569–97.
46. Capel AJ, Rimington RP, Lewis MP, Christie SDR. 3D printing for chemical, pharmaceutical and biological applications. *Nat Rev Chem.* 2018;2(12):422–36.
47. Basit AW, Gaisford S. *3D Printing of Pharmaceuticals.* 1 ed. Springer International Publishing; 2018. DOI: 10.1007/978-3-319-90755-0.
48. Nair A, Morsy MA, Jacob S. Dose translation between laboratory animals and human in preclinical and clinical phases of drug development. *Drug Dev Res.* 2018;79(8):373–82.

49. Agoram BM. Use of pharmacokinetic/pharmacodynamic modelling for starting dose selection in first-in-human trials of high-risk biologics. *Br J Clin Pharmacol.* 2009;67(2):153–60.
50. Hammond T, Allen P, Birdsall H. Is there a space-based technology solution to problems with preclinical drug toxicity testing? *Pharm Res.* 2016;33(7):1545–51.
51. Gómez-Lado N, Seoane-Viaño I, Matiz S, Madla CM, Yadav V, Aguiar P, et al. Gastrointestinal tracking and gastric emptying of coated capsules in rats with or without sedation using CT imaging. *Pharmaceutics.* 2020;12(1):81.
52. Genina N, Boetker JP, Colombo S, Harmankaya N, Rantanen J, Bohr A. Anti-tuberculosis drug combination for controlled oral delivery using 3D printed compartmental dosage forms: From drug product design to in vivo testing. *J Control Release.* 2017;268:40–8.
53. Arafat B, Qinna N, Cieszynska M, Forbes RT, Alhnan MA. Tailored on demand anti-coagulant dosing: An in vitro and in vivo evaluation of 3D printed purpose-designed oral dosage forms. *Eur J Pharm Biopharm.* 2018;128:282–9.
54. Goyanes A, Fernandez-Ferreiro A, Majeed A, Gomez-Lado N, Awad A, Luaces-Rodriguez A, et al. PET/CT imaging of 3D printed devices in the gastrointestinal tract of rodents. *Int J Pharm.* 2018;536(1):158–64.
55. Shin S, Kim TH, Jeong SW, Chung SE, Lee DY, Kim DH, et al. Development of a gastroretentive delivery system for acyclovir by 3D printing technology and its in vivo pharmacokinetic evaluation in Beagle dogs. *PLoS One.* 2019;14(5):e0216875.
56. Charoenying T, Patrojanasophon P, Ngawhirunpat T, Rojanarata T, Akkaramongkolporn P, Opanasopit P. Fabrication of floating capsule-in-3D-printed devices as gastro-retentive delivery systems of amoxicillin. *J Drug Deliv Sci Tec.* 2020;55:101393.
57. Chai X, Chai H, Wang X, Yang J, Li J, Zhao Y, et al. Fused deposition modeling (FDM) 3D printed tablets for intragastric floating delivery of domperidone. *Sci Rep.* 2017;7(1):2829.
58. Bellinger AM, Jafari M, Grant TM, Zhang S, Slater HC, Wenger EA, et al. Oral, ultra-long-lasting drug delivery: Application toward malaria elimination goals. *Sci Transl Med.* 2016;8(365):365ra157.
59. Kong YL, Zou X, McCandler CA, Kirtane AR, Ning S, Zhou J, et al. 3D-printed gastric resident electronics. *Adv Mater Technol.* 2019;4(3):1800490.
60. Awad A, Madla CM, McCoubrey LE, Ferraro F, Gavins FKH, Buanz A, et al. Clinical translation of advanced colonic drug delivery technologies. *Adv Drug Deliv Rev.* 2022;181:114076.
61. Rezaei Nejad H, Oliveira BCM, Sadeqi A, Dehkharghani A, Kondova I, Langermans JAM, et al. Ingestible osmotic pill for in vivo sampling of gut microbiomes. *Adv Intell Syst.* 2019;1(5):1900053.
62. Seoane-Viaño I, Gómez-Lado N, Lázare-Iglesias H, Barreiro-de Acosta M, Silva-Rodríguez J, Luzardo-Álvarez A, et al. Longitudinal PET/CT evaluation of TNBS-induced inflammatory bowel disease rat model. *Int J Pharm.* 2018;549(1–2):335–42.
63. van der Vossen AC, Al-Hassany L, Buljac S, Brugma JD, Vulto AG, Hanff LM. Manipulation of oral medication for children by parents and nurses occurs frequently and is often not supported by instructions. *Acta Paediatr (Oslo, Norway: 1992).* 2019;108(8):1475–81.
64. Habib WA, Alanizi AS, Abdelhamid MM, Alanizi FK. Accuracy of tablet splitting: Comparison study between hand splitting and tablet cutter. *Saudi Pharm J: SPJ.* 2014;22(5):454–9.
65. Hill S, Varker AS, Karlage K, Myrdal PB. Analysis of drug content and weight uniformity for half-tablets of 6 commonly split medications. *J Manage Care Pharm.* 2009;15(3):253–61.

66. Zheng Z, Lv J, Yang W, Pi X, Lin W, Lin Z, et al. Preparation and application of subdivided tablets using 3D printing for precise hospital dispensing. *Eur J Pharm Sci.* 2020;149:105293.
67. Januskaite P, Xu X, Ranmal SR, Gaisford S, Basit AW, Tuleu C, et al. I spy with my little eye: A paediatric visual preferences survey of 3D printed tablets. *Pharmaceutics.* 2020;12(11). DOI: 10.3390/pharmaceutics12111100.
68. Mennella JA, Roberts KM, Mathew PS, Reed DR. Children's perceptions about medicines: individual differences and taste. *BMC Pediatr.* 2015;15:130.
69. Scoutaris N, Ross SA, Douroumis D. 3D printed "Starmix" drug loaded dosage forms for paediatric applications. *Pharm Res.* 2018;35(2):34.
70. Rycerz K, Stepien KA, Czapiewska M, Arafat BT, Habashy R, Isreb A, et al. Embedded 3D printing of novel bespoke soft dosage form concept for pediatrics. *Pharmaceutics.* 2019;11(12):630.
71. Sestili M, Logrippo S, Cespi M, Bonacucina G, Ferrara L, Busco S, et al. Potentially inappropriate prescribing of oral solid medications in elderly dysphagic patients. *Pharmaceutics.* 2018;10(4). DOI: 10.3390/pharmaceutics10040280.
72. Goyanes A, Scarpa M, Kamlow M, Gaisford S, Basit AW, Orlu M. Patient acceptability of 3D printed medicines. *Int J Pharm.* 2017;530(1):71–8.
73. Eleftheriadis GK, Fatouros DG. Haptic evaluation of 3D-printed braille-encoded intraoral films. *Eur J Pharm Sci.* 2021;157:105605.
74. Awad A, Yao A, Trenfield SJ, Goyanes A, Gaisford S, Basit AW. 3D printed tablets (printlets) with braille and moon patterns for visually impaired patients. *Pharmaceutics.* 2020;12(2):172.
75. Maher RL, Hanlon J, Hajjar ER. Clinical consequences of polypharmacy in elderly. *Expert Opin Drug Saf.* 2014;13(1):57–65.
76. Murray MD, Kroenke K. Polypharmacy and medication adherence: Small steps on a long road. *J Gen Intern Med.* 2001;16(2):137–9.
77. Windolf H, Chamberlain R, Breitkreutz J, Quodbach J. 3D printed mini-floating-polypill for Parkinson's disease: Combination of levodopa, benserazide, and pramipexole in various dosing for personalized therapy. *Pharmaceutics.* 2022;14(5). DOI: 10.3390/pharmaceutics14050931.
78. Alayoubi A, Zidan A, Asfari S, Ashraf M, Sau L, Kopcha M. Mechanistic understanding of the performance of personalized 3D-printed cardiovascular polypills: A case study of patient-centered therapy. *Int J Pharm.* 2022;617:121599.
79. Pereira BC, Isreb A, Forbes RT, Dores F, Habashy R, Petit JB, et al. 'Temporary Plasticiser': A novel solution to fabricate 3D printed patient-centred cardiovascular 'Polypill' architectures. *Eur J Pharm Biopharm.* 2019;135:94–103.
80. Keikhosravi N, Mirdamadian SZ, Varshosaz J, Taheri A. Preparation and characterization of polypills containing aspirin and simvastatin using 3D printing technology for the prevention of cardiovascular diseases. *Drug Dev Ind Pharm.* 2020;46(10):1665–75.
81. Pereira BC, Isreb A, Isreb M, Forbes RT, Oga EF, Alhnan MA. Additive manufacturing of a point-of-care "Polypill:" Fabrication of concept capsules of complex geometry with bespoke release against cardiovascular disease. *Adv Healthc Mater.* 2020;9(13):e2000236.
82. Beg S, Almalki WH, Malik A, Farhan M, Aatif M, Rahman Z, et al. 3D printing for drug delivery and biomedical applications. *Drug Discov Today.* 2020;25(9):1668–81.
83. Xu X, Awad A, Robles-Martinez P, Gaisford S, Goyanes A, Basit AW. Vat photopolymerization 3D printing for advanced drug delivery and medical device applications. *J Control Release.* 2021;329:743–57.

84. Sjöholm E, Mathiyalagan R, Wang X, Sandler N. Compounding tailored veterinary chewable tablets close to the point-of-care by means of 3D printing. *Pharmaceutics.* 2022;14(7):1339.
85. Wotring VE. Chemical potency and degradation products of medications stored over 550 earth days at the international space station. *AAPS J.* 2016;18(1):210–6.
86. Prater T, Werkheiser N, Ledbetter F, Timucin D, Wheeler K, Snyder M. 3D Printing in zero G technology demonstration mission: Complete experimental results and summary of related material modeling efforts. *Int J Adv Manuf Technol.* 2019;101(1–4):391–417.
87. Ong JJ, Castro BM, Gaisford S, Cabalar P, Basit AW, Pérez G, et al. Accelerating 3D printing of pharmaceutical products using machine learning. *Int J Pharm X.* 2022;4:100120.
88. Trenfield SJ, Tan HX, Goyanes A, Wilsdon D, Rowland M, Gaisford S, et al. Non-destructive dose verification of two drugs within 3D printed polyprintlets. *Int J Pharm.* 2020;577:119066.
89. Awad A, Trenfield SJ, Basit AW. Chapter 19-Solid oral dosage forms. In: Adejare A, editor. *Remington* (23 Edition). Academic Press; 2021. pp. 333–58.
90. Melocchi A, Briatico-Vangosa F, Uboldi M, Parietti F, Turchi M, von Zeppelin D, et al. Quality considerations on the pharmaceutical applications of fused deposition modeling 3D printing. *Int J Pharm.* 2021;592:119901.

3 3D Printing for *In Vitro* Drug Release Analysis and Cell Culture Applications

Daniel Andrés Real and Marcelo Javier Kogan
Universidad de Chile and Advanced Center for Chronic Diseases

Santiago Daniel Palma and Juan Pablo Real
Unidad de cg y Desarrollo en Tecnología Farmacéutica (UNITEFA), CONICET and Universidad Nacional de Córdoba

CONTENTS

3.1 INTRODUCTION

3D printing (3DP) refers to various flexible manufacturing techniques for three-dimensional solid object production. Following instructions stored in a digital file, printers transform different materials into successive layers of a geometric element [1,2]. Based on this, 3DP has generated enormous interest in different industries, including the pharmaceutical, where the number of publications related to this

DOI: 10.1201/9781003274568-3

subject is increasing yearly [3]. In the pharmaceutical field, 3DP technology represents a versatile tool that has the potential to bring about a paradigm shift in the way drugs are produced. At a general level, 3DP allows the following distinguishing features for pharmaceutical formulation:

- Combine materials with different physicochemical properties (hydrophobicity/hydrophilicity) and inks with different active ingredients. The different inks can even be placed, without being mixed, on different layers or surfaces of the structure.
- Obtain innovative geometries, challenging to achieve with traditional methods, such as hollow or porous structures.
- Create solid structures of different shapes and sizes without loss of precision, using the same equipment and without changes in assembly.

Several 3DP methods have been developed, described, and patented for solid dosage form (SDF) production. Thus, 3DP techniques distinguish three main groups: printing systems based on inkjet, extrusion methods from nozzles, and systems based on electromagnetic radiation [3]. The rationale behind 3DP is always the same: The material is added layer by layer until the desired 3D shape is obtained. However, each of the techniques mentioned above uses completely different methodologies and presents characteristics with advantages and disadvantages when used in the production of pharmaceutical systems. In all cases, 3D printers fall short of competing with traditional drug manufacturing techniques. In large-scale drug production, production times per 3DP are 60 times longer, and costs are much higher [1]. Nevertheless, 3DP offers the possibility of obtaining SDF with unique and differential potentialities, which are challenging to achieve with industrial manufacturing:

- Design SDF customized to the patient's pharmacotherapy, adapting the dosage to the body mass and metabolic needs specific to the individualized treatment [4].
- Adjust drug release kinetics. By changing the shape, the composition of the materials, or how they are arranged in the dosage forms, immediate release [5], delayed release [6], extended release [7], dual release [8], and site-specific release [9] systems have been obtained.
- To create floating structures capable of being retained at the stomach level to favor the release of weak bases (whose absorption is favored by acidic conditions) or actives with specific action at this level [10–12].
- To obtain SDF loaded with nanoparticulate systems of different nature that traditional methods cannot obtain [13].
- To group numerous active pharmaceutical ingredients (API), even incompatible ones, in the same SDF [14]. This POLYPILL combination differs from industrially produced fixed-dose drug combinations in its ability to customize dosage and composition.

Although the direct manufacturing of pharmaceutical forms using 3D technology is an exciting topic, it does not exhaust the possibilities of 3DP for pharmaceutical technology. The capabilities of 3DP related to the fabrication of complex geometries, with no material waste and with the ability to regulate micron-sized shapes, can find a range of applications in the development of analytical equipment and models dedicated to specific non-standard dosage forms. Several pharmaceutical research groups have also applied this technology to developing *in vitro* drug testing analysis and cell culture applications. Additionally, due to the diversity of materials feasible, it is possible to create 3D cell culture models and organ-on-a-chip (OoC) platforms. These cultures can be generated with heterogeneous human cells mimicking the mechanical, physiological, and chemical characteristics of *in vivo* tissues providing a promising solution to overcome the shortcomings of both conventional 2D cell culture and animal testing [15].

Moreover, due to the flexibility of this technique and the speed with which models can be modified, 3DP also has the advantage of allowing iterative design. This involves applying a sequence of steps that can be repeated several times until the optimal shape and functionality of the printed object are achieved (Figure 3.1). This way, optimizing the *in vitro* models is possible until those with the highest degree of correlation to the *in vivo* results are achieved. Moreover, quality by design techniques could be applied to optimize these processes rationally [16,17].

To gain a deeper understanding of the developments achieved through 3DP related to these topics, the following sections discuss the use of 3DP in obtaining physical models for *in vitro* drug testing (without the incorporation of cells into the ink matrix) and the applications, limitations, and expectations of using 3DP in cell cultures and OoCs' development. Undoubtedly, these issues will be helpful for those students or research groups who want to introduce the world of 3DP applied to the development of *in vitro* pharmaceutical characterization techniques.

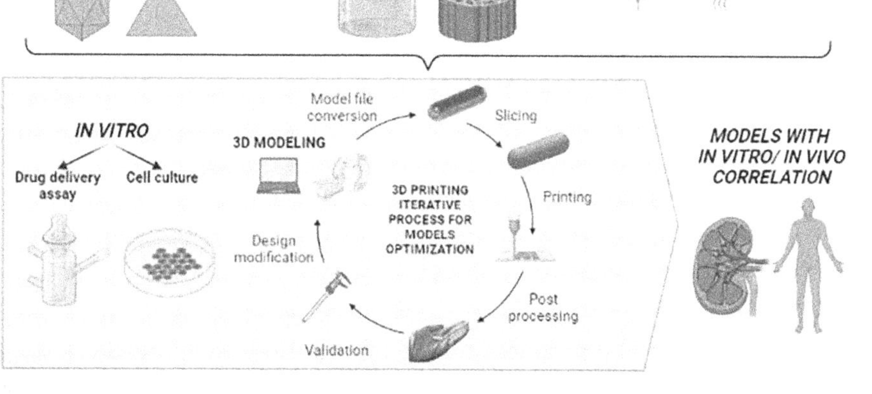

FIGURE 3.1 Main advantages of 3D printing for *in vitro* drug release analysis and cell culture applications.

3.2 3D PRINTING FOR *IN VITRO* DRUG TESTING SYSTEMS DEVELOPMENT

Developing new pharmaceutical products involves a series of research stages to evaluate the new product's safety and effectiveness. While animal testing remains the gold standard as a step prior to human testing, there are bioethical, legal, economic, and scientific reasons to develop technologies to reduce the number of *in vivo* tests [18]. From a scientific point of view, *in vitro* studies are conducted before clinical trials to optimize drug delivery methods or to demonstrate *in vitro* guidance. *In vitro* models can be used at the early stages, allowing elucidation of properties and mechanisms that contribute to the system evaluation. The more significant the correlation between the *in vitro* and *in vivo* models, the less likely candidates will fail in clinical trials, that is, be filtered out by the models, which translates into reduced I+D costs [19,20].

3D printing, like every aspect of science and technology, has advanced over the years. The increased resolution and lower costs associated with printers have provided the necessary resources to make it possible and affordable to convert any digital image created by a computer-aided design (CAD) package, a 3D scanner, or medical equipment (e.g., a computed tomography (CT) scanner) into a solid element [21]. Thus, 3DP makes it possible to obtain three-dimensional models that mimic the geometry of human organs, with their different cavities and chambers, but it is also possible to obtain such models from scanned medical images of a patient. Considering that the greater the degree of imitation the model achieves, the more valuable and predictive data it provides, it is easy to understand why 3D-printed *in vitro* models have begun to acquire relevance [22].

In vitro drug release studies are the most frequently applied biopharmaceutical tests for evaluating dosage forms [23]. These studies provide valuable information on the properties of the dosage forms tested. In many cases, they lack specificity or do not correctly reflect the physical release environment, especially in the case of non-standard dosage forms such as mucoadhesive implants, contact lenses, or nasal dosage forms. This section reviews how 3DP capabilities are used to develop analytical equipment and models dedicated to different dosage forms.

3.2.1 3D-Printed *In Vitro* Mouth Cavity Models

The first choice when establishing drug therapy is the oral route for convenience, safety, and price. However, various new drug delivery systems, such as orodispersible tablets, are administered orally but not swallowed. For example, Spritam is the first FDA-approved 3D-printed drug [24]. The powder deposition 3DP technique allowed the creation of a solid geometry without compression with a highly porous internal structure, which allows easy penetration of the dissolution medium and immediate disintegration of Spritam. This formulation is intended to be placed in the mouth to disperse the active ingredient quickly before swallowing and is ideal for people suffering from dysphagia or who experience any circumstance that prevents them from swallowing [25]. Other drug systems intended for the oral route without being swallowed are bioadhesive systems, which have been used predominantly in dental, orthopedic, and ophthalmic applications but are now beginning to arouse pharmaceutical interest. Mucoadhesive films and tablets are placed on the buccal mucosa, allowing the controlled and localized release of active ingredients.

For the *in vitro* study of these oral drug delivery systems, USP 1 or 2 dissolution apparatus loaded with different volumes typically ranging from 300 to 400 mL are generally used [26,27]. However, these volumes do not match the saliva of healthy volunteers, which usually varies between 0.87 mL in men and 0.66 mL in women, with an estimated flow rate of 0.5–1.5 mL/min [28]. On the other hand, in traditional dissolution studies, the tablets are immersed in a dissolution medium, and at different times, aliquots are sampled to evaluate the API concentration. In the case of mucoadhesive systems, the dissolution of the active ingredients is limited according to the surface that is adhered to the buccal mucosa, from where the system is hydrated, being in these cases so relevant to know how, as a function of time, the active ingredient is released from the system, and the water diffuses through it.

Considering the limitations and requirements described for dissolution studies of traditional oral delivery systems, Dorozynski et al. [29] evaluated the feasibility of the process known as fused deposition modeling (FDM) to develop an analytical kit dedicated to these specific non-standard dosage forms. Using an FDM printer and acrylonitrile–butadiene–styrene (ABS) as filament, a unique holder was created to be applied in the USP 4 apparatus equipped with a continuous flow cell. The tablet holder was designed to be attached to the flow cell and allow hydration of the single-sided buccal dosage form, which reduced the active dissolution surface, mimicking application in the oral cavity. These types of thermoplastic parts have the disadvantage of not being durable elements, but at the same time, they can be obtained quickly and customized to the geometry or functionality of the device to be evaluated. The versatility of the 3DP technique allowed the authors to introduce modifications in the geometry until they reached a satisfactory result that correctly adjusted to the tablets and the cell of the device. Finally, the thermoplastic material used, ABS, was chosen because it had been shown in previous studies to be compatible with nuclear magnetic resonance (NMR) analysis. Combining dissolution tests with imaging techniques, such as magnetic resonance imaging or Fourier transform infrared microscopy (FTIR), offers the possibility of non-invasively characterizing spatiotemporally the dosage forms during hydration and drug release. In this case, NMR was used to monitor tablet hydration as a function of time (Figure 3.2).

3.2.2 3D-Printed *In Vitro* Eye Models

Traditional ocular *in vitro* models are relatively inexpensive, easy to use, and widely available. They generally use glass vials containing a predetermined volume (usually less than 5 mL) of artificial tear fluid (e.g., phosphate-buffered saline) [30] without any fluid exchange. These models are too simplistic and do not reflect the ocular environment, which is characterized by the presence of blinking, intermittent exposure to air, and containing a very low tear volume (approximately $7 \pm 2\,\mu L$) that is renewed with a given flow (exchange rate approximately 1.6 μL/min) [31].

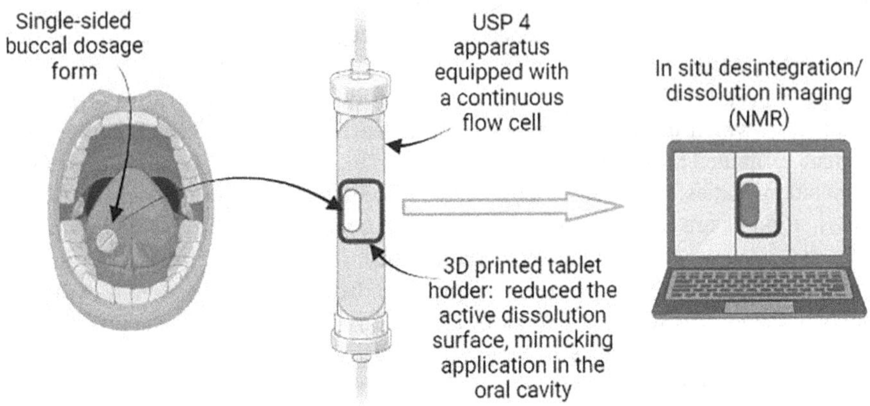

FIGURE 3.2 3D-printed tablet holder for *in vitro* drug release evaluation of single-sided buccal dosage forms.

To overcome these problems, several ocular models have been developed to physiologically mimic tear flow, volume, air exposure, and mechanical friction produced during blinking [32,33].

Bajgrowicz et al. [34] created a new *in vitro* eye model to evaluate the release of actives from disposable contact lenses. To create the model, the authors used two 3D-printed molds (one mimicking the surface of the eyeball and one functioning as a lid, the eyelid) and a microfluidic syringe pump. The final parts were created and assembled from the 3D molds, printed in polycarbonate–acrylonitrile–butadiene–styrene to allow approximately 100 µL of fluid to meet the contact lens. The model was oriented in the natural position of the eye during the day, using gravity to generate a natural flow. The model was integrated with a microfluidic syringe pump to emulate tear secretion and flow, and the flow was collected in a 12-well microliter plate (Figure 3.3). In this work, the authors proved that while drugs were released rapidly within the first hour in traditional methods, drug release was maintained over an extended observation period using the

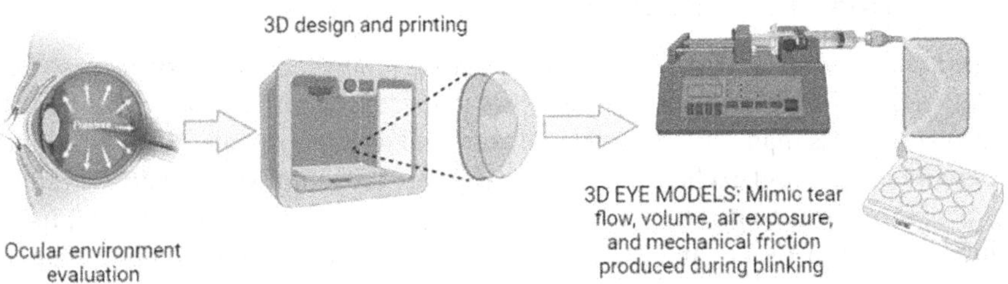

FIGURE 3.3 3D-printed *in vitro* eye models' main advantages.

in vitro model. This way, it was possible to compare the release kinetics as a function of the material from which the contact lens was made [35].

Phan CM et al. [36] used 3D design, printing, and machining techniques to obtain an advanced *in vitro* flicker model that can be used to measure topical ophthalmic drug release. The eyeballs, lower eyelid, and harvesting unit were printed with a UV-polymerizable hydrophobic resin on an SLA (stereolithography) printer (Photon S, Anycubic, Shenzhen, China). The upper lid was synthesized from polyvinyl alcohol. A syringe pump infused simulated tear fluid through a tube connected to the eyelid. The downward movement of the eyelid spreads the tear solution, which flows across the eyeball to deposit fluids in the collection unit located under the eyeball. Both the flow rate and the blinking speed can be regulated. Finally, the whole system is housed inside a chamber to maintain stable humidity during the experiment. Using this model, dye release from two commercial lenses was evaluated. The release was measured for 24 hours using a tear flow rate of 5 μL/min and a flicker rate of 1 every 10 seconds. As a result, differential lens release profiles could be observed, depending on whether the lenses were evaluated with the developed model or the traditional *in vitro* model. In both lenses, the dye release was statistically different when studied in a vial compared to the ocular model ($p < 0.05$).

Finally, mention should be made of the work done by Wang et al. [37], who created a 5× magnified eye model using 3DP, to which they added an inlet and outlet valve to simulate the fluid dynamics of the aqueous humor. Although the resolution achieved in the model was not adequate to model pores as small as 10 μm of the trabecular meshwork, advances in 3DP, especially in the field of SLA, are promising to achieve it. However, these authors used this model to study the pathophysiology and deformations that the iris could suffer because of intraocular pressure, and it can be modified, adapted, or improved in the future for the analytical study of drugs.

The models shown so far are useful to evaluate the topical ocular administration for which 90% of the ophthalmic formulations are intended [38]. However, there are a large number of drugs, approved and under development, that are administered by intravitreal injections into the posterior chamber of the eye for the treatment of retinal diseases such as age-related macular degeneration [39], diabetic retinopathy, retinitis pigmentosa (RP), or macular edema [40].

The retina is a complex tissue of specialized and neural cells that are responsible for converting light signals and transmitting them to the brain. This neurosensory retina is attached to the choroidal vessels by a membrane rich in collagen and elastin (Bruch's membrane) and a monolayer of highly specialized cells, known as the retinal pigment epithelium (RPE). This epithelium performs multiple functions, including the provision of growth factors, phagocytosis of photoreceptor outer segments, and control of molecular transport, forming what is known as the outer blood–retinal barrier. 3DP technology has made it possible to reproduce the complex and heterogeneous constructions of the retina, obtaining functional tissues that can be used for clinical application (to repair damaged retinal layers) but also for the study of disease mechanisms and drug evaluation.

Shi et al. [41] created a functional hybrid retina using a syringe 3D bioprinter. The construct was composed of an ultrathin PCL (polycaprolactone) membrane, representing Bruch's membrane, on which 3D bioprinting was applied to homogeneously seed human retinal pigment epithelium (ARPE-19) cells. After 2 weeks, cell proliferation resulted in an intact ARPE-19 cell monolayer on which photoreceptor-loaded bioink (Y79 cells) could be successfully printed. The bioprinted retinal constructs were cultured in media for 7 days, with no changes in cell configuration or viability observed. The porous bioinks used created a benign environment that allowed the transport of nutrients and debris while maintaining the biological interaction between Y79 and ARPE-19 cells. The bioretins achieved are ultimately an advanced cytocompatible structure that simulates the native retina.

Masaeli et al. [42] developed a carrier-free bioprinting method with which they were able to obtain an *in vitro* retinal model to study retinal diseases. First, a gelatin methacrylate (GelMA) solution was used to apply a coating to circular coverslips. The goal was to create an impression carrier that simulates Bruch's membrane. Then, using a piezoelectric inkjet dispenser, RPE cells (ARPE-19) were bioprinted onto the GelMA layer to obtain a fully functional and stable RPE monolayer after culture. Finally, to produce whole retinal tissues, freshly isolated photoreceptors were bioprinted onto the mature RPE cell sheets. Three days after bioprinting, the presence of positioned photoreceptors could be confirmed. The authors were able to demonstrate by protein expression analysis and microstructure imaging that both RPE cells and photoreceptors were able to perform specific retinal functions similar to native tissues in vivo. In conclusion, the bioprinted constructs exhibit functionality that would allow both clinical application and potential drug testing.

3.2.3 3D-Printed *In Vitro* Nasal Cavity Models

The nasal cavity is a route for drug delivery that has been studied extensively in pharmacy. The primary focus, for many years, has been on pulmonary inhalation and deposition of drugs or intranasal administration of drugs for treating topical nasal conditions. Currently, the nasal mucosa has emerged as a viable therapeutic route for systemic drug delivery [43].

Different specific anatomical regions within the nasal cavity are targets for drug delivery. For example, the turbinates behind the nasal vestibule are an ideal anatomical region for local corticosteroid and antibiotic administration but also for non-invasive administration of drugs with systemic effects with low stability or poor GI absorption. Administration by this route offers rapid absorption, avoiding aggressive GI conditions and presystemic metabolism. The olfactory region located in the roof of the nasal cavity is a particular area that connects to the specific area of the brain unimpeded by the blood–brain barrier and is, therefore, a candidate for brain-targeted drug delivery. Finally, the main area of nasal lymphatic drainage, the upper region of the rhinopharynx, is a target for non-invasive vaccine delivery [44].

The development of a nasal drug delivery system must consider aspects related to the formulation, the devices, and the anatomo-physiological limitations that will determine the retention and penetration of the drug in the nasal cavity. It is known that the particle size must be controlled depending on whether the aim is to favor nasal deposition or to avoid it by directing it to the lung [45]. However, there is no consensus regarding the relationship between aerosol characteristics and the specific deposition site within the nasal cavity. On the other hand, it has also been shown that two aerosols with the same particle size produced by two different delivery systems do not produce the same nasal deposition [46]. In this regard, it is helpful to have models that mimic the geometry of the upper airways as an *in vitro* tool to better understand the deposition of inhaled drugs.

Over the years, different models have been used, ranging from simplified structures built with plastic, glass tubes, or bottles [47–49] to high-precision nasal replicas with lines and volumes very close to human geometry. The enormous development of 3DP has dramatically influenced obtaining these last models. Since the first printed model in 1991 [50], this technology has gained significant interest in model making, mainly because it allows the use of anatomical images based on actual patients, which are obtained from diagnostic analysis such as CT scans or magnetic resonance imaging (MRI) scans. The combined use of image processing and 3DP allows the creation of variable models that can be influenced by age, gender, ethnicity, or the presence of pathologies or deformities (nasal septum deviation), which is an advantage over other techniques.

Different printing techniques (FDM, SLS, and SLA) have been used to construct the models, with stereolithography (SLA) being the most frequently used and achieving the most efficient models (Table 3.1).

When building the model, it is crucial to define the material from which it will be constructed. It should be inert, stable, flexible, and preferably translucent, especially if the models are not dismountable, and must be coupled with cameras and software to perform quantitative determinations of the depositions. Most of the models are washable and reusable, although, in the case of SLA resins, it is necessary to know that they deteriorate with time, in contact with solvents and UV radiation [52] (Figure 3.4).

Most models are built in separable structures (from 2 to 6 parts), allowing disassembly and quantification in specific areas. The areas of interest frequently studied are the nostrils, vestibule, turbinates, olfactory region, and rhinopharynx. A filter is usually applied to the back of the nasal casts to act as a barrier to block smaller particles (<5 μm), which could theoretically continue into the deeper airways. At the same time, it is true that mucociliary clearance, a complex parameter to be incorporated into these artificial models, is usually not included in these *in vitro* models. To avoid this problem, some studies included a step of moistening the nasal cast. Finally, it is essential to note that many factors influence drug deposition, such as particle size, formulation characteristics, type of device (and its delivery force), and delivery technique (angle of inclination of the device, depth of insertion into the nostrils, number of nostrils open and airflow applied) [44]. The value of each parameter must be correctly specified because they can be a possible source of bias, but also the influence of these variables can be studied using *in vitro* models.

TABLE 3.1
3D-Printed Nasal Cavity Models

	3D Printing		Anatomical Information			Model Type			
MODEL—Author	**Method**	**Printing Material**	**Patient Type**	**Imaging Method**	**Airways Modeled**	**Classification**	**N° parts**	**Color**	**Observation**
VIPER Model—Kelly J.T et al. (2004) [51]	SLA	Resin not described	Adult male (53 years)	Magnetic Resonance Imaging (MR)	Nares to the posterior pharynx	Closed	1	Transparent	Two printers were used, and different resolutions were obtained
Bespak Model—Hughes R. et al. [52]	SLS	Nylon Duraform PA (Medical grade)	Adult male and female	MR (male)—CT (female)	Nasal vestibule, front turbinates, olfactory region, rear turbinates and nasal pharynx + Filter	Dismountable	5	Opaque	The model was coated with glycerol and ethanol mixtures to simulate artificial mucus.
Javaheri E. et al. (2013) [53]	3D Systems Invision 3D Printer=Laminated Objected Manufacturing (LOM)	PVC	Babies from 3 to 18 months (Average geometry)	CT	Nares to the posterior pharynx	Closed	1	Opaque	The idealized structure obtained similar results to 10 replicates.
Modified VIPER model—Schroeter JD et al (2014) [54]	SLA	Not described	Adult Male (53 years). Same image as VIPER	MR	Nasal vestibule; nasal valve; anterior turbinates, olfactory, turbinates and nasopharynx.	Dismountable	6	Transparent	-

(Continued)

TABLE 3.1 (*Continued*)
3D-Printed Nasal Cavity Models

	3D Printing		Anatomical Information			Model Type			
MODEL—Author	**Method**	**Printing Material**	**Patient Type**	**Imaging Method**	**Airways Modeled**	**Classification**	**N° parts**	**Color**	**Observation**
Jinxiang Xi et al. (2015) [55]	SLA	Polypropylene	Adult Male (53 years)	MR	The two nasal cavities (right and left) are connected to the nasopharynx model. The right nasal cavity, in turn, opens into two parts.	Dismountable	5	Transparent	The division of the right nasal passage into two parts reveals the structure of the nasal turbinates and allows direct visualization of the deposition pattern within the right nasal passage.
Yarragudi SB et al. (2017) [56]	FDM	ABS	Adult male non-smoker	MR	Model designed to study the olfactory region	Dismountable	2	Opaque	For particle deposition experiments, the model was coated with a layer of mucin solution (2% w/v).
Okuda T et al. (2017) [57]	FDM	ABS	Adult Male	MR	Nasal vestibule, nasal turbinate, and nasopharynx	Dismountable	3	Opaque	The model, coated with a 10% Tween® 80 solution, was designed to study pulmonary aerosol delivery.

(*Continued*)

TABLE 3.1 (*Continued*)
3D-Printed Nasal Cavity Models

	3D Printing		Anatomical Information			Model Type			
MODEL—Author	Method	Printing Material	Patient Type	Imaging Method	Airways Modeled	Classification	N° parts	Color	Observation
Sawant and Donovan (2018) [58]	PolyJet technology—3D Objet Eden 330	Durus White Photopolymer	Child's (12-year-old)	MR	Nasal vestibule, nasal valve nasal turbinate, and nasopharynx	Dismountable	5	Opaque	The model can be coated with simulated mucus: mucin (4% and 10% w/v) in isotonic phosphate buffer (pH 6.5) containing 0.02% w/v sodium azide.
Warnken et al. (2018) [59]	SLA	Somos Watershed XC 11122-	10 Nasal models of 5 males and 5 females with varying ages	CT	Five different sections: anterior, upper turbinate region, middle turbinate region, lower turbinate region, and nasopharynx)	Dismountable	5	Transparent	Five pediatric models (9.8 ± 3.1 years old) and five adult models (40.8 ± 8.2 years old) were constructed.
SAINT (Sophia anatomical infant nose throat) Model—Janssens et al. (2001) [60]	SLA	Stereocol® Resin	Caucasian girl, 9 months old	CT	Anatomical Infant Nose Throat	Closed	1	Opaque	-

(*Continued*)

TABLE 3.1 (*Continued*)
3D-Printed Nasal Cavity Models

	3D Printing		Anatomical Information			Model Type			
MODEL—Author	Method	Printing Material	Patient Type	Imaging Method	Airways Modeled	Classification	N° parts	Color	Observation
Bishoff JS et al. (2008) [61]	LOM	PVC	11 infants from 3 to 18 months old.	CT	Nares to the posterior pharynx	Dismountable	2	Opaque	The models were constructed in two parts, with the face and throat constructed separately and then bolted together and sealed externally with putty.
Modelo PRINT—Minocchieri S et al. (2008) [62]	PolyJet technology—3D Objet Eden 330	FullCure 720® Resin	32-week gestational age premature infant	CT	One with the entire surface of the head and a smaller model consisting of the face and the air-conducting parts.	Closed	1	Transparent	The model was connected to a cascade impactor to assess lung dose.
EASYNOSE—Le Guellec S et al. (2013) [63]	FDM	ABS	Adult woman	CT	Nose and nasal valve; ostiomeatal complex (OMC), paranasal sinuses; sphenoid and rhinopharynx	Dismountable	4	Opaque	-

(*Continued*)

TABLE 3.1 (*Continued*)
3D-Printed Nasal Cavity Models

	3D Printing		Anatomical Information			Model Type			
MODEL—Author	Method	Printing Material	Patient Type	Imaging Method	Airways Modeled	Classification	N° parts	Color	Observation
Leclerc et al. (2014) [64]	SLA	Transparent, water-resistant, non-porous resin	Plastinated adult male human specimen	CT	Entire nasal cavities	Closed	1	Transparent	Nasofibroscopy and endoscopic imaging demonstrated a good correlation between the model and the plastinated human specimen.
Manniello et al. (2021) [65]	SLA (posterior section) and PolyJet Flex (anterior section)	Accura ClearVue and TANGO PLUS 27A	Adult subjects aged 21–75 years (half male and half female)	CT	Entire nasal cavities	Dismountable	2	Transparent	The airways were segmented into two regions, anterior and posterior to the internal nasal valve.

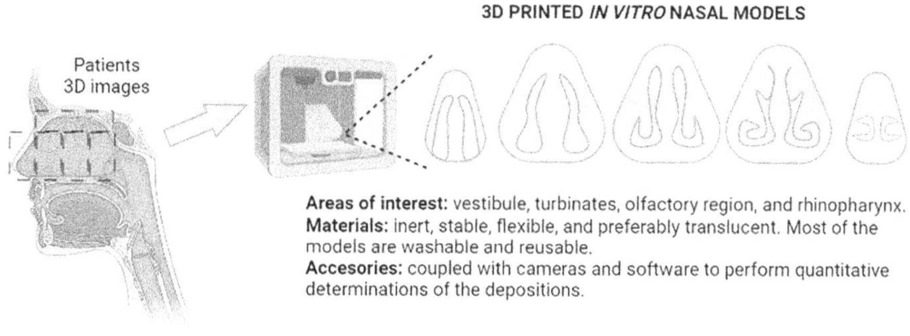

FIGURE 3.4 Application of 3D printing to nasal models' development.

3.3 3D PRINTING IN CELL CULTURE APPLICATIONS

In addition to the advantages of developing devices to analyze *in vitro* drug release, the application of 3DP to fabricate cell culture systems can provide a more realistic biomimetic environment for cells [66]. The key to the application of this technique for cell culture platforms is based on the fabrication of geometries that provide the correct mechanical signals (e.g., through perfusion flow that is guided by the geometry) and, consequently, chemical signals, which are necessary for proper cell signaling for the growth and development of specific tissues [67–69]. Using 3DP, devices can be produced with sizes relevant to the cells, where parameters such as substrate roughness, porosity, and curvature can be adjusted. Based on this, 3DP has been applied to the development of unconventional culture plates, microfluidic devices for cell encapsulation, systems for studying cell mechanics between tissues, and organ-on-chip, which will be summarized in the following sections.

3.3.1 Cost-Effective, Supply-Chain-Independent Single-Use Plastic Materials for Cell Culture

3D printing represents a democratization of manufacturing processes, and low-cost 3D-printed parts for cell culture have been tested as substitutes for single-use plastics that are currently unavailable due to supply chain issues worldwide. In addition, this decentralized manufacturing of cell culture laboratory materials helps remote areas and developing countries with limited resources. For example, the feasibility of printing shaker flasks for cell culture applications was evaluated using HEK293 cells as a model [70]. The growth curves recorded showed that biodegradable and renewable poly(lactic acid) (PLA) thermoplastic is an excellent and cost-effective substitute for single-use plastic shaker flasks, whose lead time in pandemic situations or other supply chain disruptions is more than 6 months. Additionally, it should be considered that the price was €0.60 in materials, and printers were used with prices lower than those of a box of presterilized single-use plastic shaker bottles.

3.3.2 Manufacture of Alternative Cell Culture Devices

Flat culture plates, specifically polystyrene plates for tissue culture, have been the foundation of biologically based research as they enable efficient cell expansion. As various biomedical fields grow, vigorous research efforts related to tissue/organ development and disease modeling emerge, and, therefore, so does the need for a cell culture platform that provides biomimicry, something that flat culture plates do not achieve. The transition from 2D to 3D substrate culture could improve biomimicry, thereby improving cell–cell interactions and increasing the efficiency of *in vitro* cell culture, and has driven increased interest in complex topology and choice of materials for extended and directed cell growth [71]. For this application, 3DP has been used to fabricate complex geometries with specific architecture, interconnected geometries, and microporous surfaces to facilitate tailored cellular responses [72]. The initial design of these cell culture platforms should utilize computational modeling to design the scaffold, in which fluid dynamics can be studied, and mechanical force transmission understood, thus predicting the forces acting on the cells once these acellular constructs are seeded with cells. Successful integration of modeling and part design can result in scaffolds for cell culture that balance mechanical integrity with porous structures that facilitate nutrient exchange, cell infiltration, and direct cell behavior [73–75].

3D printing provides excellent flexibility in using various chemically complex materials unavailable in traditional manufacturing environments. This includes combinations of porogens, polymers, metals, and ceramics used to mimic the mechanical and/or chemical properties of native tissues and create complex interconnected topography. Incorporating these chemically and topologically complex constructs into dynamic culture techniques improves cell infiltration and media exchange, thereby replicating the native environment. Crucial aspects of cell culture applications within 3D-printed scaffolds include cell expansion and migration, attempting to improve models to assess cell function ex vivo. The recapitulation of tissue models achieved through three-dimensionality with 3DP often provides an environment that better sustains cell proliferation and differentiation. These 3D-printed cell culture systems are often substituted for existing commercial culture platforms, providing a more cost-effective solution that suits specific interests and is customizable for specific optimized tissue applications.

3.3.3 Microfluidic Devices for Cell Encapsulation

The fabrication of conventional poly(dimethylsiloxane) (PDMS) on glass microfluidic devices begins with a complicated and time-consuming soft lithography process that requires expensive equipment in a clean room and assembly in a plasma treatment equipment [76]. Alternatively, recent advances in 3DP enable rapid, one-step fabrication of highly complex microfluidic devices while reducing the costs associated with institutional infrastructure, equipment, and physical space. Consequently, microfluidics is becoming widely accessible with the increasing availability of high-precision 3DP.

3D printing has been used to develop microfluidic devices for cell encapsulation in hydrogel droplets. For example, a 3D-printed modular microfluidic device, similar to Lego, has been developed and used to encapsulate dental pulp stem cells within alginate droplets [77]. This device was produced using FDM, with transparent PLA as the printing material, resulting in a rapidly fabricated, low-cost, transparent device that can be used for cellular imaging. Also, using digital light processing (DLP) printing, a microfluidic chip was fabricated incorporating a coaxial flow device for coextrusion of materials to generate hollow, sub-millimeter extracellular matrix (ECM)-coated alginate capsules to encapsulate cells [78]. The device created a closed microenvironment within each sphere, miming the basal membrane of the cell niche.

3.3.4 3D Printing for Cellular Mechanical Studies

In addition to the ability to fabricate microenvironments that mimic physiological tissues, the versatility of 3DP to create large, complex shapes also enables the development of culture constructs that capture the interactions of multiple tissues. This way, tissues' specific biological characteristics can be mimicked to capture cellular function and physiology within a culture platform. These features enable the study of diseases related to that tissue. For example, a dual-chamber bioreactor configuration was fabricated and fitted to a microfluidic base to represent the interactions between cartilage and subchondral bone [79]. The geometry allowed insertion into the bioreactor chamber of a biphasic osteochondral construct made of GelMA-encapsulated MSCs, which consequently exposes the chondral and bone faces of the construct to the chondrogenic and osteogenic milieu, respectively. This tissue–tissue interaction in a controlled bioreactor environment provided an avenue to investigate the physiology of osteochondral tissue and possible pathogenic mechanisms of relevant diseases in the system, such as osteoarthritis.

3.3.5 Organs-on-Chip Applications

3D printing is also being used to create models of artificial tissues and organs within microfluidic devices to provide real organs' complexity, function, and physiological responses (Figure 3.5). The field of organ-on-chip engineering has integrated 3DP technology by assembling tissues containing cells and other biomaterials with precisely controlled spatial distribution, creating organ models with a specific 3D cellular arrangement within a microfluidic chip. Incorporating other mechanical and electrical components into OoC systems is simplified in fully 3D-printed systems, enabling automated mass production and commercialization. The ease and high resolution of 3DP for OoC applications provide a promising alternative to animal studies and traditional cell culture for investigating various biomedical research questions. This section will focus on recent developments that specifically use 3DP to fabricate functional organ-like models and molds for use within microfluidic devices.

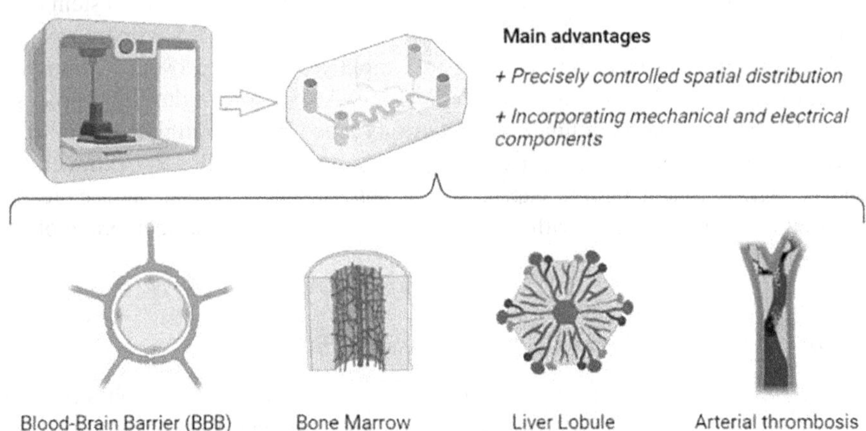

FIGURE 3.5 Application of 3D printing for organs-on-chip development.

Combining the precise geometric control features allowed by 3DP, well-defined flow patterns, and the imaging capabilities of microfluidic devices, a microfluidic perfusion platform has been developed to simulate the blood–brain barrier (BBB) environment [80]. The BBB model consists of a porous membrane on which brain microvascular endothelial cells and primary rat astrocytes are cultured on each side of the membrane. The modular chamber consists of sterilized parts assembled with a cell insert that houses two cell monolayers forming a complete closed-loop perfusion system. Characterization of the *in vitro* model reveals a high-fidelity solution for studying BBB biology due to fluid residence time, perfusion rates, model drug permeability coefficients (caffeine, cimetidine, and doxorubicin), and transendothelial electrical resistance (barrier integrity) that mimic *in vivo* values. This functionality means that BBB-on-a-chip could effectively screen brain-targeted drug candidates, overcoming the limitations of the typical transwell BBB culture, where it is challenging to achieve controlled biochemical gradients in the large volume of static fluid. Like the BBB-on-a-chip model, co-cultures relevant to other disease models are constantly being developed and optimized to capture the biological interactions that shape disease mechanisms.

A 3D bone-on-a-chip model made of PDMS, consisting of a cell growth chamber and a media reservoir separated by a membrane, has been developed to investigate the metastasis of breast cancer cells in the host bone marrow [81]. The PDMS chambers were fabricated using a 3D-printed mold (Rostock MAX V2 Desktop 3D-Printer), resulting in a transparent growth chamber allowing easy and frequent breast cancer model monitoring. The growth and phenotypic maturation of mineralized collagenous bone tissue were observed by modifying the membrane's geometric characteristics and the growth chamber, optimizing nutrient and waste transport, and providing an adequate concentration of bone matrix-building proteins. Thanks to 3DP, the geometric design of this bone-on-a-chip could be fabricated, which allows maximizing the interaction of cancer cells with the bone matrix of a concentrated surface in a high-throughput experimental manner. This serves as a reliable *in vitro* model that captures the complexity of the native bone environment and mimics *in vivo* processes, thus eliminating the need to obtain bone metastasis samples from human patients, which has been a significant limitation in the study of breast cancer bone colonization.

A DLP 3D printer was used to develop a lung model on an open-well chip [82]. The model is obtained by means of printed molds that receive a surface treatment necessary for the recurrent casting of polydimethylsiloxane (PDMS). The achieved architecture mimics the air–liquid interface under dynamic conditions of the biological microenvironment of the lung, while also facilitating cell seeding, sample collection, and parallel experiments. A human airway epithelial cell line (Calu-3) was cultured on the developed chip and maintained at an air–liquid interface. It could be observed that the cells replicated 3D morphology, retained barrier integrity, secreted mucus, and expressed P-glycoprotein, all indicative of a promising *in vitro* model for cytotoxicity assays, permeability, and drug studies. Finally, the authors were able to demonstrate, for example, how treatment with an anti-inflammatory drug significantly reduced, relative to controls, the interleukin expression of Calu-3 cells exposed to cigarette smoke extract (CSE).

A 3DP approach has been demonstrated for an on-chip perfused liver organoid model, in which the model involves the sinusoidal structure of the hepatic lobe, as enabled by 3DP (Cellbricks Bioprinter) with gelatin and poly (ethylene glycol) (PEG)-based bioinks. Characterization of HepaRG (a human hepatoma cell line) and human stellate cells cultured for 2 weeks within the liver organoid on a chip revealed increased expression of albumin and CYP3A4 proteins in 3D-printed tissues compared to monolayer culture [83]. Hepatocyte functionality was demonstrated by tight junction formation and stable overall metabolism by levels of glucose, lactate, lactate dehydrogenase, and liver-specific drug resistance-associated protein 2. This liver-on-chip model provides an alternative platform for developing complex 3D liver models, as opposed to 2D models, which are not as physiologically relevant, or 3D spheroid culture, which is the gold standard and limited by nutrient and oxygen diffusion. Using 3DP capabilities, the geometry of the liver-on-a-chip developed can be adjusted to ensure adequate nutritional delivery within larger tissue models, thus providing a new avenue for mechanistic studies in liver tissue engineering.

To fully capture the organ's functionality, the field of organs-on-a-chip shows an increasing demand for integrating other systems such as sensors, actuators, electrochemical components, and imaging systems). In particular, since 3DP requires a CAD model to produce the shapes, scanning/imaging techniques are often applied to fabricate organ models. In fabricating a 3D model of arterial thrombosis, CT angiography scans were acquired, constructed, and processed into a 3D printable model [84]. Molds for microfluidic chips containing miniaturized healthy and stenotic vascular structures were fabricated using a Perfactory 3 SLA 3D printer with PIC100 resin with a resolution of only 25 lm. Taking advantage of the printers' resolution limits, model arteries within a microfluidic device successfully recapitulated the vessel environments: confluent vessel lining with human umbilical vein endothelial cells, human whole blood flow at physiologically relevant shear stresses, and induced thrombosis in and downstream of the stenotic region were observed. The mimicry of the shape, cellular environment, and functional response of this 3D-printed OoC model underscore the superiority of 3DP over typical microfluidic fabrication employing 2D soft lithography. Traditional microfluidic manufacturing is limited to generating two-dimensional microstructures or 3D structures with minimal thickness. These design limitations, coupled with the multiple and complicated fabrication steps, highlight the advantages of 3DP. Structured light scanning has been used to capture 3D topographical data of whole organs and generate a 3D-printed microfluidic device that interacts directly with the porcine kidney as a non-invasive platform to isolate and profile whole organ biomarkers in real time [85]. The functionality of this conformal microfluidic device was demonstrated by transferring relevant metabolic and pathophysiological biomarkers from the kidney cortex to the microfluidic device while the fluid flow is present in the microchannel. This device could potentially overcome the limitations of whole organ studies by simply facilitating the transport of relevant markers from the corresponding organ to a much smaller platform and subsequent analysis. Highly complex organs require complex *in vitro* models, often incorporating many inputs and outputs within the OoC system. To investigate endocrine secretions between tissues, a microfluidic perfusion chamber with 16 channels has been developed, integrating 3DP, templating, sensors, and system automation [86]. This device is capable of precise temporal manipulation of nutrient inputs and hormone outputs, demonstrated by measuring real-time fatty acid uptake by adipose tissue exposed to a temporal mimic of postprandial insulin and glucose observed by fluorescence imaging. The flexibility demonstrated by the platforms mentioned above suggests the possibility of using 3D-printed microfluidics as building blocks for modular microfluidic devices integrated on a chip.

Further validation of these models could lead to widely accepted use, becoming the new gold standard for studies investigating mechanistic interactions of cell populations.

3.4 CONCLUSIONS AND FUTURE CHALLENGES

Technology-driven changes are known to have a substantial impact on the way things are made. 3DP has quickly gone from a manufacturing novelty to a ubiquitous manufacturing technique in Pharmaceutical Sciences research laboratories. This chapter demonstrates that 3DP technology can change not only the way drugs are produced but also the way they are researched, developed and evaluated. 3DP can increase the biomimetics of *in vitro* studies, creating specific objects to analyze specific problems. This potential will lead to changes in analytical techniques and probably reduce experimental animals' use.

Although many challenges remain for general acceptance, such as validation and repeatability, significant milestones have been reached in the 3DP revolution. However, there are several aspects of the printing technology that need to be optimized to fully meet the needs of Pharmaceutical Sciences. The main consideration is related to the choice of materials and printing techniques. For example, light-curing techniques inevitably use acrylate-based polymers, but this means that there will be a consequence on their solvent compatibility. Similarly, if strong solvent compatibility is sought, the choice of material is more restricted to very inert polymers or metals. This requires a subset of the available printing techniques. A breakthrough will likely be the ability to print glass, which has been the material of choice for chemists for approximately 200 years due to its transparency, thermal conductivity, and relative chemical inertness.

Another barrier that 3DP will have to overcome are regulatory challenges. Regulatory approval of new technologies depends on scientific validation, which takes time to obtain. Researchers are expected to resist replacing traditional models and that these prints will only be complementary tests in the early stages of adoption. However, according to a survey of researchers, the vast majority agree that, over time, these bioprinted constructs will radically reduce the need for animals/humans and that training (universities), research, and ultimately regulatory bodies will need to change to adapt to this new emerging paradigm.

ACKNOWLEDGMENTS

Daniel A. Real and Marcelo J. Kogan received funding from Agencia Nacional de Investigación y Desarrollo (ANID), Chile: FONDECYT Postdoctoral N°3200384, FONDAP N°15130011. Juan Pablo Real and Santiago D. Palma gratefully acknowledge the Universidad Nacional de Córdoba (Argentina) and CONICET (Argentina) for financial support.

REFERENCES

1. Norman J, Madurawe RD, Moore CMV, Khan MA, Khairuzzaman A. A new chapter in pharmaceutical manufacturing: 3D-printed drug products. *Adv Drug Deliv Rev.* 2017;108:39–50.
2. Coggiola VN, Real JP, Palma SD. A new method for 3D printing drugs: melting solidification printing process. *Future Med.* 2020;4(3):131–4. Available from: https://doi.org/102217/3dp-2020-0024; https://www.futuremedicine.com/doi/10.2217/3dp-2020-0024
3. Lopez-Vidal L, Real DA, Paredes AJ, Real JP, Palma SD. 3D-printed nanocrystals for oral administration of the drugs. *Drug Deliv Using Nanomater.* 2022 Jan 18;109–33. Available from: https://www.taylorfrancis.com/chapters/edit/10.1201/9781003168584-5/3d-printed-nanocrystals-oral-administration-drugs-lucía-lopez-vidal-daniel-andrés-real-alejandro-paredes-juan-pablo-real-santiago-daniel-palma
4. Cui M, Li Y, Wang S, Chai Y, Lou J, Chen F, et al. Exploration and preparation of a dose-flexible regulation system for levetiracetam tablets via novel semi-solid extrusion three-dimensional printing. *J Pharm Sci.* 2019;108(2):977–86.
5. Infanger S, Haemmerli A, Iliev S, Baier A, Stoyanov E, Quodbach J. Powder bed 3D-printing of highly loaded drug delivery devices with hydroxypropyl cellulose as solid binder. *Int J Pharm.* 2019;555:198–206.
6. Okwuosa TC, Soares C, Gollwitzer V, Habashy R, Timmins P, Alhnan MA. On demand manufacturing of patient-specific liquid capsules via co-ordinated 3D printing and liquid dispensing. *Eur J Pharm Sci.* 2018;118:134–43.

7. Zheng Y, Deng F, Wang B, Wu Y, Luo Q, Zuo X, et al. Melt extrusion deposition (MED™) 3D printing technology – a paradigm shift in design and development of modified release drug products. *Int J Pharm.* 2021;602:120639.
8. Maroni A, Melocchi A, Parietti F, Foppoli A, Zema L, Gazzaniga A. 3D printed multi-compartment capsular devices for two-pulse oral drug delivery. *J Control Release.* 2017;268:10–8.
9. Gioumouxouzis CI, Chatzitaki AT, Karavasili C, Katsamenis OL, Tzetzis D, Mystiridou E, et al. Controlled release of 5-fluorouracil from alginate beads encapsulated in 3D printed pH-responsive solid dosage forms. *AAPS PharmSciTech.* 2018;19(8):3362–75. Available from: https://pubmed.ncbi.nlm.nih.gov/29948989/
10. Real JP, Barberis ME, Camacho NM, Sánchez Bruni S, Palma SD. Design of novel oral ricobendazole formulation applying melting solidification printing process (MESO-PP): an innovative solvent-free alternative method for 3D printing using a simplified concept and low temperature. *Int J Pharm.* 2020;587:119653.
11. Barberis ME, Palma SD, Gonzo EE, Bermúdez JM, Lorier M, Ibarra M, et al. Mathematical and pharmacokinetic approaches for the design of new 3D printing inks using ricobendazole. *Pharm Res.* 2022;39(9):2277–90. Available from: https://link.springer.com/article/10.1007/s11095-022-03320-z
12. Gallo L, Peña JF, Palma SD, Real JP, Cotabarren I. Design and production of 3D printed oral capsular devices for the modified release of urea in ruminants. *Int J Pharm.* 2022;628:122353. Available from: https://linkinghub.elsevier.com/retrieve/pii/S0378517322009085
13. Lopez-Vidal L, Real JP, Real DA, Camacho N, Kogan MJ, Paredes AJ, et al. Nanocrystal-based 3D-printed tablets: semi-solid extrusion using melting solidification printing process (MESO-PP) for oral administration of poorly soluble drugs. *Int J Pharm.* 2022;611:121311.
14. Robles-Martinez P, Xu X, Trenfield SJ, Awad A, Goyanes A, Telford R, et al. 3D printing of a multi-layered polypill containing six drugs using a novel stereolithographic method. *Pharm.* 2019;11(6):274. Available from: https://www.mdpi.com/1999-4923/11/6/274/htm
15. Carvalho V, Gonçalves I, Lage T, Rodrigues RO, Minas G, Teixeira SFCF, et al. 3D printing techniques and their applications to organ-on-a-chip platforms: a systematic review. *Sensors.* 2021;21(9):3304. Available from: https://www.mdpi.com/1424-8220/21/9/3304/htm
16. Real DA, Hoffmann S, Leonardi D, Goycoolea FM, Salomon CJ. A quality by design approach for optimization of Lecithin/Span® 80 based nanoemulsions loaded with hydrophobic drugs. *J Mol Liq.* 2020;321;114743.
17. Palekar S, Nukala PK, Mishra SM, Kipping T, Patel K. Application of 3D printing technology and quality by design approach for development of age-appropriate pediatric formulation of baclofen. *Int J Pharm.* 2019;556:106–16. Available from: https://pubmed.ncbi.nlm.nih.gov/30513398/
18. Doke SK, Dhawale SC. Alternatives to animal testing: a review. *Saudi Pharm J SPJ.* 2015;23(3):223. Available from: /pmc/articles/PMC4475840/
19. Polli JE. In vitro studies are sometimes better than conventional human pharmacokinetic in vivo studies in assessing bioequivalence of immediate-release solid oral dosage forms. *AAPS J.* 2008;10(2):289–99. Available from: https://link.springer.com/article/10.1208/s12248-008-9027-6
20. Mota F, Braga L, Rocha L, Cabral B. 3D and 4D bioprinted human model patenting and the future of drug development. *Nat Biotechnol.* 2020;38(6):689–94. Available from: https://pubmed.ncbi.nlm.nih.gov/32518405/

21. Huotilainen E, Paloheimo M, Salmi M, Paloheimo KS, Björkstrand R, Tuomi J, et al. Imaging requirements for medical applications of additive manufacturing. *Acta Radiol.* 2014;55(1):78–85. Available from: https://journals.sagepub.com/doi/abs/10.1177/0284185113494198
22. Peng W, Datta P, Ayan B, Ozbolat V, Sosnoski D, Ozbolat IT. 3D bioprinting for drug discovery and development in pharmaceutics. *Acta Biomater.* 2017;57:26–46.
23. Real D, Orzan L, Leonardi D, Salomon CJ. Improving the dissolution of triclabendazole from stable crystalline solid dispersions formulated for oral delivery. *AAPS PharmSciTech.* 2020;21(1):16.
24. SPRITAM (levetiracetam) Tablets. [cited 2022 Aug 22]. Available from: https://www.accessdata.fda.gov/drugsatfda_docs/nda/2015/207958Orig1s000TOC.cfm
25. Cilurzo F, Musazzi UM, Franzé S, Selmin F, Minghetti P. Orodispersible dosage forms: biopharmaceutical improvements and regulatory requirements. *Drug Discov Today.* 2018;23(2):251–9.
26. Abdelbary A, Elshafeey AH, Zidan G. Comparative effects of different cellulosic-based directly compressed orodispersable tablets on oral bioavailability of famotidine. *Carbohydr Polym.* 2009;77(4):799–806.
27. El-Setouhy DA, El-Malak NSA. Formulation of a novel tianeptine sodium orodispersible film. *AAPS PharmSciTech.* 2010;11(3):1018–25. Available from: https://link.springer.com/article/10.1208/s12249-010-9464-2
28. Lagerlüf F, Dawes C. The volume of saliva in the mouth before and after swallowing. *J Dent Res.* 1984;63(5):618–21. Available from: https://pubmed.ncbi.nlm.nih.gov/6584462/
29. Dorożyński P, Jamróz W, Węglarz WP, Kulinowski W, Zaborowski M, Kulinowski P. 3D printing for fast prototyping of pharmaceutical dissolution testing equipment for nonstandard applications. *Dissolution Technol.* 2018;25(4):48–54. Available from: https://go.gale.com/ps/i.do?p=AONE&sw=w&issn=1521298X&v=2.1&it=r&id=GALE%7CA581867226&sid=googleScholar&linkaccess=fulltext
30. Peng CC, Kim J, Chauhan A. Extended delivery of hydrophilic drugs from silicone-hydrogel contact lenses containing Vitamin E diffusion barriers. *Biomaterials.* 2010;31(14):4032–47.
31. Qiao H, Phan CM, Walther H, Subbaraman LN, Jones L. Depth profile assessment of the early phase deposition of lysozyme on soft contact lens materials using a novel in vitro eye model. *Eye Contact Lens.* 2018;44 Suppl 2:S11–8. Available from: https://pubmed.ncbi.nlm.nih.gov/28617725/
32. Phan CM, Bajgrowicz-Cieslak M, Subbaraman LN, Jones L. Release of moxifloxacin from contact lenses using an in vitro eye model: impact of artificial tear fluid composition and mechanical rubbing. *Transl Vis Sci Technol.* 2016;5(6):1–10. Available from: https://pubmed.ncbi.nlm.nih.gov/27847690/
33. Phan CM, Walther H, Qiao H, Shinde R, Jones L. Development of an eye model with a physiological blink mechanism. *Transl Vis Sci Technol.* 2019;8(5):1–1. Available from: https://doi.org/10.1167/tvst.8.5.1
34. Bajgrowicz M, Phan CM, Subbaraman LN, Jones L. Release of ciprofloxacin and moxifloxacin from daily disposable contact lenses from an in vitro eye model. *Invest Ophthalmol Vis Sci.* 2015;56(4):2234–42. Available from: www.iovs.org
35. Phan CM, Bajgrowicz M, Gao H, Subbaraman LN, Jones LW. Release of fluconazole from contact lenses using a novel in vitro eye model. *Optom Vis Sci.* 2016;93(4):387–94. Available from: https://pubmed.ncbi.nlm.nih.gov/26641022/
36. Phan CM, Shukla M, Walther H, Heynen M, Suh D, Jones L. Development of an in vitro blink model for ophthalmic drug delivery. *Pharm.* 2021;13(3):300. Available from: https://www.mdpi.com/1999-4923/13/3/300/htm

37. Wang W, Qian X, Song H, Zhang M, Liu Z. Fluid and structure coupling analysis of the interaction between aqueous humor and iris. *Biomed Eng Online.* 2016;15(2):569–86. Available from: https://link.springer.com/articles/10.1186/s12938-016-0261-3
38. Formica ML, Real JP, Allemandi D, Palma S. Nano technological drug release approaches for the treatment of eye diseases: myth, reality or challenge? *J Pharmacol Clin Res.* 2018;5(1):555654.
39. Real JP, Luna JD, Urrets-Zavalia JA, De Santis MO, Palma SD, Granero GE. Accessibility as a conditioning factor in treatment for exudative age-related macular degeneration. *Eur J Ophthalmol.* 2013;23(6):857–64. Available from: https://pubmed.ncbi.nlm.nih.gov/23661541/
40. Formica ML, Awde Alfonso HG, Palma SD. Biological drug therapy for ocular angiogenesis: anti-VEGF agents and novel strategies based on nanotechnology. *Pharmacol Res Perspect.* 2021;9(2). Available from: https://pubmed.ncbi.nlm.nih.gov/33694304/
41. Shi P, Edgar TYS, Yeong WY, Laude A. Hybrid three-dimensional (3D) bioprinting of retina equivalent for ocular research. *Int J Bioprinting.* 2017;3(2):138–46. Available from: https://pubmed.ncbi.nlm.nih.gov/33094192/
42. Masaeli E, Forster V, Picaud S, Karamali F, Nasr-Esfahani MH, Marquette C. Tissue engineering of retina through high resolution 3-dimensional inkjet bioprinting. *Biofabrication.* 2020;12(2):025006. Available from: https://iopscience.iop.org/article/10.1088/1758-5090/ab4a20
43. Maaz A, Blagbrough IS, De Bank PA. In vitro evaluation of nasal aerosol depositions: an insight for direct nose to brain drug delivery. *Pharm.* 2021;13(7):1079. Available from: https://www.mdpi.com/1999-4923/13/7/1079/htm
44. Salade L, Wauthoz N, Goole J, Amighi K. How to characterize a nasal product. The state of the art of in vitro and ex vivo specific methods. *Int J Pharm.* 2019;561:47–65.
45. Nasal Spray and Inhalation Solution, Suspension, and Spray Drug Products--Chemistry, Manufacturing, and Controls Documentation | FDA. [cited 2022 Aug 22]. Available from: https://www.fda.gov/regulatory-information/search-fda-guidance-documents/nasal-spray-and-inhalation-solution-suspension-and-spray-drug-products-chemistry-manufacturing-and
46. Vecellio L, De Gersem R, Le Guellec S, Reychler G, Pitance L, Le Pennec D, et al. Deposition of aerosols delivered by nasal route with jet and mesh nebulizers. *Int J Pharm.* 2011;407(1–2):87–94.
47. Maniscalco M, Weitzberg E, Sundberg J, Sofia M, Lundberg JO. Assessment of nasal and sinus nitric oxide output using single-breath humming exhalations. *Eur Respir J.* 2003;22(2):323–9. Available from: https://erj.ersjournals.com/content/22/2/323
48. Möller W, Celik G, Feng S, Bartenstein P, Meyer G, Eickelberg O, et al. Nasal high flow clears anatomical dead space in upper airway models. *J Appl Physiol.* 2015;118(12):1525–32. Available from: https://journals.physiology.org/doi/10.1152/japplphysiol.00934.2014
49. Xi J, Si XA, Peters S, Nevorski D, Wen T, Lehman M. Understanding the mechanisms underlying pulsating aerosol delivery to the maxillary sinus: in vitro tests and computational simulations. *Int J Pharm.* 2017;520(1–2):254–66.
50. Swift DL. Inspiratory inertial deposition of aerosols in human nasal airway replicate casts: implication for the proposed NCRP lung model. *Radiat Prot Dosimetry.* 1991;38(1–3):29–34. Available from: https://academic.oup.com/rpd/article/38/1-3/29/3718027
51. Kelly JT, Asgharian B, Kimbell JS, Wong BA. Particle deposition in human nasal airway replicas manufactured by different methods. Part I: inertial regime particles. http://dx.doi.org/101080/027868290883360 [Internet]. 2011 Nov [cited 2023 May 30];38(11):1063–71. Available from: https://www.tandfonline.com/doi/abs/10.1080/027868290883360

52. Hughes R, Watterson J, Dickens C, Ward D, Banaszek A. Development of a nasal cast model to test medicinal nasal devices. *Proc Inst Mech Eng H.* 2008;222(7):1013–22. Available from: https://pubmed.ncbi.nlm.nih.gov/19024150/
53. Javaherin E, Golshahi L, Finlaynn WH. An idealized geometry that mimics average infant nasal airway deposition. *J Aerosol Sci.* 2013 Jan 1;55:137–48.
54. Schroeter JD, Tewksbury EW, Wong BA, Kimbell JS. Experimental measurements and computational predictions of regional particle deposition in a sectional nasal model. *J Aerosol Med Pulm Drug Deliv* [Internet]. 2015 Feb 1 [cited 2023 May 30];28(1):20–9. Available from: https://pubmed.ncbi.nlm.nih.gov/24580111/
55. Xi J, Si XA, Peters S, Nevorski D, Wen T, Lehman M. Understanding the mechanisms underlying pulsating aerosol delivery to the maxillary sinus: In vitro tests and computational simulations. *Int J Pharm.* 2017 Mar 30;520(1–2):254–66.
56. Yarragudi SB, Richter R, Lee H, Walker GF, Clarkson AN, Kumar H, et al. Formulation of olfactory-targeted microparticles with tamarind seed polysaccharide to improve nose-to-brain transport of drugs. *Carbohydr Polym.* 2017 May 1;163:216–26.
57. Okuda T, Tang P, Yu J, Finlay WH, Chan HK. Powder aerosol delivery through nasal high-flow system: In vitro feasibility and influence of process conditions. *Int J Pharm.* 2017 Nov 25;533(1):187–97.
58. Sawant N, Donovan MD. In vitro assessment of spray deposition patterns in a pediatric (12 year-old) nasal cavity model. *Pharm Res* [Internet]. 2018 May 1 [cited 2023 May 30];35(5):1–12. Available from: https://link.springer.com/article/10.1007/s11095-018-2385-6
59. Warnken ZN, Smyth HDC, Davis DA, Weitman S, Kuhn JG, Williams RO. Personalized medicine in nasal delivery: the use of patient-specific administration parameters to improve nasal drug targeting using 3D-printed nasal replica casts. *Mol Pharm* [Internet]. 2018 Apr 2 [cited 2023 May 30];15(4):1392–402. Available from: https://pubmed.ncbi.nlm.nih.gov/29485888/
60. Janssens HM, De Jongste JC, Fokkens WJ, Robben SGF, Wouters K, Tiddens HAWM. The Sophia Anatomical Infant Nose-Throat (Saint) model: a valuable tool to study aerosol deposition in infants. *J Aerosol Med* [Internet]. 2001 [cited 2023 May 30];14(4):433–41. Available from: https://pubmed.ncbi.nlm.nih.gov/11791684/
61. Storey-Bishoff J, Noga M, Finlay WH. Deposition of micrometer-sized aerosol particles in infant nasal airway replicas. *J Aerosol Sci.* 2008 Dec 1;39(12):1055–65.
62. Minocchieri S, Burren JM, Bachmann MA, Stern G, Wildhaber J, Buob S, et al. Development of the premature infant nose throat-model (PrINT-model)—an upper airway replica of a premature neonate for the study of aerosol delivery. *Pediatr Res.* 2008 642 [Internet]. 2008 Aug [cited 2023 May 30];64(2):141–6. Available from: https://www.nature.com/articles/pr2008164
63. Le Guellec S, Le Pennec D, Gatier S, Leclerc L, Cabrera M, Pourchez J, et al. Validation of anatomical models to study aerosol deposition in human nasal cavities. *Pharm Res* [Internet]. 2014 Jan [cited 2023 May 30];31(1):228. Available from: /pmc/articles/PMC3889297/
64. Leclerc L, Pourchez J, Aubert G, Leguellec S, Vecellio L, Cottier M, et al. Impact of airborne particle size, acoustic airflow and breathing pattern on delivery of nebulized antibiotic into the maxillary sinuses using a realistic human nasal replica. *Pharm Res.* 2014 Mar 4;31(9):2335–43.
65. Manniello MD, Hosseini S, Alfaifi A, Esmaeili AR, Kolanjiyil A V., Walenga R, et al. In vitro evaluation of regional nasal drug delivery using multiple anatomical nasal replicas of adult human subjects and two nasal sprays. *Int J Pharm.* 2021 Jan 25;593:120103.

66. Anton D, Burckel H, Josset E, Noel G. Three-dimensional cell culture: a breakthrough in vivo. *Int J Mol Sci.* 2015;16(3):5517–27. Available from: https://www.mdpi.com/1422-0067/16/3/5517/htm
67. Liu X, Liu R, Cao B, Ye K, Li S, Gu Y, et al. Subcellular cell geometry on micropillars regulates stem cell differentiation. *Biomaterials.* 2016;111:27–39.
68. Alias MA, Buenzli PR. Modeling the effect of curvature on the collective behavior of cells growing new tissue. *Biophys J.* 2017;112(1):193–204. Available from: http://www.cell.com/article/S0006349516342722/fulltext
69. Aizawa Y, Owen SC, Shoichet MS. Polymers used to influence cell fate in 3D geometry: new trends. *Prog Polym Sci.* 2012;37(5):645–58.
70. Satzer P, Achleitner L. 3D printing: economical and supply chain independent single-use plasticware for cell culture. *N Biotechnol.* 2022;69: 55–61.
71. Lerman MJ, Lembong J, Muramoto S, Gillen G, Fisher JP. The evolution of polystyrene as a cell culture material. *Tissue Eng - Part B Rev.* 2018;24(5):359–72. Available from: https://www.liebertpub.com/doi/10.1089/ten.teb.2018.0056
73. Lücking TH, Sambale F, Schnaars B, Bulnes-Abundis D, Beutel S, Scheper T. 3D-printed individual labware in biosciences by rapid prototyping: in vitro biocompatibility and applications for eukaryotic cell cultures. *Eng Life Sci.* 2015;15(1):57–64. Available from: https://onlinelibrary.wiley.com/doi/full/10.1002/elsc.201400094
74. Leukers B, Gülkan H, Irsen SH, Milz S, Tille C, Seitz H, et al. Biocompatibility of ceramic scaffolds for bone replacement made by 3D printing. *Materwiss Werksttech.* 2005;36(12):781–7. Available from: https://onlinelibrary.wiley.com/doi/full/10.1002/mawe.200500968
75. Roohani-Esfahani SI, Newman P, Zreiqat H. Design and fabrication of 3D printed scaffolds with a mechanical strength comparable to cortical bone to repair large bone defects. *Sci Reports.* 2016;6(1):1–8. Available from: https://www.nature.com/articles/srep19468
76. Castilho M, Dias M, Gbureck U, Groll J, Fernandes P, Pires I, et al. Fabrication of computationally designed scaffolds by low temperature 3D printing. *Biofabrication.* 2013;5(3):035012. Available from: https://iopscience.iop.org/article/10.1088/1758-5082/5/3/035012
77. Amin R, Knowlton S, Hart A, Yenilmez B, Ghaderinezhad F, Katebifar S, et al. 3D-printed microfluidic devices. *Biofabrication.* 2016;8(2):022001. Available from: https://iopscience.iop.org/article/10.1088/1758-5090/8/2/022001
78. Morgan AJL, San Jose LH, Jamieson WD, Wymant JM, Song B, Stephens P, et al. Simple and versatile 3D printed microfluidics using fused filament fabrication. *PLoS One.* 2016;11(4):e0152023. Available from: https://journals.plos.org/plosone/article?id=10.1371/journal.pone.0152023
79. Alessandri K, Feyeux M, Gurchenkov B, Delgado C, Trushko A, Krause KH, et al. A 3D printed microfluidic device for production of functionalized hydrogel microcapsules for culture and differentiation of human Neuronal Stem Cells (hNSC). *Lab Chip.* 2016;16(9):1593–604. Available from: https://pubs.rsc.org/en/content/articlehtml/2016/lc/c6lc00133e
80. Lin H, Lozito TP, Alexander PG, Gottardi R, Tuan RS. Stem cell-based microphysiological osteochondral system to model tissue response to interleukin-1B. *Mol Pharm.* 2014;11(7):2203–12. Available from: https://pubs.acs.org/doi/full/10.1021/mp500136b
81. Wang YI, Abaci HE, Shuler ML. Microfluidic blood–brain barrier model provides in vivo-like barrier properties for drug permeability screening. *Biotechnol Bioeng.* 2017;114(1):184–94. Available from: https://onlinelibrary.wiley.com/doi/full/10.1002/bit.26045

82. Hao S, Ha L, Cheng G, Wan Y, Xia Y, Sosnoski DM, et al. A spontaneous 3D bone-on-a-chip for bone metastasis study of breast cancer cells. *Small.* 2018;14(12):1702787. Available from: https://onlinelibrary.wiley.com/doi/full/10.1002/smll.201702787
83. Shrestha J, Ghadiri M, Shanmugavel M, Razavi Bazaz S, Vasilescu S, Ding L, et al. A rapidly prototyped lung-on-a-chip model using 3D-printed molds. *Organs-on-a-Chip.* 2019;1:100001.
84. Grix T, Ruppelt A, Thomas A, Amler AK, Noichl BP, Lauster R, et al. Bioprinting perfusion-enabled liver equivalents for advanced organ-on-a-chip applications. *Genes.* 2018;9(4):176. Available from: https://www.mdpi.com/2073-4425/9/4/176/htm
85. Costa PF, Albers HJ, Linssen JEA, Middelkamp HHT, Van Der Hout L, Passier R, et al. Mimicking arterial thrombosis in a 3D-printed microfluidic in vitro vascular model based on computed tomography angiography data. *Lab Chip.* 2017;17(16):2785–92. Available from: https://pubs.rsc.org/en/content/articlehtml/2017/lc/c7lc00202e
86. Singh M, Tong Y, Webster K, Cesewski E, Haring AP, Laheri S, et al. 3D printed conformal microfluidics for isolation and profiling of biomarkers from whole organs. *Lab Chip.* 2017;17(15):2561–71. Available from: https://pubs.rsc.org/en/content/articlehtml/2017/lc/c7lc00468k
87. Li X, Brooks JC, Hu J, Ford KI, Easley CJ. 3D-templated, fully automated microfluidic input/output multiplexer for endocrine tissue culture and secretion sampling. *Lab Chip.* 2017;17(2):341–9. Available from: https://pubs.rsc.org/en/content/articlehtml/2017/lc/c6lc01201a

4 3D Printing of Medical Devices

Mary B. McGuckin, Achmad Himawan, Linlin Li, Jiaqi Gao, Qonita Kurnia Anjani, Yara Naser, Ke Peng, Camila J. Picco, Anna Korelidou, Rand Ghanma, and Eneko Larrañeta
Queen's University Belfast

CONTENTS

4.1 INTRODUCTION

Additive manufacturing (also known as 3D printing) is an umbrella term used to classify a family of manufacturing techniques characterised by sequential addition of layers of material to produce 3D objects [1–3]. Additive manufacturing technologies are classified into different techniques depending on the mechanism used to add or fuse the layers of material including extrusion, sintering or vat polymerisation, among many others [2,3]. In order to produce objects using this family of techniques, computer-aided design (CAD) is required [4]. Additive manufacturing is a highly versatile technology allowing manufacturing of prototypes and geometrically complex objects [5]. Moreover, 3D printing can be applied to a wide range of materials

DOI: 10.1201/9781003274568-4

including polymers, metals, ceramics and resins [3,5]. This technique has gained popularity over the last decade in various areas of application including medical devices and pharmaceutical products [1,2].

One of the main reasons for interest is the ability of additive manufacturing techniques to prepare dosage forms and/or medical devices adapted to patients' needs [6,7]. This is highly interesting for clinicians as CAD can be directly obtained from medical imaging techniques [4]. Therefore, objects can be printed to match the anatomy of the patient at the point-of-care [8]. Studies suggest that using 3D printing for medical device manufacturing can significantly reduce supply time [9,10]. For example, it has been estimated that the production of 3D-printed stents can reduce the supply time from 150 days up to 20 min [10]. Moreover, the versatility of 3D printing allows the manufacture of drug-loaded medical devices capable of providing added therapeutic benefits to the patient [11]. Currently, applications of 3D printing for the manufacturing of medical devices range from production of surgical tools [12] or catheters [13] to the production of implantable devices [14].

Despite the numerous advantages, there remain unanswered regulatory questions that limit the application of this technology within a clinical environment. This is a complex issue considering the diversity of medical devices that have been produced using additive manufacturing technologies. Some of the regulatory issues involve the materials used, the need for sterilisation and quality control tests. Firstly, some of the materials used in different 3D-printing applications are not FDA-approved despite their biocompatible properties. Moreover, there are regulatory issues surrounding sterility and quality control of 3D-printed medical devices. However, regulatory bodies such as the FDA or MHRA are working intensively to provide guidance to research institutions and companies to enable translation of this technology for patient benefit.

This chapter will describe current developments in the field of 3D printing for medical device manufacturing. The areas covered include 3D-printing techniques and the materials used to develop 3D-printing applications. Additionally, the areas of application of this technology will be discussed in detail. Finally, this chapter will include a section discussing regulatory aspects associated with 3D printing of medical devices.

4.2 3D-PRINTING TECHNIQUES USED FOR MEDICAL DEVICE MANUFACTURING

Additive manufacturing technique known as 3D printing is a process in which a three-dimensional solid object is generated starting from a digital model, either through fusing or through depositing the starting material. 3D printing can create physical objects of virtually any shape from a geometrical representation. Thus, the printed object can be personalised based on patients' medical imaging data. This unique property enables the production of medical devices (like anatomical models, surgical guides and instruments, and custom implants), including any intricate anatomical shapes through 3D printing [15–17].

Despite the diversity of 3D-printing techniques, there are general steps in which the 3D-printed objects are prepared. For the biomedical application, the first step involves selecting the anatomical target area. The design is then imported to CAD software to optimise the 3D geometry by processing the medical images from a

CT/MRI scan, exporting the 3D model to a printer-specific recognisable format (like ".stl" or ".obj"), and selecting the 3D printer and materials appropriately. This file represents the guidance for the subsequent printing, "slicing" the digital design model into cross-sections. The "sliced" design is then sent to a 3D printer, which manufactures the object by starting at the base layer and building a series of layers until the object is built using the raw materials needed for its composition [18,19].

Different printing techniques and materials are available to reproduce objects than can be customised to match patients' needs. Most of the available printing materials are rigid, like metal and some resin, which can be used to produce objects like surgical instruments [20] or instruments used in orthopaedic trauma surgery [21]. However, some applications, such as replicating organs or soft tissue, demand flexibility and elasticity. Recent studies have discovered several material options with similar characteristics to anatomical tissues and organs that can be replicated through 3D-bioprinting technology [22]. Materials used in 3D printing are transformed during the production of the specific model by changing their physical properties. Three general means to transform the material are melting a rigid filament to give the desired form to the model by material distortion, liquid solidification through heating or photo-curing, and melting/sintering a powder material to a solid structure [23].

Techniques used in 3D printing have grown in recent decades, starting from 1986 when the first stereolithographic (SLA) systems were introduced into practice as the first commercially available technology. The technology has evolved very quickly, and research has already reported various 3D-printed pharmaceutical preparations and fully functioning printed organs [19]. According to ISO/ASTM standards, there are seven generalised standard terminologies related to 3D printing [24]. Information on various technologies that has been recently reported is provided in Table 4.1, where the technologies are grouped according to their standard term.

TABLE 4.1
Summary of 3D-Printing Technology Used for Medical Devices

ISO/ASTM Terminology	Commercial/ Other Terms	Suitable Material	Example of Medical Application	Advantageous	Disadvantageous
Binder Jetting	ProJet Color Jet Printing	Stainless steel, polymers, ceramic	Pre-operative medical model [29], bone regeneration [30]	Variety of colours, support for a variety of materials, fast process, different binder/powder combinations for different mechanical qualities	Not necessarily ideal for structural parts, cleaning the 3D-printing product takes time and adds to the procedure time

(Continued)

TABLE 4.1 (*Continued*)
Summary of 3D-Printing Technology Used for Medical Devices

ISO/ASTM Terminology	Commercial/ Other Terms	Suitable Material	Example of Medical Application	Advantageous	Disadvantageous
Directed Energy Deposition	Laser engineered net shape, electron beam additive manufacture	Metal	Knee implant [31]	High grain structure control, high quality depending on speed, high accuracy depending on accuracy, fast manufacture with rapid material deposition, fully dense parts; no supports required, the best procedure for part repair	A limited selection of materials is available, the surface quality is poor, and the wiring process is less precise
Material Extrusion	FDM, fused filament fabrication	Thermoplastic polymer	Medical instruments [32], vascular graph [33]	ABS plastic is widely used, has high structural characteristics and is inexpensive to produce	Quality is dependent on the nozzle radius and nozzle thickness. A wider nozzle results in lower quality and low accuracy. Low speed process and increased contact pressure are required to improve quality
MJ	Nanoparticle jetting, drop-on-demand, PolyJet, ProJet Multijet printing	Plastic, polymer	Medical model [34], arterial phantom prototyping [35]	High precision, minimal material waste, multiple material pieces and colours in a single process	Support material is required, materials are limited as only polymers and waxes are supported

(*Continued*)

TABLE 4.1 (*Continued*)
Summary of 3D-Printing Technology Used for Medical Devices

ISO/ASTM Terminology	Commercial/ Other Terms	Suitable Material	Example of Medical Application	Advantageous	Disadvantageous
Powder Bed Fusion	SLS, SLM, direct metal printing, direct metal laser sintering, electron beam melting, multi jet fusion	Metal, nylon	Orthopaedic implants [36], bone tissue reconstruction [37]	Low-cost, small technology as it is an office-sized machine with a wide choice of material options	Slow in terms of speed, as it lacks structural properties in materials, the sizes are limited and it depends on the powder grain size
Sheet Lamination	Laminated object manufacturing	Plastic, metal	Model of the medical implant [38]	Fast, cost-effective materials are easy to handle	Relies on paper and plastic as a material, requires further processing and has a limited material range
Vat Photo-polymerisation	SLA, DLP, continuous liquid interface production	Photopolymer resin	Dental model [39], dental surgical guide [40], hearing aid [41], indwelling bladder device [42], vascular graph [43]	High resolution and accuracy enables complex printing, good surface finishing, flexible printing setup	Inadequate strength and durability, UV light still affects the print, not suitable for heavy use.

Source: Adapted from Ref. [18].

- *Binder Jetting.* Liquid binder agents are selectively dropped/sprayed from an inkjet print head onto a thin layer of powder media through a motion-controlled print head, followed by subsequent infiltration or heating (if applicable) [25].
- *Directed Energy Deposition.* This technology utilises a focused application of energy to a coaxially feed material (metal powder) that is selectively melted and fused on a build platform or part, region by region [26].
- *Material Extrusion.* Material is mechanically dispensed, often through a heated nozzle, onto a build platform as the nozzle moves in the x and y directions to form each layer. To print the object correctly, materials used need to satisfy thermoplasticity, mechanical and rheological requirements [23].
- *Material Jetting (MJ).* This method is also known as inkjet printing. Droplets of photopolymer material are precisely jetted using a piezo-printing head

onto a build platform, where each layer is cured into a solid structure. This technique requires an entirely dense structure to support the printed object [23].

- *Powder Bed Fusion*. In this method, powder materials are deposited on a build platform and subsequently bonded together layer-by-layer using a laser or an electron beam that induces a thermal melting/sintering process. The rapid sintering process is enabled by maintaining the printing chamber at an elevated temperature, slightly below the material softening temperature. The powder particle size dramatically affects the printing resolution [23].
- *Sheet Lamination*. Discrete pre-formed layers of material are fused or glued together to form a solid 3D object. This method allows the use of different materials for different layers and enables the inclusion of pre-fabricated components between the laminated sheets [27].
- *Vat Photopolymerisation*. This technique involves the solidification of liquid resin. Liquid photopolymer or photopolymer solution is selectively exposed to a light source, such as UV light, that allows pixel-by-pixel or layer-by-layer curing to form a solid structure. The resolution will depend on the optical properties of the resin, the type of light source used and the printer configuration [23].

The material selection is directly linked to the desired properties of the 3D-printed object, choice of 3D-printing process, printer and the printers' model requirements. Individual structures necessitate different mechanical properties of materials to fulfil the required performance of the printed object. There are two main characteristics of materials which need to be considered if the printing purpose is to replicate anatomical objects, rigid and soft structures. Human bones are an example of rigid tissue, whereas ligaments or articular cartilages are examples of soft materials. Bones are the simplest and easiest biological tissue to manufacture *via* 3D printing as most materials are rigid, while softer structures are harder to replicate [18]. Organ/soft tissue bioprinting possesses the most significant technical challenge as it needs to replicate the intricate structure of the vascular network of the organ/tissue [28].

4.3 MATERIALS USED FOR 3D PRINTING OF MEDICAL DEVICES

High-quality materials are required for 3D printing to fabricate high-quality medical devices. The development of biomaterials is vital for the development of 3D-printed medical devices. The material selected varies according to the application or fabrication process. Biomaterials used in the manufacturing of medical devices can be divided into polymeric materials, metal materials, ceramic materials, composite materials and derived materials [14].

4.3.1 Polymers

Polymers are the most widely used materials in the 3D-printing industry due to their versatility and simplicity of application to various 3D-printing techniques. Polymers are macromolecules comprising a specific number of repeated monomer units. They can be synthetic or of natural origin. Based on their properties, biomedical polymer materials may be divided into two categories, namely nondegradable and degradable polymers. Degradable polymers such as collagen, poly(lactic acid), poly(caprolactone) or poly(lactic-co-glycolic acid) can be absorbed or eliminated in the biological environment of the human body [44], whereas nondegradable polymer materials such as polyethylene, polypropylene and polyformaldehyde remain stable in biological environments for a long period of time [45]. As a result, nondegradable polymers play an important role in providing mechanical support to 3D-printed devices. Biomedical polymers are widely used in fabricating orthopaedic implants or repairing cardiovascular stents [46]. Thermoplastic filaments, reactive monomers, resin and powder are all forms of polymers used in additive manufacturing [47].

4.3.2 Metals

Metal materials used in the fabrication of medical devices include stainless steel, titanium and titanium alloys, cobalt chromium–molybdenum alloys, and medical precious metals [46]. Metal 3D printing has shown excellent potential in medical applications due to its advantages and versatility. Owing to the high fatigue resistance and biocompatibility of metal materials, they have been widely used for 3D-printing medical devices such as bone and joint substitutes [14]. Cobalt-based alloys have high mechanical strength, and titanium alloys have exclusive properties such as corrosion resistance, rendering them suitable for 3D printing of dental devices [48].

4.3.3 Biomedical Ceramic Materials

Biomedical ceramics have been explored recently and represent a new variation of biomedical inorganic nonmetallic materials. Ceramics have been extensively used as a biomedical raw material since the early 18th century. At present, biomedical ceramics are mainly used as fillers for bone defects, dental implants and artificial valves. Biomedical ceramics can be subdivided into three main categories according to their bioactivity: biologically inert ceramics, biologically active ceramics and biodegradable ceramics. The first generation of biomedical ceramics refers to biologically inert ceramics based on metal oxides such as zirconia and alumina. These materials possess structural stability, strength and stable chemical properties. The second generation of biomedical ceramics are bioactive ceramics including bioactive glass [49] and also calcium phosphate, which is the most common [50]. Bioactive ceramics have the ability to release bioactive components while inducing reactions in a physiological environment. The third generation of biomedical ceramic materials are biodegradable ceramics, such as β-tricalcium phosphate. With their bioactivity, they are able to stimulate specific cellular responses or tissue repair processes at a molecular level, thus further regulating the body's spontaneous repair function and promoting new bone formation [51]. Third-generation biomedical ceramic materials are therefore the main research target for biomedical ceramics. Currently, biomedical ceramic materials suffer from low strength and low toughness in clinical practice.

4.3.4 Biomedical Composite Materials

Biomedical composite materials consist of two or more different materials, mainly including bone cement, coating materials and nanophosphoric lime [52]. Biomedical composites are widely used in the synthesis, repair, replacement and strengthening of human tissues and organs [53]. As composites are made from multiple materials, they can significantly improve the properties of certain materials. The composite material will have unique and improved properties compared to the component materials alone. Such new properties may be beneficial to humans or harmful. As a result, it is important to achieve biomechanical properties, desirable physiochemical properties while maintaining biocompatibility.

4.4 APPLICATIONS OF 3D PRINTED MEDICAL DEVICES

4.4.1 Vascular Stents and Vascular Grafts

Atherosclerosis has become a major cause of vascular disease and death [54]. This chronic arterial disease is triggered by fat or lipid deposition on the arterial wall, which forms fatty plaques, leading to arterial blockage, resulting in the disruption of blood circulation through the artery [55]. In most cases, a severely narrowed atherosclerotic coronary artery requires vascular stent implantation, which can help to widen the artery to unblock and restore the blood flow [56]. Stenting is performed *via* a procedure called percutaneous coronary intervention (PCI) or coronary angioplasty, which involves delivery of the stent to the target area in the artery. During the insertion process, the stent is equipped with a balloon, which enables the stent to open and expand by balloon inflation. The balloon is then deflated and removed, while the stent remains open within the artery.

3D printing has been used extensively in fabricating vascular stents and grafts, particularly for patient-personalised treatments, when the stents are tailored specifically to the patient's need. This can be achieved as 3D-printing technology allows stent fabrication to be made based on the results of assessments and imaging of patient-specific parameters. The personalised stent can then be printed on-the-spot before the PCI procedure. Furthermore, 3D-printing technology is widely used to generate coronary artery models which are highly precise and can be accurately compared to the initial coronary artery morphology [57]. This model can then be adapted for designing and personalising the stent as well as supporting the healthcare workers to determine the best plan for the PCI procedure.

There are several techniques available for manufacturing stents, namely SLA, selective laser melting (SLM), fused deposition modelling (FDM) and MJ. van Lith et al. made use of the SLA technique to print stents from methacrylated poly(1,12 dodecamethylene citrate) for peripheral artery disease [58]. In this work, the researchers showed that the printed stents had similar mechanical properties to bare metal stents and had an ability to expand porcine arteries following stent deployment. Despite the promising results of this study, several extensive studies need to be conducted, such as stability evaluation, *in vivo* application and biocompatibility tests.

The SLM technique has been used by Demir and Previtali to produce cardiovascular stents from cobalt-chrome (CoCr) alloy powder [61]. In this study, the researchers designed two stent models which were compared to investigate the geometric versatility of the SLM technique. They found that different geometries required specific strategies and supporting structures during printing. Furthermore, SLM can be considered as an alternative technique to prepare microtubes for additive features in stent manufacturing. The printed stents prepared using this technique have an accurate geometrical accuracy; however, the surface roughness needs to be electrochemically polished [61]. Flege et al. used the same technique to print biodegradable coronary stent prototypes from poly-L-lactic acid (PLLA) and PLLA-co-poly-ε-caprolactone powder [62]. In this study, they also designed an expandable Y-shaped stent for bifurcation application. After printing, the stents were coated and sprayed using the dip coating technique to polish the surface. Moreover, the researchers demonstrated that both polymers used to print the stent prototype were compatible with human coronary artery smooth muscle cells, endothelial progenitor cells and umbilical vein endothelial cells [62].

A different technique that has featured in stent manufacture is FDM. This approach has been used widely in many industries due to its lower production cost compared to other 3D-printing techniques [63–65]. Park et al. used FDM to prepare a 3D-printed stent fabricated from poly(caprolactone) (PCL) (Figure 4.1a) [59]. The printed stent was then coated with sirolimus in poly-(lactide-*co*-glycolide) (PLGA) and polyethylene glycol (PEG) mixture *via* spraying in order to achieve sustained release (Figure 4.1b). The results showed that the coated stent had a smoother surface compared to the uncoated stent. *In vitro* release studies on sirolimus-coated stents highlighted that 20% of the drug was released over 4 days and up to 50% of the drug released over 31 days afterwards. This release was slower compared to the commercially available Cypher® stent, which released 80% sirolimus at 31 days. The stent was implanted successfully into the porcine femoral artery, and the fibrin score was also effectively reduced.

In addition to vascular stents, 3D-printing technology has been used for the production of cardiovascular grafts. These devices are used in bypass surgery to divert blood flow around clogged or narrowed sections of an artery [66]. For this purpose, autologous grafts are commonly used; however, there are some circumstances where synthetic vascular grafts are necessary [66]. In order to prepare synthetic vascular grafts adapted to the anatomy of the patient, 3D printing can be used. Moreover, these devices can be combined with drugs to provide added functionality to the devices such as antiplatelet or antibacterial properties [67].

Melchiorri et al. developed vascular grafts using direct light processing (DLP) [43]. Poly(propylene fumarate), a biodegradable polymer, was used to prepare the vascular grafts. The resulting material showed similar mechanical properties to native blood vessels and was successfully implanted into mice. These grafts maintained their functionality and patency for at least 6 months. On the other hand, Dominguez-Robles et al. used extrusion-based 3D-printing (semisolid extrusion and FDM) to prepare cardiovascular grafts using biodegradable (PCL) and non-biodegradable (thermoplastic polyurethane, TPU) polymers [60,68,69]. PCL vascular grafts were combined with acetylsalicylic acid and dipyridamole (DIP) to add

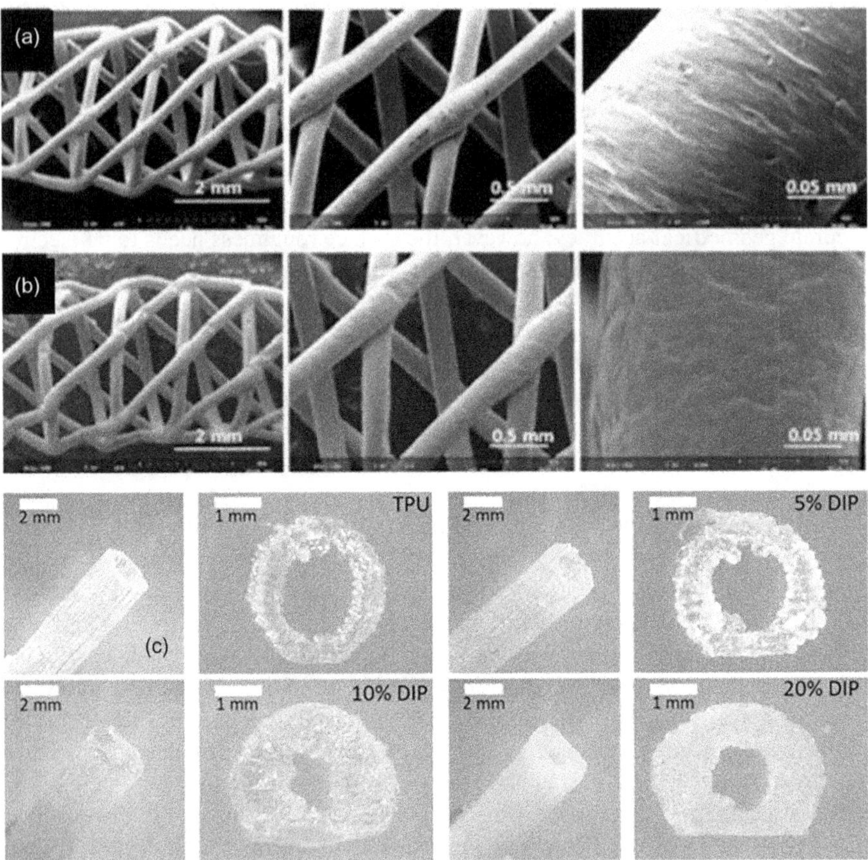

FIGURE 4.1 SEM images of PCL-based cardiovascular stents (a). SEM images of PCL-based cardiovascular stents coated with sirolimus (b). Vascular grafts prepared using TPU loaded with different amounts of DIP (c). Reproduced with permission from Refs. [59,60].

antiplatelet properties to the grafts. Another study conducted used FDM to combine TPU with DIP to obtain nonbiodegradable vascular grafts with antiplatelet properties (Figure 4.1c) [60].

If research in the future continues to develop and prove the value of 3D printing to produce vascular stents and vascular grafts, it is envisioned that this technology may emerge as a promising approach to support and enhance treatment options for vascular diseases. However, significant research is required before this technique can be translated into clinical application. One translational hurdle of particular importance arises as biodegradable polymeric materials have inferior mechanical properties which will affect application. The discovery of new biodegradable materials which have acceptable mechanical strength is paramount in order to move the field forwards to a clinical setting.

4.4.2 Prosthetic Cardiac Valves

Heart valves play a significant role in maintaining the correct direction of blood flow within the heart. Any dysfunction or illness in heart valves could put human health at risk, consequently affecting the patient's quality of life. In the elderly, myocardial infarction and senile valve disease are common and occur due to ageing [70]. Many adults are predisposed to hyperlipidaemia, hypertension and chronic renal disease, which can damage heart valves. In modern medicine, heart valve disease is a frequent illness, and valve defects can obstruct normal blood flow, increasing stress on the heart, resulting in impaired cardiac function and heart failure.

There are three treatment options for cardiac valve disease. These include either pharmacological therapy, external surgical therapy or interventional therapy. External surgical therapy involves using an artificial heart valve substitute or valvuloplasty for treatment. This is considered an effective treatment option for patients at high risk, and it is a radical cure for cardiac valve disease. Cardiac valves may be made specifically for different patients using 3D printing to enhance precision and stability, reduce the chance of the patient's body rejecting the cardiac valve and boost the success rate of heart valve replacement [71].

Mechanical valves, biological valves, interventional valves and tissue-engineered valves have all been used to construct artificial heart valves [72,73]. Tissue valves are functioning heart valves created using 3D-printing technology [14]. China commenced researching artificial cardiac valves in the 1960s. In 1999, a successful mitral valve replacement with a domestic cage valve was performed by Professor Yongzhi Cai [74]. Afterwards, a biomaterial artificial heart valve, produced by the Beijing Fuwai Hospital, was successfully used in an aortic valve replacement surgery. Furthermore, Duan et al. reported the effective use of hydrogel composite fabricated from hyaluronic acid and methacrylate, to load human valve interstitial cells [75]. This was performed by raising the concentration of methacrylate in the hydrogel to increase its viscosity and thus trigger information transmission between cells, while also preserving the human fibre cell phenotype. Figure 4.2 shows an aortic valve model and a 3D-printed product [75].

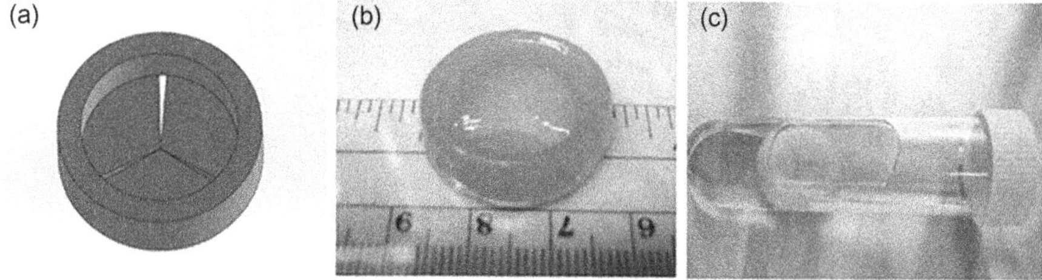

FIGURE 4.2 Hyaluronic acid-based 3D-printed cardiac valve loaded with human valve interstitial cells: heart valve model (a), freshly printed cardiac valve (b) and 3D-printed cardiac valve intact in culture tube after 7 days. Reproduced with permission from Ref. [75].

Flaws can occur in the preparation of aortic valves as there are variations between the designed aortic valve and the real aortic valve. Furthermore, the non-Newtonian properties of the hydrogel are somewhat ignored during the aortic valve printing process. Swelling phenomena could potentially occur, posing detrimental effects on the surface and dimensional accuracy of the aortic valve [14].

4.4.3 Orthopaedic Implants and Joint Prostheses

Bone is living osseous tissue that makes up the body's skeleton, providing shape and support for the body as well as protection for some organs. It is also a storage site for minerals and marrow, and for the development and storage of blood cells. Bone tissue can readily regenerate, repair and heal itself. This process involves osteoblasts forming new bone while osteoclasts resorb old bone [76]. However, in most cases, large-scale bone defects, which cannot be healed completely by the body, require external interventions to restore normal function [77].

Treatment options to repair bone defects include autografts (bone tissues taken from one location to another in the same individual), allografts (bone tissue from a deceased donor) and bone tissue engineering using artificial bone substitute materials such as polymers or metals. Autografts require two complicated and painful operation procedures and are restrained by the limited bone sources in the patients. Allografts have the risk of immune rejection and infectious diseases from the donor [78]. Thus, bone tissue engineering especially using 3D printing to synthesise and/or regenerate bone to restore, maintain or improve its functions *in vivo* is becoming popular [76].

Traditional methods of artificial bone scaffold preparation, such as gas foaming [79], fibre bonding, freeze-drying, phase separation [80] and particle leaching, are unable to reproducibly control the cell pore shape and pore size of the artificial bone scaffold. As a result, the artificial bone scaffold prepared by these methods poses difficulties for clinical use. Taking the aforementioned factors into consideration, 3D-printing technology has become a popular method for creating artificial bone scaffolds, offering a great deal of potential allowing the preparation of patient-specific devices. Figure 4.3 shows an example of a patient-specific 3D-printed titanium bone implant.

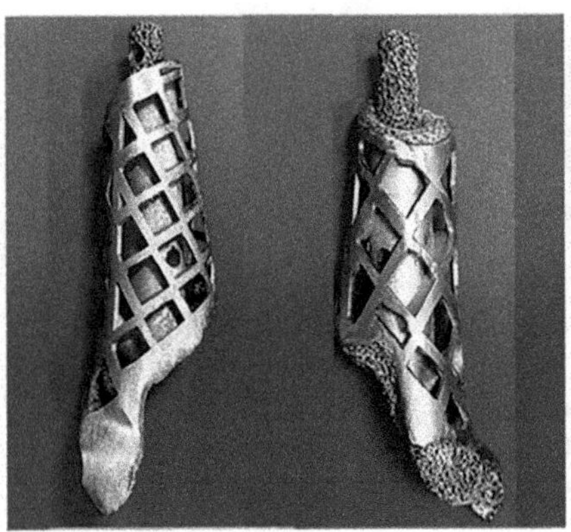
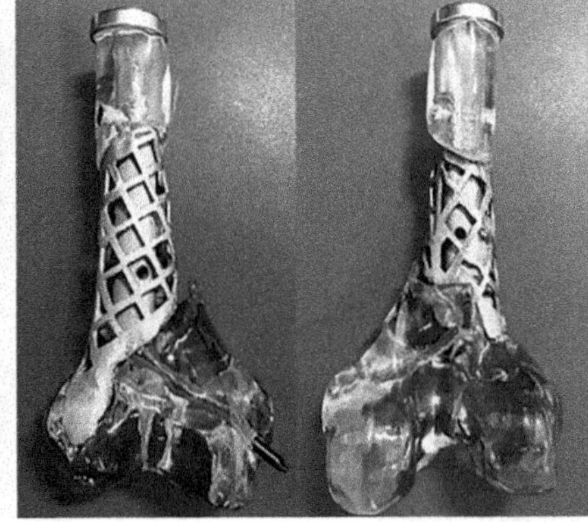

FIGURE 4.3 3D-printed titanium femoral implant. Reproduced with permission from Ref. [81].

Three patients with bone malignancies were fitted with 3D-printed titanium alloy shoulder blade prostheses, clavicular prostheses, and pelvic prostheses at the First Affiliated Hospital of the Fourth Military Medical University of Chinese PLA (Xijing Hospital) in March 2014 [14]. The first two examples were first in the world, while the third one was the first in Asia, which marks a significant step forwards in the use of 3D-printing technology in bone tissue engineering. Fan et al. used 3D-printing technology to create titanium alloy clavicles, pelvis and scapula that were successfully transplanted into three patients, with satisfactory clinical results [82]. Dai Kerong and colleagues used 3D-printing technology to prepare metal materials into an artificial pelvis. Satisfactory results in clinical practice were observed following completion of the artificial pelvis replacement [83]. Similarly, Saijo et al. used 3D-printing technology to prepare tricalcium phosphate powder into a personalised prosthesis and achieved satisfactory results in clinical applications [84].

With the current advancements in this research field, 3D printing in orthopaedics is becoming increasingly popular. However, the use of 3D-printing technology in orthopaedics remains in early stages, and suitable technological materials are still being established. Other issues which need to be resolved include the fact that 3D-printed bone implants lack extensive sample data and follow-up data, there are concerns with material selection due to the high clinical criteria for implant materials, the structure of human tissues and organs are complicated, and printing accuracy needs to be enhanced [14].

A joint is the structure where two bones connect to enable the skeleton to move. Arthritis is a common condition that causes pain and inflammation in joints. Osteoarthritis (OA) is also termed degenerative arthritis. By destroying the articular cartilage, degenerative joint disease of the whole joint occurs, resulting in loss of normal joint mobility and joint dysfunction. Joint replacement surgery is a very challenging procedure in orthopaedics and is still employed in the therapeutic practice of joint dysfunction to restore the joint's structure and function [14].

Total hip arthroplasty is a surgery to replace a defective hip joint with an artificial hip prosthesis [85]. A hip joint prosthesis is recommended for the elderly with fresh or old femoral neck fractures, middle-aged and elderly individuals with severe degenerative OA, and avascular necrosis of the femoral head. Conventional prostheses and 3D-printed titanium alloy bones have been employed to conduct artificial total hip replacement surgery for patients with femoral neck fractures, primary hip joints and secondary OA in the clinic.

The most useful operation for treating moderate-to-severe knee arthritis is total knee arthroplasty (TKA) [86]. Knee joint prostheses are surgical implants that replace the femur and tibia articular surfaces on both sides of the knee.

In the clinic, finger joint trauma is a frequent orthopaedic problem. Joint transplantation, arthroplasty, joint fusion, and artificial joint replacement are all effective treatments for finger joint dysfunction. Artificial joint replacement is widely regarded for its benefits in restoring finger function and hand knuckle stability. Burman pioneered the alloy metacarpal head hemi-joint replacement procedure in 1940, which is considered the paradigm for hand facet joint replacement [18]. The clinical use of total joint replacement prosthesis proposed by Brannon and Klein in 1959 contributed to the widespread application of artificial joint replacement [87]. Swanson and

Peltier introduced a revolutionary concept of prosthetic finger joint prosthesis in 1962 [88], which was improved in 1969 by Niebauer et al. [89] and ChiaRi and Trieb [90]. The design of the prosthesis in the 1970s was more in line with biomechanics, and application of the prosthesis was closer to normal joint anatomy. Recently, various types of human manual articular surface replacement prostheses have been in clinical use [91].

3D-printing technology has been extensively applied in joint replacement surgery. However, there is a need to enhance the stability and effectiveness of the prosthesis in the body by innovation of the material and manufacturing processes [14].

4.4.4 Implantable Devices for Drug Delivery

The use of 3D-printing technology for the development of implantable devices in drug delivery has increasingly gained relevance over the last years due to its remarkable flexibility, which allows for designing formulations in a customised approach [92,93]. Implantable devices have been widely explored to improve the treatment of multiple diseases, especially those which require treatment for long periods (more than 1 month). When loading low drug concentrations, these devices can achieve effective delivery and increase patient compliance by simplifying dose regimes and minimising potential side effects [46,94,95]. This section describes the use of 3D-printed polymeric implantable devices for controlled drug release.

Implantable devices are being investigated for different sites of administration such as subcutaneous, intravaginal, intranasal, intratumoural, intracranial and intravesical [46,96,97]. One key aspect associated with patient compliance is the design of the implant since the shape of the device must suit the anatomical features of the application site and therapeutic needs, such as systemic versus local effect, required plasma levels and dose frequency. The shape of 3D-printed objects is adjustable from simple to complex geometries using CAD software compatible with each printer [98]. The most commonly available designs enable printing of shapes including cylinders, discs and cuboids, whereas more complex implants incorporate a combination of multiple morphologies and intricacies to ensure time- and site-specific drug delivery. These implants are usually made of biodegradable materials, such as PLA, PCL, PEG and polyurethanes, among others [99,100]. Polymers provide a matrix for the drug, releasing it in a sustained manner with the advantage of polymer degradation over time into nontoxic by-products, rendering them biocompatible [101].

Holländer et al. prepared T-shaped intrauterine implants containing indomethacin as a model drug using FDM [102]. These implants were loaded with 5%, 15% and 30% (w/w) of the drug and were capable of providing 30 days of drug release. Moreover, polymeric implants can be accompanied by a membrane to control the drug release. This strategy was followed by Stewart et al. using PCL-based membranes [103]. 3D-printed implants were prepared and coated with a PCL-based formulation. These implants were loaded with model molecules such as methylene blue. The coated implants were capable of providing sustained release for up to 200 days. Similarly, Picco et al. have developed a polymeric membrane, surrounding cylindric implants of olanzapine and poly(ethylene)oxide. In this work, implant devices were formulated using a robocasting 3D-printing technique combined with a pre-formed controlling PCL membrane [104]. The implants enabled *in vitro* drug release for 190 days, achieving sustained delivery of the drug. Finally, Korelidou et al. developed a similar type of porous membranes based on PLA and low-molecular-weight PCL, which were included in 3D-printed implants as rate-controlling membranes. The resulting devices were capable of providing sustained drug release of a model antibiotic (tetracycline) for up to 4 weeks [105].

More complex implants can be fabricated with 3D-printing technology. A study of biodegradable polymer implants containing soluble "windows" made of poly(vinyl alcohol) uses FDM technology (Figure 4.4) [95]. Methylene blue, ibuprofen sodium and ibuprofen acid were used as model drugs and tested for several days depending

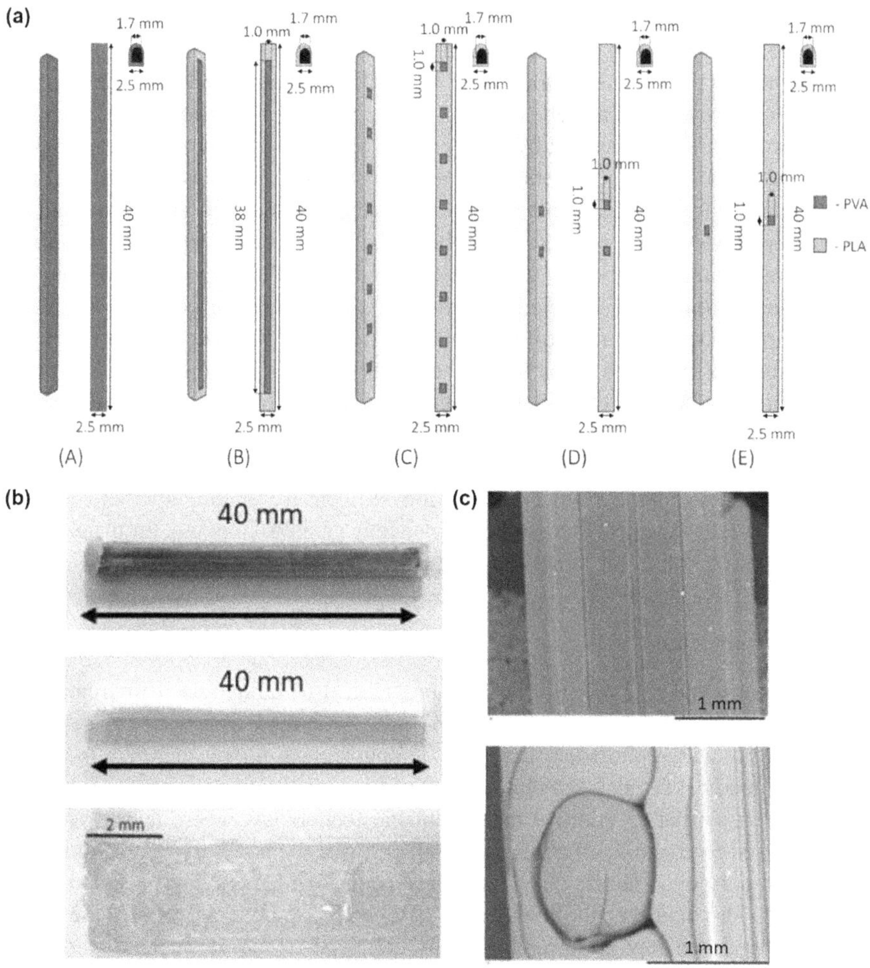

FIGURE 4.4 CAD designs of implants with soluble "windows" for drug release (a). 3D-printed implants containing methylene blue (top panel), ibuprofen (middle panel) and empty implants (bottom panel) (b). SEM image of the implant soluble "windows" (c). Reproduced with permission from Ref. [95].

on the design of the implant. The release rate was proportional to the "window" size. In another study, implants were fabricated using flexible coaxial printing [106]. This technology prints devices consisting of a core and a shell made with different materials. Therefore, it is possible to formulate devices containing more than one drug. This is interesting to explore in some diseases, such as retinal vascular diseases, where drugs used for the treatment present a short half-life, leading to more frequent administration.

Selection of materials is crucial for the release properties of drug delivery implants, as demonstrated by Kempin et al. [107]. In this work, four different polymers were used to formulate cylindrical devices printed by FDM technology. Quinine was used as a model drug for the release study in concentrations ranging from 2.5% to 15%. The results showed that releases with a PCL or PLA matrix were faster than those with EC or Eudragit® RS. Not only does the amount of drug loaded in the device have an influence on the release profiles, but it also affects the printability of the formulations. It was proved that a higher amount of drug blocked the nozzle of the printer. Similar findings were obtained by Arany et al. [108] as they analysed release behaviour by using different polymers, sizes and infill ratios. They used FDM technology to print cylindrical containers that were manually filled with diclofenac sodium. PLA, poly(ethylene)terephthalate and poly(methyl methacrylate) were tested with 16, 19 or 22 mm diameters and 0%, 5%, 10% or 15% infill percentages. The authors concluded that by increasing the diameter, the release rate was faster due to the larger surface area, whereas if the infill percentage is increased the drug release is lower.

The findings discussed above reveal the potential of 3D-printing technology when formulating implantable devices for drug delivery. Not only is the awareness of the disease and application sites crucial, but it is also important to choose suitable drugs and materials to enable selection of the most appropriate printing approach. Taking these parameters into careful consideration will ensure an implant with optimal mechanical behaviour and release performance is printed. Implants for drug release are a promising option for long-term treatments.

4.4.5 Human Organs

Three-dimensional (3D) bioprinting is a biomedical technique used to create a 3D structural architecture imitating structural and functional tissues or organs [109]. The main clinical applications are in tissue engineering for regenerative medicine, prosthetic medical devices and replacement of functional tissues or organs [110]. The procedure is similar to additive manufacturing technology, where layers of bioink are deposited to create live tissues such as blood vessels, body organs and skin. The bioink category may include cells, biomaterials, growth factors, hormones and additives [111]. The induced pluripotent stem (iPS) cells are obtained from the patient's body, isolated and reprogrammed into any cell type of the particular organ [112]. Scientists who discovered the iPS methodology won a Nobel Prize, and their discovery has had a huge impact on 3D bioprinting as it may solve the lack of organ supply for transplants and eliminates the risk of rejection from the patient's immune system [109]. An additional application of the 3D bioprinted organs is to prepare model organs to improve surgical techniques, train inexperienced surgeons and achieve more patient-specific treatments [15]. Organ bioprinting can also be applied in drug development and drug toxicity testing, as it can be utilised in discovery and dosage research [110]. Furthermore, combining bioprinting and microfluidic technology can be used to develop organ-on-chips for disease modelling, imitating the natural extracellular matrix. The aforementioned techniques contribute to drug discovery with efficient and high-throughput assays, lowering the cost and demand for animal testing [113].

The first artificial organ fabricated using bioprinting and stem cells was printed by a team of scientists led by Dr Anthony Atala at the Wake Forest Institute for Regenerative Medicine [114]. The scientists printed an artificial scaffold for a human bladder and subsequently seeded the scaffold with cells from their patient. Ten years after implantation, the patient had no serious complications [115]. Since then, research has continued with successful bioprinting of other organs such as the liver and heart valves. Recent studies using the freeform reversible embedding of suspended hydrogels technique have reported bioprinting of a 3D heart. The bioprinted heart was not transplanted into a patient; however, it was the first promising approach for creating a detailed large-scale, 3D, external and internal biological structure [116,117]. In 2019, a breakthrough discovery occurred as scientists printed a rabbit-sized heart with a network of blood vessels contracting in a similar manner to natural blood vessels (Figure 4.5) [118]. Further encouraging research resulted in successful printing of a fully functional artificial human pancreas [119]. Studies have also been conducted to attempt to develop a vascular system in a liver tissue model, further highlighting the many possibilities arising from bioprinting [120]. 3D bioprinting has been used to create a miniature liver that could be used for liver transplantation [121,122]. At the University of São Paulo in Brazil, scientists have succeeded in creating miniature versions of a human liver from blood cells, where these liver organoids integrate the functionalities of the organ [123]. An American bioprinting company, Organovo, bioprinted a miniature liver with natural functions and announced the successful automated production of kidney organoids via its bioprinting platform. 3D-printing technology has also been used to prepare an *in vitro* 3D proximal tubule tissue model, which has been vitally important in organ transplantation and kidney regeneration [124].

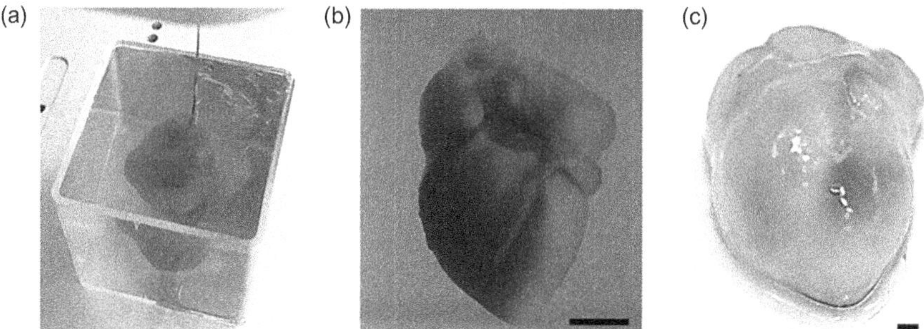

FIGURE 4.5 A printed small-scaled, cellularised human heart (a and b). After printing, the ventricles were injected with blue and red dyes to show that the heart contains hollow chambers and a septum in between them. Scale bars: B = 0.5 cm; C = 1 mm. Reproduced with permission from Ref. [118].

Researchers have developed an artificial ovary that can be transplanted into women with fertility issues. These studies reported successful implantation of a bioprinted ovary in a sterile mouse, highlighting the promising nature of these structures [125]. 3D printing has also been utilised to benefit eye research. At the University of Newcastle, a proof-of-concept project was developed with a 3D-printed artificial cornea that could be transplanted for people in need [126]. Another team from Marmara University in Turkey prepared 3D-printed artificial corneas potentially suitable for transplantation [127]. Several studies have effectively 3D-bioprinted human skin tissue structures and analogues, which provided a reliable source for skin transplantation [128,129]. Interestingly, researchers in New York could 3D-print "living" skin patches with blood vessels [130]. The first proof of concept of having 3D-printed lungs was conducted by Jordan Miller and his team. Even though the printed vasculature was just 300 μM in diameter, it is a significant step towards creating therapeutically useful lung tissues [131].

3D printing of human organs necessitates improvement in the resolution, accuracy and flexibility of biomaterials that meet the functional, biological and economic requirements for clinical applications [132]. A significant challenge remains the vasculature required to keep the organs alive and functional over a long period of time [14]. Additionally, ethical approval from the country's government is required for human organ culture and utilisation. Impressive progress has been made recently in the bioprinting sector; therefore, regulation and ethical considerations should be established [135]. Intellectual property and ownership also need to be regulated as they can impact issues such as piracy and quality control for manufacturing [133,136]. Before bioprinted organs become widely available, extensive research must be conducted including sourcing sustainable cell and development of large-scale manufacturing processes.

4.4.6 Medical Apparatus and Instruments

3D printing can vastly enhance health facilities' surgical capacity where access to basic surgical needs might be limited, like in developing countries or space missions [137]. 3D-printing technologies provide a cost-effective solution to provide needed medical supplies in a direct, on-demand fashion on-site, to further enhance the physicians' interventional capacity to render surgical services [138]. Figure 4.6 shows some examples of a 3D-printed surgical tools. Printing essential medical equipment can significantly reduce the functional burden of disease in developing countries, quick prototyping to improve and expand the existing toolkits, and allow a certain degree of customisation for case-by-case needs. These surgical toolkits, referred to as the "integrative surgical toolkits" or ISTs, provide a feasible solution for direct access to primary and customised surgical instruments. A core principle behind the fabrication of these medical/surgical toolkits is that they must provide real, functional utility (comparable to the original instrument they are trying to mimic) and encompass a variety of medical instruments/tools' designs [12]. In this chapter, we summarise attempts that have been made to fabricate surgical instruments grouped into several categories based on their functionality.

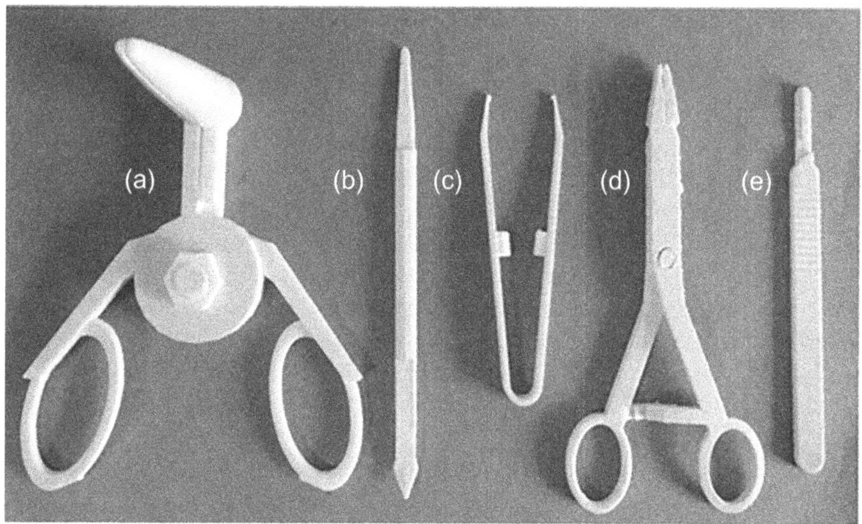

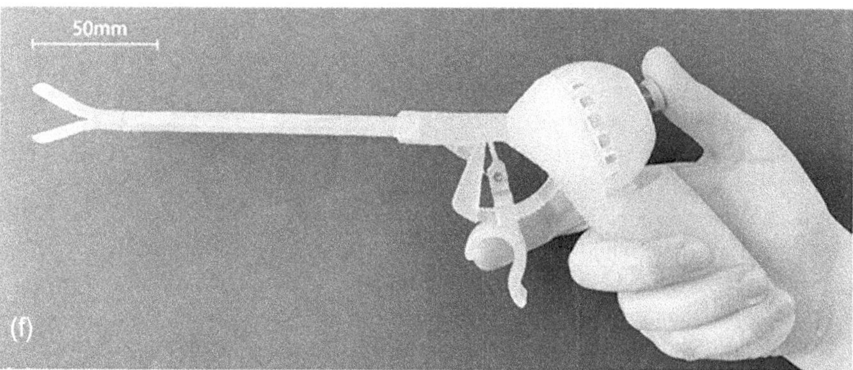

FIGURE 4.6 3D-printed surgical tools for septoplasty (a–e). 3D-printed tool for minimally invasive surgery (b). Reproduced with permission from Refs. [138,139].

- *Cutting and Dissecting Surgical Instruments.* This group contains both disposable and nondisposable instruments. Blades and scalpels are disposable, while knives and scissors are reusable. No 3D-printed materials can replace metal blades and knives in surgery, but the scalpel' handle can be 3D-printed using FDM [139] or selective laser sintering (SLS) printer [140]. A softer mucosal tissue can be cut using a Cottle elevator (commonly used in septoplasty) produced using an FDM 3D printer [139].
- *Grasping and Handling Surgical Instruments.* These instruments are used to grasp or hold tissues to get a closer view of the surgical field. Tools such as forceps, tenaculum and bone holders fall into this category. A toothed forceps can be printed using an FDM printer [139] and an SLS printer [140].
- *Clamping and Occluding Surgical Instruments.* These instruments help the surgeon clamp blood vessels or tissue to get them away from the surgical area during the procedure. This group includes hemostatic forceps,

hemostats, crushing clamps and noncrushing vascular clamps. A surgical hemostat printed using SLS technology can be used to occlude hernia sac for excision and handling of tissue plane for slit opening [140].

- *Retracting and Exposing Instruments.* Surgeons retract tissue away from the surgical field using retractors to get better visualisation. Retractors are designed to minimise the trauma to the tissue being retracted. An Army Navy retractor can be fabricated using an SLS printer on a plastic substrate. This retractor provides adequate exposure during the procedure tested against a human cadaver [140].
- *Instruments for Improving Visualisation.* Special instruments such as speculums, endoscopes, anoscopes and proctoscopes can be used to view deep structures that cannot be seen externally. Killian's speculum can be printed and shows functionality when tested using a cadaver to perform a septoplasty [139]. A bi-valve vaginal speculum high-dose-rate interstitial gynaecologic brachytherapy applicator can be made from resin and printed using an SLA printer. This hybrid instrument enables both viewings of the cervix and image-guided brachytherapy applicator placement [141].
- *Suturing and Stapling Surgical Instruments.* Sutures and staples in surgery are used to bring the skin and/or soft tissue adjacent together. Typical suturing kits comprise a needle, a needle holder, a forceps and a fine suturing scissor. 3D-printed needle holders can be produced using two-step printing with an FDM printer that allows a hinge formation [139].
- *Suctioning and Aspiration Instruments.* This group of tools aid the surgeon in clearing fluids around the surgical area. Different tips are used for different purposes. A clog-free tip design was printed using an SLA printer using medical-grade liquid photo-resin. The design was proposed, developed and tested by orthopaedic surgeons, highlighting the end-user friendliness of clinical adaptation of 3D-printing techniques [142].
- *Dilating and Probing Instruments.* Dilating instruments are used to expand the size of orifices while probes are inserted into natural openings. A low-cost urethral dilator can be produced using an FDM printer. When comparing it with a conventional metal dilator, the cost difference becomes less if the scale of the production economy is considered [143].

3D-printed instruments should not (yet) be considered as a replacement for conventional manufacturing. It still can be used to adapt to patients' specific needs, prototyping or manufacturing complex parts with additional functionality [143].

4.5 REGULATORY ASPECTS

Recent advancements in 3D printing have significantly enhanced the biomedical field, enabling rapid fabrication of patient-specific devices. Unfortunately, the lack of defined regulatory requirements remains the largest obstacle for 3D-printed products to reach the market, and the lack of established legal status prevents their frequent use in clinical settings.

According to Regulation (EU) 2017/745 of the European Parliament and of the Council of 5 April 2017, all 3D-printed products are classified as custom-made devices, designed for the sole use of a particular individual according to their condition and needs. It is the authorised prescriber's responsibility to provide a prescription outlining specific design characteristics for the custom-made device, which may be implantable or nonimplantable [144]. Article 2 of Regulation (EU) 2017/745 outlines conditions whereby a device would not be considered as custom-made. Any device which is mass-produced *via* industrial manufacturing processes would not be regarded as custom-made, even if it needs to be adapted to accommodate the particular needs of a patient [145]. Any device which falls outside the custom-made or investigational device categories must affix the CE marking of conformity which indicates that the product is deemed to meet EU safety, health and environmental protection requirements [146]. Contrastingly, custom-made devices do not have to undergo the constraining process to attain CE approval, and they do not require the unique device identification system which enables identification and facilitates the traceability of the device.

A different strategy is applied to custom-made implants. An "implantable device" is defined as those that are intended to be totally introduced into the human body or to replace an epithelial surface or surface of the eye. If a device is partially introduced into the body during a procedure and remains in place for at least 30 days, it is also considered implantable [147]. In order for custom-made implants to be commercialised and used, it is essential that a CE mark is affixed. However, custom-made nonimplantable devices do not require the CE mark provided that safety and performance requirements are met before use.

Similar to many other products on the market, it is very important to avoid misleading users when labelling and advertising medical devices. Article 7 of Regulation (EU) 2017/745 describes conditions which are prohibited including ascribing functions and properties to the device which the device does not have, creating a false impression regarding treatment properties which the device does not have, failing to inform the user of any potential risks associated with the device and indicating uses for the device that differ from the intended purpose for which the conformity assessment was carried out.

Ongoing work by the EU has been carried out in recent years to improve the medical devices directive by supporting innovation. To enable continuous progress in the 3D-printing field, clear guidance in relation to safe usage of 3D-printing technology is required. Although the current regulatory approach covers various components such as supervision of notified bodies, clinical investigations and clinical evaluation, there is a need to establish transparency and traceability regarding medical devices in order to improve health and safety for patients, and in turn, increase the use of medical devices in medicine.

4.6 CONCLUSIONS

3D printing, as a new type of digital printing technology, offers numerous advantages and potential uses in medicine, prompting every country to devote greater resources to its research and development. 3D-printing technology has been used in a variety of clinical settings, particularly in the use of implantable medical devices, which has gotten greater interest among scholars in various countries. Even though 3D-printing technology is already in full swing, it nevertheless confronts many challenges such as developing different 3D-printing raw materials. The second issue is that there are no industry standards for 3D-printing implanted medical devices. The third issue is that the product technology chain is still in its infancy. The key to the advancement and development of 3D-printing technology is the research on materials. In the future, biomaterials should have the best mechanical characteristics, diffusion coefficient and biocompatibility as these are the foundation and guidance for 3D-printing technology to advance in the medical field. Furthermore, if the problem of combining different cells' types and functions into a three-dimensional structure can be solved by combining biomaterials and printing technology, it will be a breakthrough. This technology will lead to a massive change in 3D-printing technology and biological tissue engineering. Also, the repair of human tissues and the transplantation of tissues and organs will be entirely addressed by biological printing technology. Independent 3D-printing manufacturing centres for human organs could be established in the future. These centres could allow complex diseases encountered in clinical practice to be rapidly resolved and patients' pain to be properly managed by producing suitable implants in a timely manner based on the disease's requirements.

In order to get better tissue regeneration while preventing immune rejection and infection, in situ 3D printing was proposed. This addition represents the implantation of original tissues in original body parts. In comparison with bioprinted implants, in situ 3D printing is more precise in size and shape, and it also eliminates the challenges of hard implantation. The optimisation and cross linking of inks used in the development of 3D printing in situ is one of the outstanding hurdles.

Investigation, characterisation and standardisation should be done for different formulas of silk-based inks in order to achieve shape accuracy while avoiding potential *in vivo* harmful effects of photoinitiators during photopolymerisation and enlarging the production scale to be employed in clinical practice [148]. Smart materials, also known as programmable materials, are materials that can be transformed by external stimuli, opening up intriguing new possibilities for 3D printing. This combination has given rise to a new domain known as 4D printing. The potential for 4D bioprinting to produce bones on a large scale is captivating. Another milestone in this field is the 5D printing in which the print head and the printable object have five degrees of freedom. 5D printing can save up to 25% of materials in the printing process when compared to 3D printing. Another advantage of 5D printing is its capability to produce curved layers instead of the flat layer because in this technique the print part moves while the printer head is printing. This curved structure will lead to an enhanced strength. This in turn will increase the possibility of using 5D printing to make artificial curved bones with high strength for surgery. This technology has a lot of potential to meet this fundamental need. In the future, 3D printing will become an important way of precise medicine and personalised treatment, as it is very promising for the medical sector. Multidimensional printing will become a bright point in the medical area, and it will help a country's medical biology research progress.

REFERENCES

1. Kholgh Eshkalak S, Rezvani Ghomi E, Dai Y, Choudhury D, Ramakrishna S. The role of three-dimensional printing in healthcare and medicine. *Mater Des.* 2020;194:108940. Available from: https://linkinghub.elsevier.com/retrieve/pii/S0264127520304743

2. Seoane-Viaño I, Trenfield SJ, Basit AW, Goyanes A. Translating 3D printed pharmaceuticals: From hype to real-world clinical applications. *Adv Drug Deliv Rev.* 2021;174:553–75. Available from: https://linkinghub.elsevier.com/retrieve/pii/S0169409X21001599
3. Detamornrat U, McAlister E, Hutton ARJ, Larrañeta E, Donnelly RF. The role of 3D printing technology in microengineering of microneedles. *Small.* 2022;18(18):2106392. Available from: https://onlinelibrary.wiley.com/doi/10.1002/smll.202106392
4. Abdullah KA, Reed W. 3D printing in medical imaging and healthcare services. *J Med Radiat Sci.* 2018;65(3):237–9. Available from: https://onlinelibrary.wiley.com/doi/10.1002/jmrs.292
5. Jandyal A, Chaturvedi I, Wazir I, Raina A, Ul Haq MI. 3D printing – A review of processes, materials and applications in industry 4.0. *Sustain Oper Comput.* 2022;3:33–42. Available from: https://linkinghub.elsevier.com/retrieve/pii/S2666412721000441
6. Goyanes A, Madla CM, Umerji A, Duran Piñeiro G, Giraldez Montero JM, Lamas Diaz MJ, et al. Automated therapy preparation of isoleucine formulations using 3D printing for the treatment of MSUD: First single-centre, prospective, crossover study in patients. *Int J Pharm.* 2019;567:118497. Available from: https://linkinghub.elsevier.com/retrieve/pii/S0378517319305393
7. De La Peña A, De La Peña-Brambila J, Pérez-De La Torre J, Ochoa M, Gallardo GJ. Low-cost customized cranioplasty using a 3D digital printing model: A case report. *3D Print Med.* 2018;4(1):4. Available from: https://threedmedprint.biomedcentral.com/articles/10.1186/s41205-018-0026-7
8. Calvo-Haro JA, Pascau J, Asencio-Pascual JM, Calvo-Manuel F, Cancho-Gil MJ, Del Cañizo López JF, et al. Point-of-care manufacturing: A single university hospital's initial experience. *3D Print Med.* 2021;7(1):11. Available from: https://threedmedprint.biomedcentral.com/articles/10.1186/s41205-021-00101-z
9. Larrañeta E, Dominguez-Robles J, Lamprou DA. Additive manufacturing can assist in the fight against COVID-19 and other pandemics and impact on the global supply chain. *3D Print Addit Manuf.* 2020 Jun 1;7(3):100–3. Available from: https://www.liebertpub.com/doi/10.1089/3dp.2020.0106
10. Moore SS, O'Sullivan KJ, Verdecchia F. Shrinking the supply chain for implantable coronary stent devices. *Ann Biomed Eng.* 2016;44(2):497–507. Available from: http://link.springer.com/10.1007/s10439-015-1471-8
11. Mathew E, Pitzanti G, Larrañeta E, Lamprou DA. 3D printing of pharmaceuticals and drug delivery devices. *Pharmaceutics.* 2020;12(3):266.
12. Bhatia SK, Ramadurai KW. 3-dimensional printing of medical devices and supplies. In *3D Printing and Bio-Based Materials in Global Health*, 2017. pp. 63–93. Available from: http://link.springer.com/10.1007/978-3-319-58277-1_4
13. Mathew E, Domínguez-Robles J, Stewart SA, Mancuso E, O'Donnell K, Larrañeta E, et al. Fused deposition modeling as an effective tool for anti-infective dialysis catheter fabrication. *ACS Biomater Sci Eng.* 2019;5(11):6300–10. Available from: https://doi.org/10.1021/acsbiomaterials.9b01185
14. Wang Z, Yang Y. Application of 3D printing in implantable medical devices. Chen X, editor. *Biomed Res Int.* 2021;2021:6653967.
15. Ventola CL. Medical applications for 3D printing: Current and projected uses. *P T.* 2014;39(10):704–11.
16. Shahrubudin N, Lee TC, Ramlan R. An overview on 3D printing technology: Technological, materials, and applications. *Procedia Manuf.* 2019;35:1286–96.
17. Tack P, Victor J, Gemmel P, Annemans L. 3D-printing techniques in a medical setting: A systematic literature review. *Biomed Eng Online.* 2016;15(1):115.
18. Aimar A, Palermo A, Innocenti B. The role of 3D printing in medical applications: A state of the art. *J Healthc Eng.* 2019 Mar 21;2019:1–10. Available from: https://www.hindawi.com/journals/jhe/2019/5340616/

19. Jamroz W, Szafraniec J, Kurek M, Jachowicz R. 3D printing in pharmaceutical and medical applications – Recent achievements and challenges. *Pharm Res.* 2018;35(9):176.
20. Mekata E, Yamada A, Shimagaki M, Kajiyama T, Tani T. Lightweight carbon-reinforced resin surgical instruments. In *Surgery and Operating Room Innovation*, 2022: pp. 3–16.
21. Lal H, Patralekh MK. 3D printing and its applications in orthopaedic trauma: A technological marvel. *J Clin Orthop Trauma.* 2018;9(3):260–8.
22. Wang X. Advanced polymers for three-dimensional (3D) organ bioprinting. micromachines. *Micromachines (Basel).* 2019;10(12):814.
23. Zhou LY, Fu J, He Y. A review of 3D printing technologies for soft polymer materials. *Adv Funct Mater.* 2020;30(28):2000187.
24. Alexander AE, Wake N, Chepelev L, Brantner P, Ryan J, Wang KC. A guideline for 3D printing terminology in biomedical research utilizing ISO/ASTM standards. *3D Print Med.* 2021;7(1):8.
25. Mostafaei A, Elliott AM, Barnes JE, Li F, Tan W, Cramer CL, et al. Binder jet 3D printing – Process parameters, materials, properties, modeling, and challenges. *Prog Mater Sci.* 2021;119:100707.
26. Oh WJ, Lee WJ, Kim MS, Jeon JB, Shim DS. Repairing additive-manufactured 316L stainless steel using direct energy deposition. *Opt Laser Technol.* 2019;117:6–17.
27. Bhatt PM, Kabir AM, Peralta M, Bruck HA, Gupta SK. A robotic cell for performing sheet lamination-based additive manufacturing. *Addit Manuf.* 2019;27:278–89.
28. Yan Q, Dong H, Su J, Han J, Song B, Wei Q, et al. A review of 3D printing technology for medical applications. *Engineering.* 2018;4(5):729–42.
29. Salmi M. Possibilities of preoperative medical models made by 3D printing or additive manufacturing. *J Med Eng.* 2016;2016:1–6.
30. Bandyopadhyay A, Mitra I, Bose S. 3D printing for bone regeneration. *Curr Osteoporos Rep.* 2020;18(5):505–14.
31. Ryu DJ, Ban HY, Jung EY, Sonn CH, Hong DH, Ahmad S, et al. Osteo-compatibility of 3D titanium porous coating applied by direct energy deposition (DED) for a cementless total knee arthroplasty implant: In vitro and in vivo study. *J Clin Med.* 2020;9(2):478.
32. Azila TN, Rahim T, Manaf A, Hazizan A&, Akil M, Noraihan T, et al. Recent developments in fused deposition modeling-based 3D printing of polymers and their composites. *Polym Rev.* 2019;59(4):589–624. Available from: https://doi.org/10.1080/15583724.2019.1597883
33. Basile S, Mathew E, Genta I, Conti B, Dorati R, Lamprou DA. Optimization of FDM 3D printing process parameters to produce haemodialysis curcumin-loaded vascular grafts. *Drug Deliv Transl Res.* 2021;1–14.
34. Ibrahim D, Broilo TL, Heitz C, de Oliveira MG, de Oliveira HW, Nobre SMW, et al. Dimensional error of selective laser sintering, three-dimensional printing and PolyJet™ models in the reproduction of mandibular anatomy. *J Cranio-Maxillofacial Surg.* 2009;37(3):167–73.
35. Biglino G, Verschueren P, Zegels R, Taylor AM, Schievano S. Rapid prototyping compliant arterial phantoms for in-vitro studies and device testing. *J Cardiovasc Magn Reson.* 2013;15(1):1–7.
36. Sing SL, An J, Yeong WY, Wiria FE. Laser and electron-beam powder-bed additive manufacturing of metallic implants: A review on processes, materials and designs. *J Orthop Res.* 2016;34(3):369–85.
37. Yang J, Jin X, Gao H, Zhang D, Chen H, Zhang S, et al. Additive manufacturing of trabecular tantalum scaffolds by laser powder bed fusion: Mechanical property evaluation and porous structure characterization. *Mater Charact.* 2020;170:110694.

38. Dermeik B, Travitzky N. Laminated object manufacturing of ceramic-based materials. *Adv Eng Mater.* 2020 Sep;22(9):2000256.
39. Cohen A, Laviv A, Berman P, Nashef R, Abu-Tair J. Mandibular reconstruction using stereolithographic 3-dimensional printing modeling technology. *Oral Surg Oral Med Oral Pathol Oral Radiol Endodontol.* 2009;108(5):661–6.
40. Whitley D, Eidson RS, Rudek I, Bencharit S. In-office fabrication of dental implant surgical guides using desktop stereolithographic printing and implant treatment planning software: A clinical report. *J Prosthet Dent.* 2017;118(3):256–63.
41. Vivero-Lopez M, Xu X, Muras A, Otero A, Concheiro A, Gaisford S, et al. Anti-biofilm multi drug-loaded 3D printed hearing aids. *Mater Sci Eng C.* 2021;119:111606.
42. Xu X, Goyanes A, Trenfield SJ, Diaz-Gomez L, Alvarez-Lorenzo C, Gaisford S, et al. Stereolithography (SLA) 3D printing of a bladder device for intravesical drug delivery. *Mater Sci Eng C.* 2021;120:111773. Available from: https://linkinghub.elsevier.com/retrieve/pii/S0928493120336924
43. Melchiorri AJ, Hibino N, Best CA, Yi T, Lee YU, Kraynak CA, et al. 3D-printed biodegradable polymeric vascular grafts. *Adv Healthc Mater.* 2016;5(3):319–25.
44. Stewart AS, Domínguez-Robles J, Donnelly RF, Larrañeta E. Implantable polymeric drug delivery devices: Classification, manufacture, materials, and clinical applications. *Polymers (Basel).* 2018;10(12):1379.
45. Tan WS, Chua CK, Chong TH, Fane AG, Jia A. 3D printing by selective laser sintering of polypropylene feed channel spacers for spiral wound membrane modules for the water industry. *Virtual Phys Prototyp.* 2016;11(3):151–8.
46. Utomo E, Stewart SA, Picco CJ, Domínguez-Robles J, Larrañeta E. Classification, material types, and design approaches of long-acting and implantable drug delivery systems. In: *Long-Acting Drug Delivery Systems.* Elsevier; 2022. pp. 17–59. Available from: https://linkinghub.elsevier.com/retrieve/pii/B9780128217498000124
47. Ngo TD, Kashani A, Imbalzano G, Nguyen KTQ, Hui D. Additive manufacturing (3D printing): A review of materials, methods, applications and challenges. *Compos Part B Eng.* 2018;143:172–96.
48. Hitzler L, Alifui-Segbaya F, Williams P, Heine B, Heitzmann M, Hall W, et al. Additive manufacturing of cobalt-based dental alloys: Analysis of microstructure and physicomechanical properties. Yao Z, editor. *Adv Mater Sci Eng.* 2018;2018:8213023.
49. Hench LL, Splinter RJ, Allen WC, Greenlee TK. Bonding mechanisms at the interface of ceramic prosthetic materials. *J Biomed Mater Res.* 1971;5(6):117–41.
50. Oonishi H. Orthopaedic applications of hydroxyapatite. *Biomaterials.* 1991;12(2):171–8.
51. Hench LL, Polak JM. Third-generation biomedical materials. *Science.* 2002;295(5557):1014–7.
52. Lu H, Yu K, Sun S, Liu Y, Leng J. Mechanical and shape-memory behavior of shape-memory polymer composites with hybrid fillers. *Polym Int.* 2010;59(6):766–71.
53. Sherwood JK, Riley SL, Palazzolo R, Brown SC, Monkhouse DC, Coates M, et al. A three-dimensional osteochondral composite scaffold for articular cartilage repair. *Biomaterials.* 2002;23(24):4739–51.
54. Herrington W, Lacey B, Sherliker P, Armitage J, Lewington S. Epidemiology of atherosclerosis and the potential to reduce the global burden of atherothrombotic disease. *Circ Res.* 2016;118(4):535–46. Available from: https://www.ahajournals.org/doi/10.1161/CIRCRESAHA.115.307611
55. Pan C, Han Y, Lu J. Structural design of vascular stents: A review. *Micromachines* [Internet]. 2021;12(7):770. Available from: https://www.mdpi.com/2072-666X/12/7/770
56. Sarjeant JM, Rabinovitch M. Understanding and treating vein graft atherosclerosis. *Cardiovasc Pathol.* 2002;11(5):263–71. Available from: https://linkinghub.elsevier.com/retrieve/pii/S1054880702001254

57. Huang C, Lan Y, Chen S, Liu Q, Luo X, Xu G, et al. Patient-specific coronary artery 3D printing based on intravascular optical coherence tomography and coronary angiography. *Complexity*. 2019;2019:1–10. Available from: https://www.hindawi.com/journals/complexity/2019/5712594/
58. van Lith R, Baker E, Ware H, Yang J, Farsheed AC, Sun C, et al. 3D-printing strong high-resolution antioxidant bioresorbable vascular stents. *Adv Mater Technol*. 2016;1(9):1600138. Available from: https://onlinelibrary.wiley.com/doi/10.1002/admt.201600138
59. Park SA, Lee SJ, Lim KS, Bae IH, Lee JH, Kim WD, et al. In vivo evaluation and characterization of a bio-absorbable drug-coated stent fabricated using a 3D-printing system. *Mater Lett*. 2015;141:355–8. Available from: https://linkinghub.elsevier.com/retrieve/pii/S0167577X14021223
60. Domínguez-Robles J, Utomo E, Cornelius VA, Anjani QK, Korelidou A, Gonzalez Z, et al. TPU-based antiplatelet cardiovascular prostheses prepared using fused deposition modelling. *Mater Des*. 2022;220:110837. Available from: https://linkinghub.elsevier.com/retrieve/pii/S0264127522004592
61. Demir AG, Previtali B. Additive manufacturing of cardiovascular CoCr stents by selective laser melting. *Mater Des*. 2017;119:338–50. Available from: https://linkinghub.elsevier.com/retrieve/pii/S0264127517301156
62. Flege C, Vogt F, Höges S, Jauer L, Borinski M, Schulte VA, et al. Development and characterization of a coronary polylactic acid stent prototype generated by selective laser melting. *J Mater Sci Mater Med*. 2013;24(1):241–55. Available from: http://link.springer.com/10.1007/s10856-012-4779-z
63. Guerra E, de Lara J, Malizia A, Díaz P. Supporting user-oriented analysis for multi-view domain-specific visual languages. *Inf Softw Technol*. 2009;51(4):769–84. Available from: https://linkinghub.elsevier.com/retrieve/pii/S0950584908001304
64. Tofail SAM, Koumoulos EP, Bandyopadhyay A, Bose S, O'Donoghue L, Charitidis C. Additive manufacturing: Scientific and technological challenges, market uptake and opportunities. *Mater Today*. 2018;21(1):22–37. Available from: https://linkinghub.elsevier.com/retrieve/pii/S1369702117301773
65. Turner BN, Gold SA. A review of melt extrusion additive manufacturing processes: II. Materials, dimensional accuracy, and surface roughness. *Rapid Prototyp J*. 2015;21(3):250–61. Available from: https://www.emerald.com/insight/content/doi/10.1108/RPJ-02-2013-0017/full/html
66. Kimicata M, Swamykumar P, Fisher JP. Extracellular matrix for small-diameter vascular grafts. *Tissue Eng Part A*. 2020;26(23–24):1388–401. Available from: https://www.liebertpub.com/doi/10.1089/ten.tea.2020.0201
67. Martin NK, Domínguez-Robles J, Stewart SA, Cornelius VA, Anjani QK, Utomo E, et al. Fused deposition modelling for the development of drug loaded cardiovascular prosthesis. *Int J Pharm*. 2021;595:120243. Available from: https://linkinghub.elsevier.com/retrieve/pii/S0378517321000478
68. Domínguez-Robles J, Diaz-Gomez L, Utomo E, Shen T, Picco CJ, Alvarez-Lorenzo C, et al. Use of 3D printing for the development of biodegradable antiplatelet materials for cardiovascular applications. *Pharmaceuticals*. 2021;14(9):921. Available from: https://www.mdpi.com/1424-8247/14/9/921
69. Domínguez-Robles J, Shen T, Cornelius VA, Corduas F, Mancuso E, Donnelly RF, et al. Development of drug loaded cardiovascular prosthesis for thrombosis prevention using 3D printing. *Mater Sci Eng C*. 2021;129:112375. Available from: https://linkinghub.elsevier.com/retrieve/pii/S0928493121005154
70. Yazdanyar A, Newman AB. The burden of cardiovascular disease in the elderly: morbidity, mortality, and costs. *Clin Geriatr Med*. 2009 Nov;25(4):563–77, vii. https://doi.org/10.1016/j.cger.2009.07.007. PMID: 19944261; PMCID: PMC2797320.

71. Wang Z, Yang Y. Application of 3D Printing in Implantable Medical Devices. *Biomed Res Int.* 2021 Jan 12;2021:6653967. https://doi.org/10.1155/2021/6653967. PMID: 33521128; PMCID: PMC7817310.
72. Hoerstrup SP, Kadner A, Melnitchouk S, Trojan A, Eid K, Tracy J, et al. Tissue engineering of functional trileaflet heart valves from human marrow stromal cells. *Circulation.* 2002;106(13 SUPPL.):143–50.
73. Hoerstrup SP, Sodian R, Daebritz S, Wang J, Bacha EA, Martin DP, et al.. Functional living trileaflet heart valve grown in vitro. *Circulation.* 2000;102(19 SUPPL. 3): 11144–9.
74. Baoren Z, Zhu J. *Artificial Heart Valve and Valve Replacement.* People's Medical Publishing House, Beijing; 1999.
75. Duan B, Kapetanovic E, Hockaday LA, Butcher JT. Three-dimensional printed trileaflet valve conduits using biological hydrogels and human valve interstitial cells. *Acta Biomater.* 2014;10(5):1836–46.
76. Bose S, Vahabzadeh S, Bandyopadhyay A. Bone tissue engineering using 3D printing. *Mater Today.* 2013;16(12):496–504.
77. Mouriño V, Boccaccini AR. Bone tissue engineering therapeutics: Controlled drug delivery in three-dimensional scaffolds. *J R Soc Interface.* 2010;7(43):209–27.
78. Reichert JC, Saifzadeh S, Wullschleger ME, Epari DR, Schütz MA, Duda GN, et al. The challenge of establishing preclinical models for segmental bone defect research. *Biomaterials.* 2009;30(12):2149–63.
79. Lee YH, Lee JH, An IG, Kim C, Lee DS, Lee YK, et al. Electrospun dual-porosity structure and biodegradation morphology of Montmorillonite reinforced PLLA nanocomposite scaffolds. *Biomaterials.* 2005;26(16):3165–72.
80. Fan H, Tao H, Wu Y, Hu Y, Yan Y, Luo Z. TGF-β3 immobilized PLGA-gelatin/chondroitin sulfate/hyaluronic acid hybrid scaffold for cartilage regeneration. *J Biomed Mater Res Part A.* 2010;95(4):982–92.
81. Wong KW, Wu CD, Chien CS, Lee CW, Yang TH, Lin CL. Patient-specific 3-dimensional printing titanium implant biomechanical evaluation for complex distal femoral open fracture reconstruction with segmental large bone defect: A nonlinear finite element analysis. *Appl Sci.* 2020;10(12):4098. Available from: https://www.mdpi.com/2076-3417/10/12/4098
82. Fan H, Fu J, Li XX, Pei Y, Li XX, Pei G, et al. Implantation of customized 3-D printed titanium prosthesis in limb salvage surgery: A case series and review of the literature. *World J Surg Oncol.* 2015;13(1):1–10.
83. Li T, Zhou X, Deng C, Yang X, Yang H, Ma Z, et al. Research center of 3D bioprinting in Shanghai Ninth people's hospital. *Bio-Design Manuf.* 2019;2(3):213–20.
84. Saijo H, Igawa K, Kanno Y, Mori Y, Kondo K, Shimizu K, et al. Maxillofacial reconstruction using custom-made artificial bones fabricated by inkjet printing technology. *J Artif Organs.* 2009;12(3):200–5.
85. Hosalkar H. CORR insights ® : Is age or surgical approach associated with osteonecrosis in patients with developmental dysplasia of the hip? A meta-analysis. *Clin Orthop Relat Res.* 2016;474(5):1178–9.
86. Fuchs M, Effenberger B, Märdian S, Berner A, Kirschbaum S, Pumberger M, et al. Mid-term survival of total knee arthroplasty in patients with posttraumatic osteoarthritis. *Acta Chir Orthop Traumatol Cech.* 2018;85(5):319–24.
87. Brannon, EW, Klein G. Experiences with a finger-joint prosthesis. *Plast Reconstr Surg.* 1959;Publish Ah(2):224.
88. Swanson AB. Silicone rubber implants for replacement of arthritis or destroyed joints in the hand. *Surg Clin North Am.* 1968;48(5):1113–27.
89. Niebauer JJ, Shaw JL, Doren WW. Silicone-Dacron hinge prosthesis. Design, evaluation, and application. *Ann Rheum Dis.* 1969;28(5):56.

90. Chiari C, Trieb K, Goldfarb CA, Stern PJ. Metacarpophalangeal joint arthroplasty in rheumatoid arthritis. *J Bone Jt Surg*. 2004;86(8):1832–3.
91. Linscheid RL, Murray PM, Vidal MA, Beckenbaugh RD. Development of a surface replacement arthroplasty for proximal interphalangeal joints. *J Hand Surg Am*. 1997;22(2):286–98.
92. Goole J, Amighi K. 3D printing in pharmaceutics: A new tool for designing customized drug delivery systems. *Int J Pharm*. 2016;499(1–2):376–94.
93. Pons-Faudoa FP, Ballerini A, Sakamoto J, Grattoni A. Advanced implantable drug delivery technologies: Transforming the clinical landscape of therapeutics for chronic diseases. *Biomed Microdevices*. 2019;21(2):47. Available from: https://link.springer.com/article/10.1007/s10544-019-0389-6
94. Santos A, Sinn Aw M, Bariana M, Kumeria T, Wang Y, Losic D. Drug-releasing implants: current progress, challenges and perspectives. *J Mater Chem B*. 2014;2(37):6157–82. Available from: http://xlink.rsc.org/?DOI=C4TB00548A
95. Stewart S, Domínguez-Robles J, McIlorum V, Mancuso E, Lamprou D, Donnelly R, et al. Development of a biodegradable subcutaneous implant for prolonged drug delivery using 3D printing. *Pharmaceutics*. 2020;12(2):105. Available from: https://www.mdpi.com/1999-4923/12/2/105
96. Kotta S, Nair A, Alsabeelah N. 3D printing technology in drug delivery: Recent progress and application. *Curr Pharm Des*. 2018;24(42):5039–48.
97. Salerno A, Netti PA. Review on computer-aided design and manufacturing of drug delivery scaffolds for cell guidance and tissue regeneration. *Front Bioeng Biotechnol*. 2021;9(June):1–19.
98. Domsta V, Seidlitz A. 3D-printing of drug-eluting implants: An overview of the current developments described in the literature. *Molecules*. 2021;26:4066.
99. Prajapati SK, Jain AA, Jain AA, Jain S. Biodegradable polymers and constructs: A novel approach in drug delivery. *Eur Polym J*. 2019;120(August):109191.
100. Ulery BD, Nair LS, Laurencin CT. Biomedical applications of biodegradable polymers. *J Polym Sci Part B Polym Phys*. 2011;49(12):832–64.
101. Water JJ, Bohr A, Boetker J, Aho J, Sandler N, Nielsen HM, et al. Three-dimensional printing of drug-eluting implants: Preparation of an antimicrobial polylactide feedstock material. *J Pharm Sci*. 2015;104(3):1099–107.
102. Holländer J, Genina N, Jukarainen H, Khajeheian M, Rosling A, Mäkilä E, et al. Three-dimensional printed PCL-based implantable prototypes of medical devices for controlled drug delivery. *J Pharm Sci*. 2016;105(9):2665–76.
103. Stewart SA, Domínguez-Robles J, McIlorum VJ, Gonzalez Z, Utomo E, Mancuso E, et al. Poly(caprolactone)-based coatings on 3D-printed biodegradable implants: A novel strategy to prolong delivery of hydrophilic drugs. *Mol Pharm*. 2020;17(9):3487–500. Available from: https://pubs.acs.org/doi/10.1021/acs.molpharmaceut.0c00515
104. Picco CJ, Domínguez-Robles J, Utomo E, Paredes AJ, Volpe-Zanutto F, Malinova D, et al. 3D-printed implantable devices with biodegradable rate-controlling membrane for sustained delivery of hydrophobic drugs. *Drug Deliv*. 2022;29(1):1038–48. Available from: https://www.tandfonline.com/doi/full/10.1080/10717544.2022.2057620
105. Korelidou A, Domínguez-Robles J, Magill E, Eleftheriadou M, Cornelius VA, Donnelly RF, et al. 3D-printed reservoir-type implants containing poly(lactic acid)/poly(caprolactone) porous membranes for sustained drug delivery. *Biomater Adv*. 2022;139:213024. Available from: https://linkinghub.elsevier.com/retrieve/pii/S2772950822003016
106. Won JY, Kim JJ, Gao G, Kim JJ, Jang J, Park Y-H, et al. 3D printing of drug-loaded multi-shell rods for local delivery of bevacizumab and dexamethasone: A synergetic therapy for retinal vascular diseases. *Acta Biomater*. 2020;116:174–85.

107. Kempin W, Franz C, Koster LC, Schneider F, Bogdahn M, Weitschies W, et al. Assessment of different polymers and drug loads for fused deposition modeling of drug loaded implants. *Eur J Pharm Biopharm.* 2017;115:84–93.
108. Arany P, Papp I, Zichar M, Csontos M, Elek J, Regdon G, et al. In vitro tests of FDM 3D-printed diclofenac sodium-containing implants. *Molecules.* 2020;25(24):5889.
109. Munoz-Abraham AS, Rodriguez-Davalos MI, Bertacco A, Wengerter B, Geibel JP, Mulligan DC. 3D printing of organs for transplantation: Where are we and where are we heading? *Curr Transplant Reports.* 2016;3(1):93–9.
110. Dey M, Ozbolat IT. 3D bioprinting of cells, tissues and organs. *Sci Rep.* 2020;10:14023.
111. Gopinathan J, Noh I. Recent trends in bioinks for 3D printing. *Biomater Res.* 2018;22:11.
112. Robinton DA, Daley GQ. The promise of induced pluripotent stem cells in research and therapy. *Nature.* 2012;481:295–305.
113. Zhang B, Gao L, Ma L, Luo Y, Yang H, Cui Z. 3D bioprinting: A novel avenue for manufacturing tissues and organs. *Engineering.* 2019;5:777–94.
114. Chia HN, Wu BM. Recent advances in 3D printing of biomaterials. *J Biol Eng.* 2015;9(1):4.
115. Atala A. Tissue engineering of human bladder. *Br Med Bull.* 2011 Mar;97(1):81–104.
116. Hinton TJ, Jallerat Q, Palchesko RN, Park JH, Grodzicki MS, Shue HJ, et al. Three-dimensional printing of complex biological structures by freeform reversible embedding of suspended hydrogels. *Sci Adv.* 2015;1(9):e1500758.
117. Lee A, Hudson AR, Shiwarski DJ, Tashman JW, Hinton TJ, Yerneni S, et al. 3D bioprinting of collagen to rebuild components of the human heart. *Science.* 2019;365:482–7.
118. Noor N, Shapira A, Edri R, Gal I, Wertheim L, Dvir T. 3D printing of personalized thick and perfusable cardiac patches and hearts. *Adv Sci.* 2019;6(11):1900344.
119. Wszoła M, Nitarska D, Cywoniuk P, Gomółka M, Klak M. Stem cells as a source of pancreatic cells for production of 3D bioprinted bionic pancreas in the treatment of type 1 diabetes. *Cells.* 2021;10:1544.
120. Kang D, Hong G, An S, Jang I, Yun WS, Shim JH, et al. Bioprinting of multiscaled hepatic lobules within a highly vascularized construct. *Small.* 2020;16(13):1905505.
121. Perica ER, Sun Z. A systematic review of three-dimensional printing in liver disease. *J Dig Imaging.* 2018;31:692–701.
122. Zein NN, Hanouneh IA, Bishop PD, Samaan M, Eghtesad B, Quintini C, et al. Three-dimensional print of a liver for preoperative planning in living donor liver transplantation. *Liver Transplant.* 2013;19(12):1304–10.
123. Goulart E, De Caires-Junior LC, Telles-Silva KA, Araujo BHS, Rocco SA, Sforca M, et al. 3D bioprinting of liver spheroids derived from human induced pluripotent stem cells sustain liver function and viability in vitro. *Biofabrication.* 2019;12(1):015010.
124. Turunen S, Kaisto S, Skovorodkin I, Mironov V, Kalpio T, Vainio S, et al. 3D bioprinting of the kidney – Hype or hope? *AIMS Cell Tissue Eng.* 2018;2(3):119–62.
125. Laronda MM, Rutz AL, Xiao S, Whelan KA, Duncan FE, Roth EW, et al. A bioprosthetic ovary created using 3D printed microporous scaffolds restores ovarian function in sterilized mice. *Nat Commun.* 2017;8:15261.
126. Isaacson A, Swioklo S, Connon CJ. 3D bioprinting of a corneal stroma equivalent. *Exp Eye Res.* 2018;173:188–93.
127. Ulag S, Ilhan E, Sahin A, Karademir Yilmaz B, Kalaskar DM, Ekren N, et al. 3D printed artificial cornea for corneal stromal transplantation. *Eur Polym J.* 2020;133:109744.
128. Koch L, Deiwick A, Schlie S, Michael S, Gruene M, Coger V, et al. Skin tissue generation by laser cell printing. *Biotechnol Bioeng.* 2012;109(7):1855–63.
129. Weng T, Zhang W, Xia Y, Wu P, Yang M, Jin R, et al. 3D bioprinting for skin tissue engineering: Current status and perspectives. *J Tissue Eng.* 2021;12:20417314211028574.

130. Baltazar T, Merola J, Catarino C, Xie CB, Kirkiles-Smith NC, Lee V, et al. Three dimensional bioprinting of a vascularized and perfusable skin graft using human keratinocytes, fibroblasts, pericytes, and endothelial cells. *Tissue Eng Part A*. 2020; 26(5–6):227–38. Available from: https://www.liebertpub.com/doi/10.1089/ten.tea.2019.0201
131. Grigoryan B, Paulsen SJ, Corbett DC, Sazer DW, Fortin CL, Zaita AJ, et al. Multivascular networks and functional intravascular topologies within biocompatible hydrogels. *Science*. 2019;364(6439):458–64.
132. Wragg NM, Burke L, Wilson SL. A critical review of current progress in 3D kidney biomanufacturing: Advances, challenges, and recommendations. *Ren Replace Ther.* 2019;5:18.
133. Vijayavenkataraman S, Lu WF, Fuh JYH. *3D bioprinting – An Ethical, Legal and Social Aspects (ELSA) framework*. Vols. 1–2, Bioprinting. Elsevier B.V.; 2016. pp. 11–21.
134. Panja N, Maji S, Choudhuri S, Ali KA, Hossain CM. 3D bioprinting of human hollow organs. *AAPS PharmSciTech*. 2022;23(5):139.
135. Gilbert F, O'Connell CD, Mladenovska T, Dodds S. Print me an organ? Ethical and regulatory issues emerging from 3D bioprinting in medicine. *Sci Eng Ethics*. 2018;24(1):73–91.
136. Wolinsky H. Printing organs cell-by-cell. *EMBO Rep*. 2014;15(8):836–8.
137. Cornejo J, Cornejo-Aguilar JA, Vargas M, Helguero CG, Milanezi De Andrade R, Torres-Montoya S, et al. Anatomical engineering and 3D printing for surgery and medical devices: International review and future exponential innovations. *Biomed Res Int*. 2022;2022:6797745.
138. Culmone C, Lussenburg K, Alkemade J, Smit G, Sakes A, Breedveld P. A fully 3D-printed steerable instrument for minimally invasive surgery. *Materials (Basel)*. 2021;14(24):7910. Available from: https://www.mdpi.com/1996-1944/14/24/7910
139. Zaidi S, Naik P, Ahmed S. Three-dimensional printed instruments used in a septoplasty: A new paradigm in surgery. *Laryngoscope Investig Otolaryngol*. 2021;6(4):613–8.
140. George M, Aroom KR, Hawes HG, Gill BS, Love J. 3D printed surgical instruments – The design and fabrication process. *World J Surg*. 2017;41(1):314.
141. Kunogi H, Yamaguchi N, Sasai K. Evaluation of a new bi-valve vaginal speculum applicator design for gynecologic interstitial brachytherapy. *J Contemp Brachytherapy*. 2020;12(1):27.
142. Wang J, Yang L, Ma M, Li G, Xu S, Li Q, et al. Development and application of a no-clog surgical suction tip using 3D printing technology. *Med Sci Monit*. 2018;24:6765.
143. Chen MY, Skewes J, Daley R, Woodruff MA, Rukin NJ. Three-dimensional printing versus conventional machining in the creation of a metal urethral dilator: Development and mechanical testing. *Biomed Eng Online*. 2020;19(1):1–11.
144. Regulation (EU) 2017/745 of the European Parliament and of the Council of 5 April 2017 on medical devices, amending Directive 2001/83/EC, Regulation (EC) No 178/2002 and regulation (EC) No 1223/2009 and repealing Council Directive 90/985/EEC and 93/42/EEC. 2017.
145. Article 2, Comma 3 of the Regulation (EU) 2017/745. 2017.
146. Article 10 of the Regulation (EU) 2017/745. 2017.
147. Article 2, Comma 5 of the Regulation (EU) 2017/745. 2017.
148. Agostinacchio F, Mu X, Dirè S, Motta A, Kaplan DL. In situ 3D printing: Opportunities with silk inks. *Trends Biotechnol*. 2021;39(7):719–30. Available from: https://linkinghub.elsevier.com/retrieve/pii/S0167779920302985

5 Polymers for Bioinks Development

Patricia Diaz-Rodriguez and Luis Diaz-Gomez
Universidad de Santiago de Compostela

CONTENTS

DOI: 10.1201/9781003274568-5

5.1 INTRODUCTION: DEFINITION AND CLASSIFICATION OF POLYMERS

Polymers are, by definition, macromolecules formed by repeated units of monomers. As gathered from the above-mentioned definition, the term polymer encompasses a family of organic biomaterials with a wide range of properties and functionalities. These macromolecules are typically classified based on their origin in natural or synthetic polymers. Proteins such as collagen, gelatin, and silk fibroin, and polysaccharides such as alginate, carrageenan, chitosan, and hyaluronic acid are the most widely used natural polymers for biomedical applications. Despite the numerous advantages of natural polymers, including reactivity for chemical modification associated with the presence of numerous functional groups (amine, hydroxyl, carboxylic acid…), bioactivity, biodegradability, and biocompatibility, several features hinder their use as bioink components, namely high batch-to-batch variability, poor mechanical performance, and stability [1,2].

Among natural polymers suitable for bioprinting, alginate and collagen are most frequently used [3,4]. Alginate is a polysaccharide obtained from brown algae formed by repeated units of β-D-mannuronic acid and α-L-guluronic acid. Alginate hydrogels can be easily obtained by the addition of divalent ions to the polymer solutions. This mild and fast crosslinking trigger together with its biocompatibility and the ability to be combined with other polymers makes alginate the gold standard for cell encapsulation [5]. The use of alginate for bioprinting takes advantage of the previous knowledge obtained from this application. Several studies have been focused on elucidating the effect of alginate molecular weight, mannuronic/guluronic ratio, degradation rate and concentration on cell survival, mechanical properties, and cell distribution. These factors can be modulated to obtain bioinks with desirable properties [6].

Collagen is a natural component of the connective tissue extracellular matrix (ECM) in mammals. Therefore, collagen is usually incorporated in bioinks to confer ECM-like properties. Moreover, this polymer tends to form hydrogels in physiological conditions derived from self-assembled fibril structures. However, the poor mechanical properties of plain collagen hydrogels require its combination with other materials [7].

One step further in mimicking ECM to promote cell attachment and proliferation is the use of a new type of natural polymer that is gaining attention in the last years, namely decellularized extracellular matrix (dECM). Bioinks based on dECM present a distinctive composition, containing most of the ECM components present in the original tissue, including collagens, glycosaminoglycans, and growth factors. This mixture of components is obtained after the removal of the tissue cellular constituents by biological, chemical, or physical methods [8]. The application of dECM is limited by its poor mechanical stability, reproducibility, and control during bioprinting.

Regarding synthetic polymers, polylactic-co-glycolic acid (PLGA), poly(ethylene glycol) (PEG), poly(L-lactic acid) (PLA), and poly(ε-caprolactone) (PCL) are the most frequently used components for bioink development [4]. Moreover, a new class within synthetic polymers called smart polymers are getting attention in biomedical applications. These macromolecules allow the obtaining of structures endorsed with distinct properties depending on the surrounding environment. These changes can be triggered by numerous stimuli such as pH, temperature, and electric or magnetic field [9]. These stimuli-sensitive polymeric bioinks allow for obtaining 4D constructs where the time variable is the fourth dimension and will be further described in Section 5.4. In this approach, dynamic systems are obtained, where the structure is modified over time by external stimuli. Although synthetic polymers are mainly used for this method, natural polymers can also be employed, including collagen, a stimuli-sensitive molecule responding to pH and temperature [10]. Frequently, natural and synthetic polymers are combined during bioink formulation to obtain 3D constructs with the desired properties.

5.2 POLYMERS FOR BIOINK DEVELOPMENT

5.2.1 General Requirements

The availability, specifications, and cost effectiveness of 3D printers have significantly improved in the past few years, which is directly translated into the range of materials that can be used for bioink development. Materials for biomedical applications, also known as biomaterials, are those components intended to interact with cells and tissues to repair, replace, or enhance their function [11]. Therefore, their main requirements are biocompatibility, biodegradability, adequate mechanical properties, non-immunogenicity, functionalization ability, and sterilizability [12]. Initially, biomaterials as a whole, and in particular polymers, were designed to not interact with the surrounding tissue and cells, behaving as inert systems. However, nowadays polymers for biomedical applications are intended to promote their interaction with cells controlling cell attachment, ECM production, proliferation, and differentiation [13].

A bioink is a combination of biomaterials, bioactive molecules, and cells handled using bioprinting devices [14]. In short, bioinks are the raw materials in bioprinting. Polymers for bioinks are used as tools to reach the main purposes of bioprinting, specifically control over cell location, and ability to obtain scaffolds with high resolution and reproducibility. Over the general requirements of biomaterials, polymers for bioink development should also present the characteristics summarized in Figure 5.1. First, the polymeric systems must show good printability. This property is defined as the appropriateness of a bioink to manufacture stable three-dimensional structures showing high fidelity to the original template and structural integrity [15]. This feature is related to the ability of the printed material to maintain its defined structure and sustain their shape during bioprinting.

Polymers are generally used in bioinks as aqueous solutions or dispersions that undergo gelation through different mechanisms before, during, or after printing, leading to the formation of hydrogels. Several crosslinking mechanisms can be used based on electrostatic interactions, covalent bonds, or enzymatic reactions. These mechanisms will be further described in Section 5.3.1. However, neither the designed trigger nor the chemical modification of the polymers or reagents should be cytotoxic [4]. Moreover, the polymers selected for bioprinting should provide cell support and present adequate gelation kinetics to indeed ensure the mechanical stability of the construct [3].

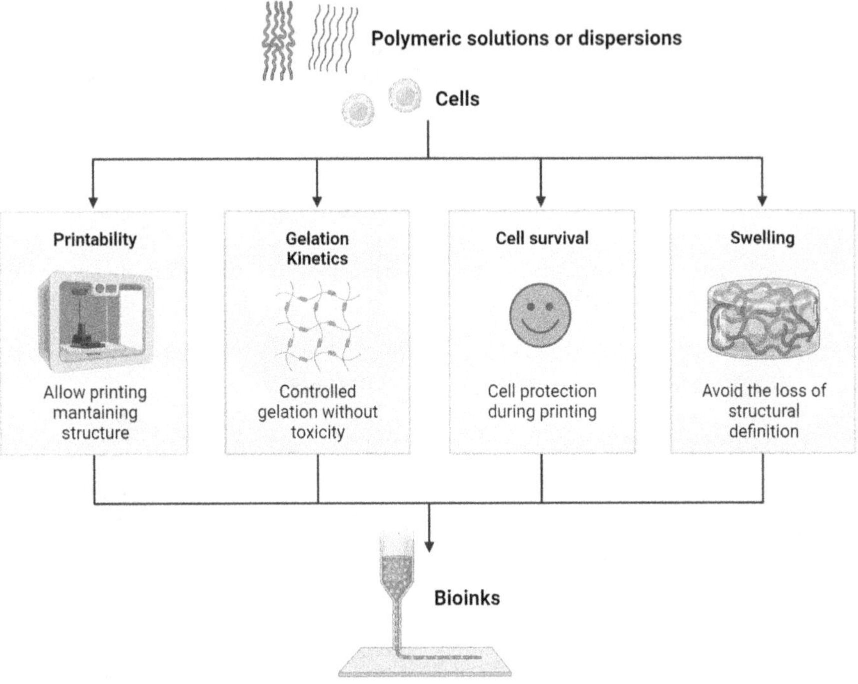

FIGURE 5.1 Polymer requirements for bioink development.

The main role of bioprinting for tissue engineering is to obtain systems able to restore, replace, or regenerate the damaged tissue. In this scenario, a crucial function of polymers as bioink components is to protect cells during printing and establish an adequate cell–polymer interaction to support cell attachment and survival after printing. Therefore, a suitable bioink used in a specific printing strategy should ensure high cell viability throughout the entire biofabrication process [16]. Moreover, bioink swelling is another factor to keep in mind to avoid the loss of the structural definition on the construct while guaranteeing nutrient and oxygen diffusion essential for cell survival [16]. This swelling is controlled by the crosslinking density and the ionic charge of the polymeric chain.

Nowadays, several polymer-based bioinks commercialized for biomedical applications are prepared using both natural and synthetic polymers including gelatin, alginate, fibronectin, collagen, and PEG [16–18]. In fact, there are open-source tools and databases to select the most appropriate polymeric bioink composition and printing conditions for the desired application [19–21].

5.2.2 Required Specific Features Based on the Selected Printing Strategy

Bioprinting entails the incorporation of live cells suspended in different carriers, and, therefore, only cell-friendly printing strategies can be used in this process, including extrusion-based bioprinting, droplet-based bioprinting, laser-induced forward

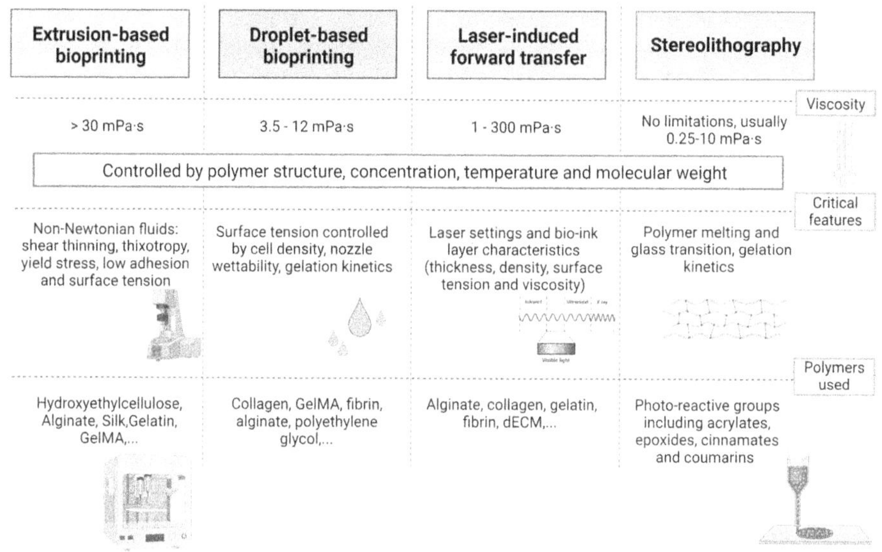

FIGURE 5.2 Polymer characteristics of each of the selected bioprinting strategies. GelMA, methacrylated gelatin; dECM, decellularized extracellular matrix.

transfer (LIFT) bioprinting, and stereolithography (SLA) [22]. The required specific features are summarized in Figure 5.2. The bioink viscosity is critical, conditioning the printing process related to the flow of the material (especially for extrusion-based and droplet-based bioprinting) and the post-printing stability of the construct. The requirements regarding this property are dependent on the selected bioprinting method. Extrusion-based bioprinting requires viscosity values higher than 30 mPa·s, whereas droplet-based bioprinting entails the use of less viscous solutions (3.5–12 mPa·s). On the other hand, LIFT bioprinting allows polymeric solutions with a wider range of viscosities (1–300 mPa·s), and (SLA) has no viscosity limitations [23]. The viscosity of the polymeric solution or dispersion is determined by the temperature, the polymer structure itself, the concentration, and its molecular weight [24]. Most of these parameters can be tailored to obtain the desired bioink viscosity.

5.2.2.1 Extrusion-Based Bioprinting

Extrusion-based bioprinting is the most used technology in tissue engineering, allowing for the combination of different materials, cells, and signaling molecules on the same construct while being relatively simple and affordable [14]. This printing strategy is based on forcing the flow of the bioink through a nozzle by applying pressure, and the subsequent deposition of the ink with the desired structure in a substrate [25]. In this procedure, the rheological behavior of the bioink is crucial to avoid spreading after printing together with cell sedimentation, nozzle clogging, and high shear stress during extrusion. The ideal bioink for this technology should behave as a non-Newtonian fluid where the viscosity is dependent on the shear rate. Preferably, they should present a shear-thinning behavior, which means that at a high shear rate the polymer chains align in a favorable direction during extrusion, thus decreasing the viscosity and the shear stress of the fluid and increasing cell survival. Moreover, thixotropy, a time-dependent shear-thinning behavior, is also desirable. This property allows the bioink to recover the initial viscosity, hence ensuring shape fidelity after printing. Bioinks with an adequate yield stress (minimum stress to initiate the bioink flow), low adhesion, and adequate surface tension properties are also preferred [26].

Since extrusion-based bioprinting is the most used bioprinting strategy, it is not hard to imagine the wide variety of polymers that have been used for this application. The combination of hydroxyethylcellulose and sodium alginate have shown adequate shear thinning and thixotropy allowing for high cell viability [27]. Another natural polymer widely used in biomedical applications is silk fibroin. This natural polymer is ideal for extrusion-based bioprinting as it presents a shear-thinning behavior at low concentrations and its mechanical properties can be modulated by modifying the secondary conformation of the protein. However, the shear-thinning behavior disappears at high concentrations due to the lower mobility of the molecules. To overcome this issue, silk can be combined with other polymers, such as gelatin, that also presents a shear-thinning behavior and displays a high bioactivity [28]. However, gelatin should be chemically modified with photocrosslinkable reactive groups to be used as the sole component of bioinks, such as gelatin methacryloyl (GelMA) due to its low mechanical stability [29].

5.2.2.2 Droplet-Based Bioprinting

Droplet-based bioprinting is based on the layered deposition of picolitre drops on top of a substrate. Unlike extrusion-based bioprinting, this technology often uses bioinks with lower viscosities [22]. However, the low bioink viscosity limits the cell density that can be used for bioprinting due to cell sedimentation and surface tension modifications. The bioink surface tension and the wettability of the nozzle control the drop formation [30]. At the same time, surface tension is controlled by the cell density, where high cell densities are associated with a decrease in the surface tension, leading to the formation of a jet instead of drops [16].

The control over polymer gelation kinetics is desired to avoid the spreading of the droplets and, therefore, the loss of the construct structure. Thus, fast gelation is required in this bioprinting strategy. At the same time, an adequate drop impact velocity should be reached to increase cell survival while avoiding drop splashing and high shear stress [16,31]. Unlike for extrusion-based bioprinting, few polymers have been used in droplet-based bioprinting, including collagen, GelMA, fibrin, alginate, and PEG [32].

5.2.2.3 Laser-Induced Forward Transfer (LIFT) Bioprinting

LIFT bioprinting is based on a pulsed laser beam that is scanned over a substrate coated with a laser-absorbing layer and a bioink layer. The application of the laser between both layers results in the vaporization of a portion of the donor layer and the subsequent formation of a high-pressure bubble leading to the jet formation [23,33]. This strategy avoids the use of a nozzle and the associated risk of clogging and shear stress [34]. The process is highly dependent on the laser settings and the bioink layer features, including thickness, density, surface tension, and viscosity. Therefore, it is important to characterize and control these properties. Different polymers have been used in LIFT, where alginate, collagen, gelatin, fibrin, and dECM are the most used in the tissue engineering field [35].

5.2.2.4 Stereolithography

SLA is based on the use of light to precisely control the crosslinking of a photosensitive polymer. Derived from the base of the technique, the crosslinking mechanism entails the use of photoinitiators that can be toxic to cells [36]. SLA is less layer dependent compared with other printing methods, thus reducing the difficulty of the printing [23]. Different bioink requirements should be considered for adequate construct performance, including the selection of non-toxic photoinitiators. Other aspects that should be considered are the melting and glass transition temperatures of the polymers. These temperatures should be lower than the printing temperature to allow for high chain mobility. Moreover, usually low viscosity solutions are used (0.25–10 mPa·s) to allow for fast construct formation and easy removal of the non-polymerized bioink. Fast crosslinking rates are also desirable, which can be achieved using multifunctional polymer chains, including reactive groups such as acrylates, epoxides, cinnamates, and coumarins [37].

5.2.3 Tissue-Dependent Polymer Requirements

5.2.3.1 Skin Regeneration

Skin is a layered tissue formed from top to bottom by epidermis, dermis, and hypodermis. Epidermis is the outside hydrophobic layer, composed mainly of keratinocytes, that controls molecule diffusion, and protects the body from external environment. Dermis is formed by a hydrophilic connective tissue of collagenous ECM. Hypodermis, composed by elastin and collagen fibers, contains sweat glands, hair follicle roots, and blood and lymphatic vessels. The use of bioprinting for skin regeneration entails the mimicking of these layers while ensuring printability. Until now, most of the developed skin constructs are based on fibrinogen, collagen, hyaluronic acid, alginate, gelatin, silk, cellulose-derived materials, chitosan, and poly(γ-glutamic acid), either alone or in combination. Despite the high cell viability observed in most of the developed systems, the addition of the epidermis layer is usually performed in further steps after bioprinting by the deposition of keratinocytes on top of the constructs [28,38].

5.2.3.2 Bone Regeneration

Bone is an anisotropic mineralized tissue characterized by high strength and compressive properties [39]. Therefore, one of the main requirements for bone tissue regeneration is to deliver biomaterials with an adequate mechanical performance. This is particularly relevant for polymer-based bioprinted constructs as they are mainly composed of water. Different strategies have been assessed to achieve adequate mechanical properties, such as the chemical modification of polymeric chains, thus enhancing the crosslinking density. Another strategy is based on specific non-covalent reactions, including reversible Diels–Alder reactions, disulfide bonding, boronate ester, or aldimine formation to generate supramolecular networks. A third alternative is the development of interpenetrating networks (IPNs). These systems are created by the interaction of two independent polymeric networks. The incorporation of nanoparticles in the bioink or the use of thermoplastic mesh reinforcements has been also explored to improve the hydrogel mechanical properties in bone regeneration [40]. Polymers used for bone bioprinting include polyurethane, PLGA, and PLA together with collagen, gelatin, and alginate [41].

5.2.3.3 Cartilage Regeneration

Cartilage is characterized by low vascularization and innervation, which limits its self-repairing capacity. Moreover, the morphology of cartilage, formed by rounded-shape chondrocytes embedded in ECM, makes this tissue adequate for bioprinting. In this sense, the modification of the construct stiffness by modulating the crosslinking density can control chondrocyte phenotype and proliferation, showing adequate results when 17 kPa stiffness scaffolds are used [42]. However, constructs should ensure the stability when subjected to the mechanical requirements of the cartilage. Different polymers have been used for this purpose, including PCL, hyaluronic acid, fibrin, collagen, gelatin, agarose, GelMA, hyaluronic acid methacrylic anhydride (HAMA), dECM, and alginate [43,44].

5.2.3.4 Vascular Regeneration

Despite the progress on the vascularization of tissue scaffolds, this step remains a big challenge for bioprinting to ensure long-term cell survival [45]. Vasculature is formed by concentric layers of distinct cellular and ECM compositions. These characteristics confer each of them with specific functionalities. In this sense, the inner layer or intima works as an anti-thrombogenic surface, while the second layer or media provides contractility. On the other hand, the last layer or adventitia serves as the union with the surrounding tissue. Consequently, polymers used to resemble the intima layer will be in contact with the blood stream and, therefore, should not be thrombogenic. On the other hand, polymers designed for media mimicking should present adequate mechanical performance to withstand the mechanical changes during beating. Indirect printing is widely used to obtain hollow tubular scaffolds able to mimic the structure of vasculature. This strategy is based on the use of sacrificial inks, generally gelatin, that are printed as cylindrical tubes followed by the bioprinting of the layers around them. After crosslinking, the sacrificial ink is removed rendering in hollow tubular structures [33]. Polymers used for vascular tissue regeneration include alginate, collagen, gelatin, fibrin, PCL, and PLA [46].

5.3 CROSSLINKABLE POLYMERIC BIOINKS

Bioink crosslinking is a crucial step during the biofabrication process to obtain self-supportive tridimensional structures. The mechanical and physicochemical properties of the bioinks and, by extension the cells encapsulated in the scaffolds, are significantly impacted by crosslinking [47–50]. Crosslinking strategies include, alone or in combination, physical, chemical, and enzymatic crosslinking (Figure 5.3). Although it is frequently applied during or after the printing process, crosslinking strategies could also be considered during pre-printing. For instance, a certain degree of crosslinking is beneficial when the bioink is contained in the

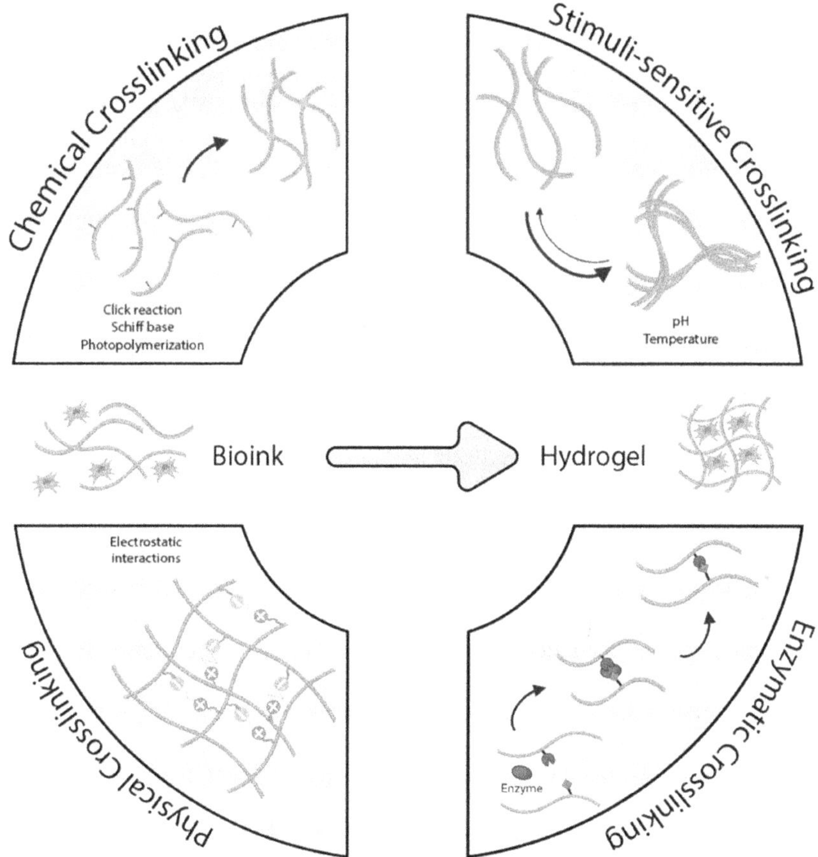

FIGURE 5.3 Scheme of the main crosslinking strategies used for 3D printing of bioinks.

cartridge to prevent cell sedimentation and damage. Pre-crosslinked printable bioinks can be obtained by physical crosslinking of one or more polymeric components or by introducing a small density of covalent linkages [51].

Although layer-by-layer crosslinking is generally applied, if the bioink retains and maintains its shape after printing, a one-step post-crosslinking can be applied to the printed construct, reducing the biofabrication time and, therefore, preserving the bioactivity of the encapsulated cells.

5.3.1 Crosslinking Methods

5.3.1.1 Covalent Crosslinking

This crosslinking strategy consists in the irreversible covalent bonding of precursors. To crosslink the tridimensional bioink network, the precursors should exhibit reciprocal reactive functionalities. Contrary to physically crosslinked hydrogels, the covalent crosslinked structures are generally degraded over time by hydrolytic processes [52,53]. Although polymer concentration is important to control the viscosity and, therefore, the printability of the bioink, the concentration of reactive moieties present in the structure of the polymer chains is crucial to control the degree of crosslinking and determine the mechanical properties of the resulting structure [52]. While covalent crosslinking usually enables the biofabrication of mechanically stable and tunable structures, the limited cytocompatibility of chemically modified precursors and crosslinking initiators restricts their use. Covalent crosslinking approaches include chemical crosslinking, photocrosslinking, Schiff's base crosslinking, and click chemistry [54–56].

5.3.1.1.1 Chemical Crosslinking

One of the most used chemical crosslinking strategies is the formation of amide or ester bonds between carboxylic acids and amines or hydroxyls via 1-ethyl-3-(3-dimethylaminopropyl)carbodiimide (EDC) catalysis. Specifically, EDC activates carboxyl groups such as those present in glutamic or aspartic acid residues of proteins to couple them to amino groups in proteins and polysaccharides. Although this crosslinking reaction is considered safe and biocompatible, the use of the carboxyl group in the glutamic acid has detrimental effects on cell adhesion, proliferation, and spreading [57]. EDC-based crosslinking has been widely used in collagen bioinks, resulting in lower degradation rates and preventing scaffold contraction [58].

While the use of synthetic crosslinking agents, such as glutaraldehyde, is very extended in hydrogel preparation, its use in bioink development is limited due to their high cytotoxicity and the potential induction of inflammatory response. As an alternative, natural crosslinking agents are attractive in the development of bioprinted constructs. Among them, genipin is widely used for crosslinking of amine-containing polymers, such as gelatin, collagen, and chitosan. The cytotoxicity of genipin is remarkably lower, compared with other aldehyde-based crosslinkers [59].

5.3.1.1.2 Photocrosslinking

Photocrosslinking is a very extended approach for obtaining mechanically stable constructs. The photocrosslinking rapid reaction can result in high-resolution structures while avoiding collapse or spreading [60]. The control over light intensity and exposure time expands the range of materials and cells that can be incorporated in the bioinks. On the contrary, the limited availability of cell-friendly precursors and photoinitiators limit their use in bioink development. In addition, the exposure of cells to UV light can damage DNA and lead to cell mutations and death [61,62].

The selection of the photoinitiator is critical in preventing cell damage and maintaining the bioink as cell friendly as possible. Wavelengths in the UVA range (320–400 nm) have a pronounced effect on genomic damage and carcinogenesis, while UVB range (290–320 nm) impacts cell survival by triggering apoptotic mechanisms. Therefore, visible light photoinitiators maintain high cell viability. The most used visible light photoinitiators include lithium phenyl-2,4,6-trimethylbenzoylphosphinate (LAP), eosin Y (EY), ruthenium/sodium persulfate, and riboflavin [61,63,64].

Acrylated biomaterials are commonly used photocrosslinkable precursors and can be synthesized from natural or synthetic polymers via conjugation with methyl methacrylate or glycidyl methacrylate [65]. The presence of acryl groups in bioinks has several implications in terms of safety, since unreacted radicals can lead to inflammatory effects. As gathered from Section 5.2, GelMA is the most common acrylated polymer used in bioink development due to its cell adhesion, proliferation, and migration properties related to the presence of RGD motifs [66,67]. Other acrylated materials include HAMA, pectin methacrylate (PECMA), poly(ethylene glycol) diacrylate (PEGDA), or galactoglucomannan methacrylate. Among them, HAMA has shown excellent printing properties and high printing resolution [3,68].

5.3.1.1.3 Schiff's Base

Schiff's base crosslinking is a linkage between amine and aldehyde groups by means of a dynamic covalent imine bond. These linkages can be generated under physiological conditions and in the presence of cells, tissues, and labile bioactive molecules [69]. Moreover, the dynamic networks formed by this crosslinking method can also render hydrogels with self-healing properties and pH sensitivity. Amino-rich polymers, such as chitosan and polyacrylamide, are combined with polymers with abundant aldehydes, such as hyaluronic acid, oxidized alginate, or dextran, to form Schiff's base linkages. Therefore, stable hydrogel networks can be formed without the need of a cytotoxic chemical crosslinking agent [70]. Some examples include the combination of oxidized dextran or alginate with gelatin to develop cell-laden hydrogels with excellent printing properties and pH sensitivity [71,72].

5.3.1.1.4 Click Chemistry

Recent advances in click reaction enabled versatile, fast, and selective reactions carried out under mild conditions. Moreover, the crosslinking process can be carried out in aqueous conditions and in a bio-orthogonal manner. Ideally, click chemistry is ideal for bioink development since crosslinking reactions spontaneously develop upon combining two or more reactive precursors without the application of external energy sources or crosslinkers. Additionally, this approach enables the tuning of the mechanical properties of the printed constructs by modifying the gelation and degradation time, leading to controlled network formation [51,73].

Although the most extended reactions are based on copper-catalyzed azide–alkyne cycloadditions, the toxicity related to the metal catalyst has prevented its use in bioink development. Several cytocompatible click reactions have been proposed for direct crosslinking in the presence of cells, such as thiol–vinyl sulfone and thiol–maleimide. Other examples are Michael addition reactions, azide–alkyne cycloaddition reactions, and thiol–ene photocoupling reaction [52,53]. Michael addition and thiol–ene click chemistry have been widely used due to their high selectivity, the absence of toxic byproducts, and the availability of functional precursors. However, thiol–ene click chemistry requires photoirradiation for the creation of initial radicals [56]. Thiolated HA and gelatin, or acrylated PEG has been used to develop bioinks with high cell viability and rapid crosslinking rates. Moreover, the mechanical properties and degradation rate of the printed constructs can be precisely tuned by controlling the crosslinking reaction [74,75].

5.3.1.2 Physical Crosslinking

Physical crosslinking consists in the entanglement of polymer chains through non-covalent linkages, including hydrogen bonds, electrostatic or hydrophobic interactions, and ionic crosslinking [76]. In general, physical crosslinking is reversible and precursors are commercially available. Besides, gelation usually completes in short times and no additional reagents are required. However, the mechanical properties and structural stability of the resulting hydrogels are limited, and degradation is significantly faster than other crosslinking approaches [47,77,78].

The electrostatic interactions between multivalent cations and anions have been extensively used for hydrogel development. The main advantages of this method are the low toxicity of the crosslinking agents, the fast gelation rate, and the mild conditions of the process. Moreover, hydrogels prepared via ionic crosslinking present self-healing abilities, which is remarkably beneficial for biomedical applications. However, the poor mechanical properties and the fast degradation rate of the printed structures can compromise the performance of the scaffolds for certain applications. Among the large variety of crosslinking agents, calcium and phosphate ions are regarded as the most attractive molecules for polyanionic or polycationic polymers, respectively [79].

Calcium cations are commonly used as crosslinkers in alginate-based bioinks due to their high affinity to guluronate residues. Calcium concentration should be precisely controlled to obtain a homogeneously crosslinked structure, avoiding uneven gelation. Moreover, cell viability and function could be impacted with high calcium concentrations [80,81].

Electrostatic crosslinking could also be attained by the interaction of ionic groups present in the components of the bioinks, thus reducing the cytotoxicity associated with multivalent ions. The method consists in the use of two oppositely charged polymers leading to the formation of a crosslinked network. Interestingly, several bioinks presenting electrostatic interactions show shear-thinning properties during the extrusion process. Once extruded, the fast recovery of the electrostatic interactions allows for the mechanical stability of the printed structure. Bioinks containing natural polysaccharides such as alginate (negatively charged) and chitosan or polylysine (positively charged) showed tunable rheological properties and improved printability, compared with plain alginate bioinks [82–84].

5.3.1.3 Enzymatic Reactions

Enzymes can be used as catalysts for site-directed coupling of proteins or protein-modified polymers, generally by amide bonds. The main advantage of this method is the mild conditions needed for the enzymatic reactions to happen, which allows for high cell survival. However, the need for expensive specific reactants may limit their use in bioink applications. Transglutaminase, phosphopantetheinyl transferase, lysyl oxidase, and horseradish peroxidase have been applied for bioink crosslinking [58,85,86]. Inspired by blood clotting mechanism, several studies have used thrombin to crosslink fibrinogen-based bioinks to develop fibrin networks. Some studies have reported fibrinogen bioinks containing collagen, alginate, or gelatin and encapsulating one or more cell types. After extrusion, the further incubation of the constructs in thrombin solution led to scaffolds with high structural integrity and bioactivity [87–90].

Enzyme-driven crosslinking can also be used to precisely control the rheological properties of the bioink. As an example, Zhou et al. used transglutaminase to partially catalyze the covalent bond formation between chains of a GelMA bioink.

The control of the reaction time and enzyme concentration and activity allowed for the tuning of MSC-laden bioinks printability without affecting cell survival and bioactivity [91].

5.3.2 Hybrid Crosslinking

Hybrid crosslinking includes the combination of two distinct crosslinking mechanisms and is usually employed in multimaterial bioinks [92,93]. Normally, this method comprises two crosslinking steps: (i) an ionic crosslinking with a divalent cation (i.e., calcium chloride) is applied to each layer immediately after printing; and (ii) once printed, the whole structure is crosslinked by UV light. This method ensures tridimensional structures with high precision, avoiding UV overexposure to the encapsulated cells. Other studies have used hydrogen bonds to obtain adequate printing properties, followed by a post-printing secondary crosslinking with multivalent ions [94]. Das et al. encapsulated MSCs in a gelatin–silk fibroin bioink. Gelation was then induced by sonication (physical crosslinking) followed by tyrosinase-mediated enzymatic crosslinking. The obtained scaffolds supported multilineage differentiation of the encapsulated MSCs, opening this approach to several tissue targets [95]. Hybrid crosslinking has also been used to print dECM or multimaterial bioinks, prepared with GelMA, alginate, or hyaluronic acid, among others [51,96–98] (Table 5.1).

TABLE 5.1
Comparison of the Advantages and Disadvantages of Crosslinking Strategies for Bioink Development

Crosslinking Strategy	Advantages	Disadvantages
Chemical crosslinking	Tunable mechanical stability and degradation rate.	Toxicity of synthetic crosslinking agents, time-consuming, limited biocompatibility.
Photocrosslinking	Fast processing time, high-resolution structures, control of crosslinking extent, printing accuracy.	Limited availability of non-toxic photoinitiators, UV damage to DNA, limited UV penetration depth.
Schiff's base	Improved mechanical stability, accurate control of crosslinking degree, non-toxic.	Limited crosslinking density, slow reaction rates, need of amine groups in the polymer structure.
Click chemistry	Fast and versatile, high selectivity, mild conditions, control over degradation rate.	Requires specific functional groups, in economy.
Physical (ionic)	Reversible, short gelation time, biocompatible reagents, mild conditions.	Limited mechanical stability, fast degradation rate, high sensitivity to environmental conditions.
Enzymatic	Precise control over rheological properties, physiological conditions, high specificity.	Expensive reactants, limited enzyme stability and reaction conditions.
Hybrid	Improved mechanical stability, versatile, fine-tuning of crosslinking kinetics.	Complex methodology, high costs, difficult to optimize.

5.4 STIMULI-SENSITIVE POLYMERIC BIOINKS

Recently, stimuli-responsive polymers that undergo an in situ physicochemical change secondary to internal or external stimuli triggered by biological or pathological cues are gaining attention [10]. These triggers include physical, chemical, or biological signals.

5.4.1 pH-Responsive

The pH of the intra- and extracellular environments within the human body is broad and can be considered as a trigger for pH-responsive bioinks. Specifically, pH has a direct effect on the crosslinking strength and extent, which is attributed to the protonation of ionizable groups or to the degradation of acid-cleavable bonds present in the polymer structure. While most of the current research is focused on the precise delivery of anticancer therapies triggered by the local acidic environment of tumor tissue, there is a growing interest in the development of pH-responsive bioinks for tissue engineering applications [99,100].

Natural polymers with pH-responsive properties have been used as bioinks incorporating a wide range of cell types and tissue targets. Cardiac tissue has been printed using collagen I with high resolution thanks to its gelling properties at specific pH values. In this approach, collagen was extruded in a crosslinking bath at pH 7.4, causing the immediate hardening of the printed structure and therefore enabling the fabrication of highly precise, complex anatomical structures without significantly affecting cell viability [101].

5.4.2 Temperature-Responsive

Thermoresponsive polymers have been proposed for bioink development due to their simplicity for crosslinking. When the temperature is raised above the low critical solution temperature (LCST), the bioink solution becomes insoluble, leading to gelation. Thermoresponsive bioinks are usually prepared from natural (gelatin, collagen, chitosan…) or synthetic (PNIPAAm, PEG, and PEO-PPO-PEO) polymers. The combination of thermoresponsive polymers is a recurring strategy for improving cell viability and obtaining scaffolds with tunable mechanical properties. Bioinks containing methylcellulose, gelatin, or cyclic imino ethers have been recently reported [102,103].

In addition, recent studies evaluated the combination of different pH- and thermoresponsive materials to obtain multi-responsive bioinks, with interesting applications in the field of tissue engineering and drug delivery [104].

5.4.3 Magnetic-/Electric-Field-Responsive

Magneto-responsive materials are those materials that, as a result of their deformation when subjected to magnetic fields, are employed to print four-dimensional structures. Due to the magnetorheological effect, magneto-responsive materials can quickly and irreversibly change the mechanical characteristics of the bioink under the presence of a magnetic field [105–107]. There is a lot of promise for polymeric constructs prepared with magneto-responsive bioinks. However, the main limitation is that the printed constructs should be small and light to be impacted by the magnetic field.

Certain cell lines, including cardiomyocytes, myoblasts, or endothelial progenitor cells, can respond to electric fields. Researchers have used this property to modulate cell alignment and fate. The incorporation of electrosensitive components (such as carbon nanotubes (CNTs) and gold nanowires (GNWs)) in bioinks has emerged as a viable alternative to guide their electrical response [108–110]. Collagen-, GelMA-, or dECM-based bioinks containing electrosensitive components have been developed, leading to constructs able to induce a high degree of myoblast alignment and myotube formation [111,112].

5.5 MULTICOMPONENT POLYMERIC BIOINKS

The rapid development achieved in the 3D bioprinting field has enabled the biofabrication of complex scaffolds with intricated structures and distinct compositions. Among the strategies available to biofabricate complex constructs is the use of multicomponent bioinks. A multicomponent bioink is a single-phase homogenous bioink that is prepared from a blend of two or more distinct biomaterials. Multicomponent bioinks are often more effective than single component bioinks in creating structures that closely resemble the heterogeneous attributes of native tissues. Moreover, multicomponent bioinks allows for the incorporation of features such as graded compositions or environmental cues. A wide range of advanced materials have been designed for multimaterial bioprinting to improve the intrinsic properties of traditional bioinks, including adequate crosslinking, or enhanced mechanical and biomimetic properties [105].

As explained before, the selection of a biomaterial as bioink components depends on several key factors, including their biocompatibility and biodegradation rate, immunogenicity, swelling, mechanical stability, and printing properties. One of the earlier approaches in multicomponent bioinks is the combination of distinct biomaterials to obtain multimaterial bioinks matching the requirements for tissue-specific regeneration. An example of this approach is the increasing mechanical strength of bioprinted constructs by incorporating inorganic particles, such as silicates or apatites. Nanoparticles and nanofibers are frequently combined with polymers to create composite bioinks. Depending on the distribution and orientation of the components in the hydrogel, bioinks may exhibit isotropic or anisotropic properties [113]. Composite bioinks benefit from each individual component to produce printed objects with improved attributes. The incorporation of fibrillar biomaterials in composite bioinks can recapitulate the fibrous nature of several human tissues, such as nervous or musculoskeletal tissues [114,115].

The synthesis of building blocks from proteins, lipids, and carbohydrates components is a naturally occurring process during tissue formation and regeneration. Inspired by this, multicomponent self-assembly bioinks aim to develop materials using an array of molecular building blocks with increased structural intricacy and functionality. This strategy enables the prospect of providing cells with signals mimicking the natural ECM based on, for instance, self-assembling peptide co-assemblies. As an example, self-assembling tissue strands and peptides have been investigated as bioinks due to their resemblance of the ECM structure. Hedegaard et al. reported a novel self-assembling supramolecular bioink to develop constructs with hierarchical structure and composition, based on the co-assembly of peptide amphiphiles (PAs) with bioactive molecules naturally present in the ECM [116]. This approach enables a biofabrication platform capable of spatially distributing and encapsulating various cell types in distinct ECM-like environments. In a similar approach, custom self-assembling peptide-based bioinks were used to print constructs with tunable stiffness and structural integrity to better replicate native ECM [117].

5.6 FUTURE DIRECTIONS

The field of bioprinting has undergone exciting advancements aimed at addressing the needs of tissue regeneration and the biofabrication of functional organs and tissues. Significant advances in novel fabrication approaches have been recently developed to generate tridimensional structures with precise control over their composition and mechanical properties. This progress entails the development of new polymers, crosslinking techniques, and hybrid approaches to enhance the printability and spatial resolution of polymer-based bioinks.

However, 3D printing also presents several challenges, particularly in terms of printing structures with defined geometries that are both mechanically strong and maintain tissue function and cell viability. In this chapter, we have summarized the main strategies proposed to overcome these limitations, including a myriad of natural and synthetic polymers, bioprinting capabilities, crosslinking strategies, and stimuli-sensitive bioinks. Moreover, the distinct characteristics of each tissue has led to a portfolio of bioinks designed to mimic their structural, mechanical, and chemical properties.

Bioprinting is an emergent field with a huge potential for controlling cell distribution and structural composition. Grounding on this, the wide use of this technology in the clinical field most likely will take place in the near future. In fact, commercial bioinks for specific tissue applications are already available. In summary, bioink development is a critical step forward in the bioprinting field, as it will enable the production of more complex and functional biological structures, with applications in tissue engineering, drug discovery, and regenerative medicine.

REFERENCES

1. Puppi D, Chiellini F. Biodegradable polymers for biomedical additive manufacturing. Applied Materials Today. 2020;20:100700.
2. Teixeira MC, Lameirinhas NS, Carvalho JPF, Silvestre AJD, Vilela C, Freire CSR. A guide to polysaccharide-based hydrogel bioinks for 3D bioprinting applications. International Journal of Molecular Sciences. 2022;23(12):6564.
3. Tarassoli SP, Jessop ZM, Jovic T, Hawkins K, Whitaker IS. Candidate bioinks for extrusion 3D bioprinting—a systematic review of the literature. Frontiers in Bioengineering and Biotechnology. 2021;9:616753. Published 2021 Oct 13. doi:10.3389/fbioe.2021.616753.

4. Carrow JK, Kerativitayanan P, Jaiswal MK, Lokhande G, Gaharwar AK. Chapter 13-Polymers for Bioprinting. In: Atala A, Yoo JJ, editors. Essentials of 3D Biofabrication and Translation. Boston: Academic Press; 2015. pp. 229–48.
5. Farina M, Alexander JF, Thekkedath U, Ferrari M, Grattoni A. Cell encapsulation: overcoming barriers in cell transplantation in diabetes and beyond. Advanced Drug Delivery Reviews. 2019;139:92–115.
6. Piras CC, Smith DK. Multicomponent polysaccharide alginate-based bioinks. Journal of Materials Chemistry B. 2020;8(36):8171–88.
7. Osidak EO, Kozhukhov VI, Osidak MS, Domogatsky SP. Collagen as bioink for bioprinting: a comprehensive review. International Journal of Bioprinting. 2020;6(3):270.
8. Abaci A, Guvendiren M. Designing decellularized extracellular matrix-based bioinks for 3D bioprinting. Advanced Healthcare Materials. 2020;9(24):2000734.
9. Huang H-J, Tsai Y-L, Lin S-H, Hsu S-H. Smart polymers for cell therapy and precision medicine. Journal of Biomedical Science. 2019;26(1):73.
10. Lui YS, Sow WT, Tan LP, Wu Y, Lai Y, Li H. 4D printing and stimuli-responsive materials in biomedical aspects. Acta Biomaterialia. 2019;92:19–36.
11. Ajmal S, Athar Hashmi F, Imran I. Recent progress in development and applications of biomaterials. Materials Today: Proceedings. 2022;62(1):385–91.
12. Al-Himdani S, Jessop ZM, Al-Sabah A, Combellack E, Ibrahim A, Doak SH, et al. Tissue-engineered solutions in plastic and reconstructive surgery: principles and practice. Frontiers in Surgery. 2017;4:4. Published 2017 Feb 23. doi:10.3389/fsurg.2017.00004.
13. Bolívar-Monsalve EJ, Alvarez MM, Hosseini S, Espinosa-Hernandez MA, Ceballos-González CF, Sanchez-Dominguez M, et al. Engineering bioactive synthetic polymers for biomedical applications: a review with emphasis on tissue engineering and controlled release. Materials Advances. 2021;2(14):4447–78.
14. Gillispie G, Prim P, Copus J, Fisher J, Mikos AG, Yoo JJ, et al. Assessment methodologies for extrusion-based bioink printability. Biofabrication. 2020;12(2):022003.
15. Heinrich MA, Liu W, Jimenez A, Yang J, Akpek A, Liu X, et al. 3D Bioprinting: from benches to translational applications. Small. 2019;15(23):1805510.
16. Hölzl K, Lin S, Tytgat L, Van Vlierberghe S, Gu L, Ovsianikov A. Bioink properties before, during and after 3D bioprinting. Biofabrication. 2016;8(3):032002.
17. Liu F, Chen Q, Liu C, Ao Q, Tian X, Fan J, et al. Natural polymers for organ 3D bioprinting. Polymers. 2018;10(11):1278.
18. Theus AS, Ning L, Hwang B, Gil C, Chen S, Wombwell A, et al. Bioprintability: physiomechanical and biological requirements of materials for 3D bioprinting processes. Polymers. 2020;12(10):2262.
19. https://www.sigmaaldrich.com/ES/es/technical-documents/technical-article/cell-culture-and-cell-culture-analysis/3d-cell-culture/3d-bioprinting-bioinks
20. Mahadik B, Margolis R, McLoughlin S, Melchiorri A, Lee SJ, Yoo J, et al. An open-source bioink database for microextrusion 3D printing. Biofabrication. 2023;15(1):015008.
21. https://debbie.bsc.es/search/
22. Donderwinkel I, van Hest JCM, Cameron NR. Bio-inks for 3D bioprinting: recent advances and future prospects. Polymer Chemistry. 2017;8(31):4451–71.
23. Xu J, Zhang M, Du W, Zhao J, Ling G, Zhang P. Chitosan-based high-strength supramolecular hydrogels for 3D bioprinting. International Journal of Biological Macromolecules. 2022;219:545–57.
24. Chopin-Doroteo M, Mandujano-Tinoco EA, Krötzsch E. Tailoring of the rheological properties of bioinks to improve bioprinting and bioassembly for tissue replacement. Biochimica et Biophysica Acta (BBA) - General Subjects. 2021;1865(2):129782.
25. Michel R, Auzély-Velty R. Hydrogel-colloid composite bioinks for targeted tissue-printing. Biomacromolecules. 2020;21(8):2949–65.

26. Ozbolat IT. The Bioink. In: Ozbolat IT, editor. 3D Bioprinting. Oxford: Academic Press; 2017. pp. 41–92.
27. Gospodinova A, Nankov V, Tomov S, Redzheb M, Petrov PD. Extrusion bioprinting of hydroxyethylcellulose-based bioink for cervical tumor model. Carbohydrate Polymers. 2021;260:117793.
28. Chawla S, Midha S, Sharma A, Ghosh S. Silk-based bioinks for 3D bioprinting. Advanced Healthcare Materials. 2018;7(8):1701204.
29. Liu W, Heinrich MA, Zhou Y, Akpek A, Hu N, Liu X, et al. Extrusion bioprinting of shear-thinning gelatin methacryloyl bioinks. Advanced Healthcare Materials. 2017;6(12):1601451.
30. He B, Yang S, Qin Z, Wen B, Zhang C. The roles of wettability and surface tension in droplet formation during inkjet printing. Scientific Reports. 2017;7(1):11841.
31. Ng WL, Huang X, Shkolnikov V, Goh GL, Suntornnond R, Yeong WY. Controlling droplet impact velocity and droplet volume: key factors to achieving high cell viability in sub-nanoliter droplet-based bioprinting. International Journal of Bioprinting. 2022;8(1):424.
32. Gudapati H, Dey M, Ozbolat I. A comprehensive review on droplet-based bioprinting: past, present and future. Biomaterials. 2016;102:20–42.
33. Datta P, Ayan B, Ozbolat IT. Bioprinting for vascular and vascularized tissue biofabrication. Acta Biomaterialia. 2017;51:1–20.
34. Yusupov V, Churbanov S, Churbanova E, Bardakova K, Antoshin A, Evlashin S, et al. Laser-induced forward transfer hydrogel printing: a defined route for highly controlled process. International Journal of Bioprinting. 2020;6(3):271.
35. Ventura RD. An overview of laser-assisted bioprinting (LAB) in tissue engineering applications. Medical Lasers. 2021;10(2):76–81.
36. Derakhshanfar S, Mbeleck R, Xu K, Zhang X, Zhong W, Xing M. 3D bioprinting for biomedical devices and tissue engineering: a review of recent trends and advances. Bioactive materials. 2018;3(2):144–56.
37. Mondschein RJ, Kanitkar A, Williams CB, Verbridge SS, Long TE. Polymer structure-property requirements for stereolithographic 3D printing of soft tissue engineering scaffolds. Biomaterials. 2017;140:170–88.
38. Perez-Valle A, Del Amo C, Andia I. Overview of current advances in extrusion bioprinting for skin applications. International Journal of Molecular Sciences. 2020;21(18):6679. Published 2020 Sep 12. doi:10.3390/ijms21186679.
39. Morgan EF, Unnikrisnan GU, Hussein AI. Bone mechanical properties in healthy and diseased states. Annual Review of Biomedical Engineering. 2018;20:119–43.
40. Li N, Guo R, Zhang ZJ. Bioink formulations for bone tissue regeneration. Frontiers in Bioengineering and Biotechnology. 2021;9:630488.
41. Vanaei S, Parizi MS, Vanaei S, Salemizadehparizi F, Vanaei HR. An overview on materials and techniques in 3D bioprinting toward biomedical application. Engineered Regeneration. 2021;2:1–18.
42. Mei Q, Rao J, Bei HP, Liu Y, Zhao X. 3D bioprinting photo-crosslinkable hydrogels for bone and cartilage repair. International Journal of Bioprinting. 2021;7(3):367.
43. Matai I, Kaur G, Seyedsalehi A, McClinton A, Laurencin CT. Progress in 3D bioprinting technology for tissue/organ regenerative engineering. Biomaterials. 2020;226:119536.
44. McGivern S, Boutouil H, Al-Kharusi G, Little S, Dunne NJ, Levingstone TJ. Translational application of 3D bioprinting for cartilage tissue engineering. Bioengineering (Basel, Switzerland). 2021;8(10):144.
45. van Kogelenberg S, Yue Z, Dinoro JN, Baker CS, Wallace GG. Three-dimensional printing and cell therapy for wound repair. Advances in Wound Care. 2018;7(5):145–55.
46. Alonzo M, AnilKumar S, Roman B, Tasnim N, Joddar B. 3D bioprinting of cardiac tissue and cardiac stem cell therapy. Translational Research: The Journal of Laboratory and Clinical Medicine. 2019;211:64–83.

47. GhavamiNejad A, Ashammakhi N, Wu XY, Khademhosseini A. Crosslinking strategies for 3D bioprinting of polymeric hydrogels. Small. 2020;16(35):2002931.
48. Chimene D, Kaunas R, Gaharwar AK. Hydrogel bioink reinforcement for additive manufacturing: a focused review of emerging strategies. Advanced Materials. 2020;32(1):1902026.
49. Decante G, Costa JB, Silva-Correia J, Collins MN, Reis RL, Oliveira JM. Engineering bioinks for 3D bioprinting. Biofabrication. 2021;13(3):032001.
50. Li J, Chen M, Fan X, Zhou H. Recent advances in bioprinting techniques: approaches, applications and future prospects. Journal of Translational Medicine. 2016;14(1):271.
51. Hull SM, Brunel LG, Heilshorn SC. 3D bioprinting of cell-laden hydrogels for improved biological functionality. Advanced Materials. 2022;34(2):2103691.
52. Valot L, Martinez J, Mehdi A, Subra G. Chemical insights into bioinks for 3D printing. Chemical Society Reviews. 2019;48(15):4049–86.
53. Kharkar PM, Kiick KL, Kloxin AM. Designing degradable hydrogels for orthogonal control of cell microenvironments. Chemical Society Reviews. 2013;42(17):7335–72.
54. Mueller E, Poulin I, Bodnaryk WJ, Hoare T. Click chemistry hydrogels for extrusion bioprinting: progress, challenges, and opportunities. Biomacromolecules. 2022;23(3):619–40.
55. Stichler S, Bertlein S, Tessmar J, Jüngst T, Groll J. Thiol-ene cross-linkable hydrogels as bioinks for biofabrication. Macromolecular Symposia. 2017;372(1):102–7.
56. Unagolla JM, Jayasuriya AC. Hydrogel-based 3D bioprinting: a comprehensive review on cell-laden hydrogels, bioink formulations, and future perspectives. Applied Materials Today. 2020;18:100479.
57. Bax DV, Davidenko N, Gullberg D, Hamaia SW, Farndale RW, Best SM, et al. Fundamental insight into the effect of carbodiimide crosslinking on cellular recognition of collagen-based scaffolds. Acta Biomaterialia. 2017;49:218–34.
58. Gu L, Shan T, Ma YX, Tay FR, Niu L. Novel biomedical applications of crosslinked collagen. Trends in Biotechnology. 2019;37(5):464–91.
59. Zhu K, Chen N, Liu X, Mu X, Zhang W, Wang C, et al. A general strategy for extrusion bioprinting of bio-macromolecular bioinks through alginate-templated dual-stage crosslinking. Macromolecular Bioscience. 2018;18(9):1800127.
60. Parak A, Pradeep P, du Toit LC, Kumar P, Choonara YE, Pillay V. Functionalizing bioinks for 3D bioprinting applications. Drug Discovery Today. 2019;24(1):198–205.
61. Lim KS, Schon BS, Mekhileri NV, Brown GCJ, Chia CM, Prabakar S, et al. New visible-light photoinitiating system for improved print fidelity in gelatin-based bioinks. ACS Biomaterials Science & Engineering. 2016;2(10):1752–62.
62. Zhang W, Ye W, Yan Y. Advances in photocrosslinkable materials for 3D bioprinting. Advanced Engineering Materials. 2022;24(1):2100663.
63. Hu J, Hou Y, Park H, Choi B, Hou S, Chung A, et al. Visible light crosslinkable chitosan hydrogels for tissue engineering. Acta Biomaterialia. 2012;8(5):1730–8.
64. Zheng Z, Eglin D, Alini M, Richards GR, Qin L, Lai Y. Visible light-induced 3D bioprinting technologies and corresponding bioink materials for tissue engineering: a review. Engineering. 2021;7(7):966–78.
65. Sun M, Sun X, Wang Z, Guo S, Yu G, Yang H. Synthesis and properties of gelatin methacryloyl (GelMA) hydrogels and their recent applications in load-bearing tissue. Polymers. 2018;10(11):1290.
66. Kurian AG, Singh RK, Patel KD, Lee J-H, Kim H-W. Multifunctional GelMA platforms with nanomaterials for advanced tissue therapeutics. Bioactive Materials. 2022;8:267–95.
67. Yue K, Trujillo-de Santiago G, Alvarez MM, Tamayol A, Annabi N, Khademhosseini A. Synthesis, properties, and biomedical applications of gelatin methacryloyl (GelMA) hydrogels. Biomaterials. 2015;73:254–71.

68. Ouyang L, Armstrong JPK, Lin Y, Wojciechowski JP, Lee-Reeves C, Hachim D, et al. Expanding and optimizing 3D bioprinting capabilities using complementary network bioinks. Science Advances. 2020;6(38):eabc5529.
69. Xu J, Liu Y, Hsu S-H. Hydrogels based on Schiff base linkages for biomedical applications. Molecules. 2019;24(16):3005.
70. Nguyen NT-P, Nguyen LV-H, Tran NM-P, Nguyen DT, Nguyen TN-T, Tran HA, et al. The effect of oxidation degree and volume ratio of components on properties and applications of in situ cross-linking hydrogels based on chitosan and hyaluronic acid. Materials Science and Engineering: C. 2019;103:109670.
71. Benwood C, Chrenek J, Kirsch RL, Masri NZ, Richards H, Teetzen K, et al. Natural biomaterials and their use as bioinks for printing tissues. Bioengineering. 2021;8(2):27.
72. Musilová L, Achbergerová E, Vítková L, Kolařík R, Martínková M, Minařík A, et al. Cross-linked gelatine by modified dextran as a potential bioink prepared by a simple and non-toxic process. Polymers. 2022;14(3):391.
73. Wang LL, Highley CB, Yeh Y-C, Galarraga JH, Uman S, Burdick JA. Three-dimensional extrusion bioprinting of single- and double-network hydrogels containing dynamic covalent crosslinks. Journal of Biomedical Materials Research Part A. 2018;106(4):865–75.
74. Rutz AL, Gargus ES, Hyland KE, Lewis PL, Setty A, Burghardt WR, et al. Employing PEG crosslinkers to optimize cell viability in gel phase bioinks and tailor post printing mechanical properties. Acta Biomaterialia. 2019;99:121–32.
75. Bertlein S, Brown G, Lim KS, Jungst T, Boeck T, Blunk T, et al. Thiol–Ene clickable gelatin: a platform bioink for multiple 3D biofabrication technologies. Advanced Materials. 2017;29(44):1703404.
76. Singh YP, Bandyopadhyay A, Mandal BB. 3D bioprinting using cross-linker-free silk–gelatin bioink for cartilage tissue engineering. ACS Applied Materials & Interfaces. 2019;11(37):33684–96.
77. Gu Y, Zhang L, Du X, Fan Z, Wang L, Sun W, et al. Reversible physical crosslinking strategy with optimal temperature for 3D bioprinting of human chondrocyte-laden gelatin methacryloyl bioink. Journal of Biomaterials Applications. 2018;33(5):609–18.
78. Lee SC, Gillispie G, Prim P, Lee SJ. Physical and chemical factors influencing the printability of hydrogel-based extrusion bioinks. Chemical Reviews. 2020;120(19):10834–86.
79. Kirchmajer DM, Gorkin III R, in het Panhuis M. An overview of the suitability of hydrogel-forming polymers for extrusion-based 3D-printing. Journal of Materials Chemistry B. 2015;3(20):4105–17.
80. Demirtaş TT, Irmak G, Gümüşderelioğlu M. A bioprintable form of chitosan hydrogel for bone tissue engineering. Biofabrication. 2017;9(3):035003.
81. Li M, Tian X, Zhu N, Schreyer DJ, Chen X. Modeling process-induced cell damage in the biodispensing process. Tissue Engineering Part C: Methods. 2010;16(3):533–42.
82. Bai J, Navara AM, Zhao L, Song Y, Yang X, Lian X, et al. Harnessing electrostatic interactions for enhanced printability of alginate-based bioinks. Bioprinting. 2022;27:e00215.
83. Adhikari J, Perwez MS, Das A, Saha P. Development of hydroxyapatite reinforced alginate–chitosan based printable biomaterial-ink. Nano-Structures & Nano-Objects. 2021;25:100630.
84. Lin Z, Wu M, He H, Liang Q, Hu C, Zeng Z, et al. 3D printing of mechanically stable calcium-free alginate-based scaffolds with tunable surface charge to enable cell adhesion and facile biofunctionalization. Advanced Functional Materials. 2019;29(9):1808439.
85. Petta D, Armiento AR, Grijpma D, Alini M, Eglin D, D'Este M. 3D bioprinting of a hyaluronan bioink through enzymatic-and visible light-crosslinking. Biofabrication. 2018;10(4):044104.

86. Le Thi P, Son JY, Lee Y, Ryu SB, Park KM, Park KD. Enzymatically crosslinkable hyaluronic acid-gelatin hybrid hydrogels as potential bioinks for tissue regeneration. Macromolecular Research. 2020;28(4):400–6.
87. de Melo BAG, Jodat YA, Cruz EM, Benincasa JC, Shin SR, Porcionatto MA. Strategies to use fibrinogen as bioink for 3D bioprinting fibrin-based soft and hard tissues. Acta Biomaterialia. 2020;117:60–76.
88. Gungor-Ozkerim PS, Inci I, Zhang YS, Khademhosseini A, Dokmeci MR. Bioinks for 3D bioprinting: an overview. Biomaterials Science. 2018;6(5):915–46.
89. Ramakrishnan R, Kasoju N, Raju R, Geevarghese R, Gauthaman A, Bhatt A. Exploring the potential of alginate-gelatin-diethylaminoethyl cellulose-fibrinogen based bioink for 3D bioprinting of skin tissue constructs. Carbohydrate Polymer Technologies and Applications. 2022;3:100184.
90. Piard C, Baker H, Kamalitdinov T, Fisher J. Bioprinted osteon-like scaffolds enhance in vivo neovascularization. Biofabrication. 2019;11(2):025013.
91. Zhou M, Lee BH, Tan YJ, Tan LP. Microbial transglutaminase induced controlled crosslinking of gelatin methacryloyl to tailor rheological properties for 3D printing. Biofabrication. 2019;11(2):025011.
92. Ren P, Wei D, Liang M, Xu L, Zhang T, Zhang Q. Alginate/gelatin-based hybrid hydrogels with function of injecting and encapsulating cells in situ. International Journal of Biological Macromolecules. 2022;212:67–84.
93. Janmaleki M, Liu J, Kamkar M, Azarmanesh M, Sundararaj U, Nezhad AS. Role of temperature on bio-printability of gelatin methacryloyl bioink in two-step cross-linking strategy for tissue engineering applications. Biomedical Materials. 2021;16(1):015021.
94. Habib A, Sathish V, Mallik S, Khoda B. 3D printability of alginate-carboxymethyl cellulose hydrogel. Materials. 2018;11(3):454.
95. Das S, Pati F, Choi Y-J, Rijal G, Shim J-H, Kim SW, et al. Bioprintable, cell-laden silk fibroin–gelatin hydrogel supporting multilineage differentiation of stem cells for fabrication of three-dimensional tissue constructs. Acta Biomaterialia. 2015;11:233–46.
96. Colosi C, Shin SR, Manoharan V, Massa S, Costantini M, Barbetta A, et al. Microfluidic bioprinting of heterogeneous 3D tissue constructs using low-viscosity bioink. Advanced Materials. 2016;28(4):677–84.
97. Zhang YS, Arneri A, Bersini S, Shin S-R, Zhu K, Goli-Malekabadi Z, et al. Bioprinting 3D microfibrous scaffolds for engineering endothelialized myocardium and heart-on-a-chip. Biomaterials. 2016;110:45–59.
98. Nedunchezian S, Banerjee P, Lee C-Y, Lee S-S, Lin C-W, Wu C-W, et al. Generating adipose stem cell-laden hyaluronic acid-based scaffolds using 3D bioprinting via the double crosslinked strategy for chondrogenesis. Materials Science and Engineering: C. 2021;124:112072.
99. Ratemi E. 5-pH-responsive polymers for drug delivery applications. In: Makhlouf ASH, Abu-Thabit NY, editors. Stimuli Responsive Polymeric Nanocarriers for Drug Delivery Applications, Volume 1. Duxford: Woodhead Publishing; 2018. pp. 121–41.
100. Diamantides N, Wang L, Pruiksma T, Siemiatkoski J, Dugopolski C, Shortkroff S, et al. Correlating rheological properties and printability of collagen bioinks: the effects of riboflavin photocrosslinking and pH. Biofabrication. 2017;9(3):034102.
101. Lee A, Hudson AR, Shiwarski DJ, Tashman JW, Hinton TJ, Yerneni S, et al. 3D bioprinting of collagen to rebuild components of the human heart. Science. 2019;365(6452):482–7.
102. Cochis A, Bonetti L, Sorrentino R, Contessi Negrini N, Grassi F, Leigheb M, et al. 3D printing of thermo-responsive methylcellulose hydrogels for cell-sheet engineering. Materials. 2018;11(4):579.

103. Lorson T, Jaksch S, Lübtow MM, Jüngst T, Groll J, Lühmann T, et al. A thermogelling supramolecular hydrogel with sponge-like morphology as a cytocompatible bioink. Biomacromolecules. 2017;18(7):2161–71.
104. Badeau BA, DeForest CA. Programming stimuli-responsive behavior into biomaterials. Annual Review of Biomedical Engineering. 2019;21(1):241–65.
105. Levato R, Jungst T, Scheuring RG, Blunk T, Groll J, Malda J. From shape to function: the next step in bioprinting. Advanced Materials. 2020;32(12):1906423.
106. Vítková L, Musilová L, Achbergerová E, Kolařík R, Mrlík M, Korpasová K, et al. Formulation of magneto-responsive hydrogels from dually cross-linked polysaccharides: synthesis, tuning and evaluation of rheological properties. International Journal of Molecular Sciences. 2022;23(17):9633.
107. Ahmed A, Arya S, Gupta V, Furukawa H, Khosla A. 4D printing: fundamentals, materials, applications and challenges. Polymer. 2021;228:123926.
108. Chen C, Bai X, Ding Y, Lee I-S. Electrical stimulation as a novel tool for regulating cell behavior in tissue engineering. Biomaterials Research. 2019;23(1):25.
109. Sun H, Zhou J, Huang Z, Qu L, Lin N, Liang C, et al. Carbon nanotube-incorporated collagen hydrogels improve cell alignment and the performance of cardiac constructs. International Journal of Nanomedicine. 2017;12:3109–20.
110. Kim H, Kim M-C, Asada HH. Extracellular matrix remodelling induced by alternating electrical and mechanical stimulations increases the contraction of engineered skeletal muscle tissues. Scientific Reports. 2019;9(1):2732.
111. Kim W, Jang CH, Kim GH. A myoblast-laden collagen bioink with fully aligned au nanowires for muscle-tissue regeneration. Nano Letters. 2019;19(12):8612–20.
112. Kim W, Lee H, Lee CK, Kyung JW, An SB, Han I-B, et al. A bioprinting process supplemented with in situ electrical stimulation directly induces significant myotube formation and myogenesis. Advanced Functional Materials. 2021;31(51):2105170.
113. Ravanbakhsh H, Bao G, Luo Z, Mongeau LG, Zhang YS. Composite inks for extrusion printing of biological and biomedical constructs. ACS Biomaterials Science & Engineering. 2021;7(9):4009–26.
114. Turnbull G, Clarke J, Picard F, Riches P, Jia L, Han F, et al. 3D bioactive composite scaffolds for bone tissue engineering. Bioactive Materials. 2018;3(3):278–314.
115. Bhattacharyya A, Janarthanan G, Noh I. Nano-biomaterials for designing functional bioinks towards complex tissue and organ regeneration in 3D bioprinting. Additive Manufacturing. 2021;37: 101639.
116. Hedegaard CL, Collin EC, Redondo-Gómez C, Nguyen LTH, Ng KW, Castrejón-Pita AA, et al. Hydrodynamically guided hierarchical self-assembly of peptide–protein bioinks. Advanced Functional Materials. 2018;28(16):1703716.
117. Raphael B, Khalil T, Workman VL, Smith A, Brown CP, Streuli C, et al. 3D cell bioprinting of self-assembling peptide-based hydrogels. Materials Letters. 2017;190:103–6.

6 Decellularized Matrices for Bioink Development

Daniel P. Reis, Luca Gasperini, and Alexandra P. Marques
University of Minho and ICVS/3B's–PT
Government Associate Laboratory

CONTENTS

6.1 INTRODUCTION

Tissue engineering (TE) research aims to feed the global and constant need for artificial tissues in the context of both tissue regeneration and *in vitro* testing/screening platforms [1,2]. However, successful mimicry of the overall complexity of any living tissue is still largely incomplete, as most TE strategies fall short of accurately representing the structure and functionality of what surrounds the native cells, their extracellular matrix (ECM) [3]. The ECM combines cell-secreted molecules that offer biochemical and structural support to cells defining tissues and organs and their respective functions. In particular, the functional requirements of each tissue are modulated by the precise balance of the three main ECM components – water, proteins, and polysaccharides [4–6]. This balance accounts for the mechanical properties of the ECM, which depend on the protein content, particularly the abundance of collagen and elastin [7].

Several approaches have been steadily developed throughout the years to attain suitable alternatives to regenerate or replace human tissues or organs [8,9]. Among those, 3D printing emerged as an evident technology since it allows for the

DOI: 10.1201/9781003274568-6

free-forming, three-dimensional (3D) fabrication of structures with a high degree of shape fidelity and complexity at the microscale level [10,11]. Notwithstanding, inks capable of achieving this level of dimensional accuracy, since they are typically selected because of their processing properties, are usually pale in their biological mimicry lacking polymers found in human or even animal tissues [12]. Therefore, ECM-based inks derived from native tissues and cells [13–16], which bestow functionality due to their intrinsic biological cues, have been increasingly used to fabricate 3D constructs that may serve as substitutes for damaged or diseased tissues [17–20]. Nonetheless, the development of an appropriate ink capable of providing a suitable microenvironment to guarantee tissue-specific cellular behavior is a complex task. It requires careful and thorough selection of the extraction and processing methodologies tailored to the features of the origin tissue [21]. Moreover, the resulting ECM does not possess inherent printable characteristics, requiring further processing [22,23].

Herein, we describe the major components of the ECM, dissecting their role in the overall tissue functionality and mechanical properties. Furthermore, we provide an overview of the current methodologies for obtaining and processing ECM extracts and insight into which are more appropriate for each tissue source and what their outcomes are. Finally, we present a thorough rundown on the works being carried out to make ECM extracts printable and their influence on the printed construct's biological relevance.

6.2 EXTRACELLULAR MATRIX

6.2.1 Composition

Extracellular matrices are organized 3D microarchitectural networks with structural and functional roles in tissue organization and remodeling by directly and indirectly regulating several cellular processes [5,24]. Through integrin-mediated interactions, cells sense the surrounding ECM, transducing the overall microenvironment features into a biological response (motility, proliferation, differentiation, etc.) [5,6]. Thus, knowledge of the precise composition of the ECM of different tissues is important for understanding their structure–function relationship. The ECM is predominantly composed of structural (collagens and elastin) and specialized (fibrillin, fibronectin, and laminin) proteins, proteoglycans (PGs) (heparin (HEP) sulfate, chondroitin sulfate (CS), keratin sulfate (KS), and glycosaminoglycans (GAGs)), and an array of sequestered growth factors (GFs), tailored to the specific functions of the tissue [4,6].

Collagens are trimeric proteins comprised of three polypeptide chains – α-chains – which form a triple helix of variable length, a shared structural motif within the 28 collagen types (I–XXVIII) that have been identified so far [25,26]. Each collagen type contains at least one triple-helical domain, which is secreted and deposited into the ECM and is the building block for the assembly of any collagenous structure. Most collagens can form supramolecular aggregates and are divided into subfamilies depending on the supramolecular structure they form [27].

Large fibril-forming collagens are responsible for maintaining the 3D structure of the ECM, while smaller molecules act as signaling agents for cell adhesion, chemotaxis, and migration [24]. Intracellular biosynthesis of these collagens and their isoforms involves the transcription of messenger RNA (mRNA) molecules encoded by three-chain combinations of different α-chain genes to form pre-procollagen, which is converted into procollagen by the removal of the signal peptide [28]. Posteriorly, these chains form disulfide bonds that strongly intertwine each set of three chains, stabilizing the triple-helical formation that then propagates in a zipper-like manner from the C-terminus to the N-terminus [29]. Thus, changes in any of these steps can alter collagen structure and secretion levels, which occur in many diseases including cancer and fibrosis [30–32].

PGs are part of a superfamily containing more than 30 molecules, consisting of a protein core decorated with negatively charged GAGs. GAGs are unbranched, long polysaccharides with a repeating disaccharide structure that consist of a hexosamine (D-glucosamine or D-galactosamine) alternating with a uronic acid (D-glucuronic or L-iduronic) or a neutral sugar (D-galactose) [33,34]. Depending on the composition of the disaccharide unit and the position of the sulfate group, GAGs can be classified as heparan sulfate (HS), HEP sulfate, CS, KS, and dermatan sulfate (DS), whose location and distribution vary depending on their anatomical location [24,35]. PGs are responsible for mechanical resistance to compression due to their viscoelastic properties modulated by their water retention capability within the ECM. PGs are also linked to the ECM capacity of storing GFs due to the inherent hydrophilicity of their polysaccharide chains [36,37]. The largest class of PGs – small leucine-rich PGs – functions as a structural component and signaling molecule, particularly during tissue remodeling under non-homeostatic conditions, interacting with cell membrane receptors' regulating processes such as migration, proliferation, innate immunity, apoptosis, autophagy, and angiogenesis [38,39].

Another major component of ECM is elastin, which is the component mainly responsible for conferring elasticity to tissues and organs. In fact, it is roughly 1,000 times more deformable than collagens and does not have the pronounced hierarchical organization these have [27]. Elastin is a linearly elastic material present as long, flexible strands in the soft tissues. Its soluble precursor – tropoelastin – alternates hydrophobic and hydrophilic domains [40]. The hydrophilic domains contain either lysyl-alanine (KA) or lysyl-proline (KP) motifs and are involved in the covalent cross-linking induced by lysyl-oxidases (LOX) and/or lysyl-oxidase-like (LOXL) enzymes, forming elastin fibers [41–43]. This cross-linked elastin composes the dense core of the elastic fibers – over 90% of the fiber content – which is then covered by longitudinally aligned fibrillin-based microfibrils. The microfibrils are 10- to 12-nm-wide filaments, which have a bead-on-a-string appearance [44]. However, elastin hydrophobic domains, which are rich in valine, proline, and glycine, are responsible for elasticity and are involved in cell interactions [45]. Overall, these extracellular elastic assemblies, due to their recoiling ability, are dominant in extensible tissues that undergo reversible and repetitive deformation such as arteries, skin, tendons, or lungs [46,47].

6.2.2 Functions

Depending on the tissue's type and anatomical localization, its native ECM composition and overall complexity are modulated to answer inherent functional requirements [48]. Additionally, ECM's exact composition differs based on sex, age, and health conditions. This generates spectra of ECM types that vary in the ratios of the previously described components, whose extremes are bridged in a plethora of different tissues (Figure 6.1).

Among tissue functions, mechanical performance is the one primarily linked to the ECM composition. Being responsible for the maintenance of overall tissue integrity and macrostructure, collagen is ever-present throughout the distinct ECMs found in the human body [5]. For instance, in bone, the main function of tissue is to support most of the human body weight, and over 90% of the organic fraction of its ECM consists of collagen type I [49]. Combined with the organic fraction of bone ECM (40%) are inorganic compounds (60%), mainly calcium hydroxyapatite, responsible for the stiffness of the tissue. The combination of a collagen framework with other components that are directly correlated with tissue's mechanical performance occurs in many other human tissues. For example, articular cartilage ECM is composed mainly of a collagen-rich network (90%) enriched with PGs (10%–15%, mainly aggrecan), and a movable interstitial fluid phase, which is predominately water [50,51]. The interactions between the PGs within the organic matrix and the water in the fluid phase are responsible for the osmotic swelling and the compressibility of the tissue [51]. Interestingly, the conversion of cartilage into bone requires several processes that directly involve the presence and differential expression of PGs and collagen types [52], accounting for the smooth transition between cartilage (compressive) and bone (supportive) tissue. Collagen is also the most abundant protein in the skin dermis, accounting for approximately 70% of the total protein. Although decorated with several appendages to address all of the tissue's functions, such as hair

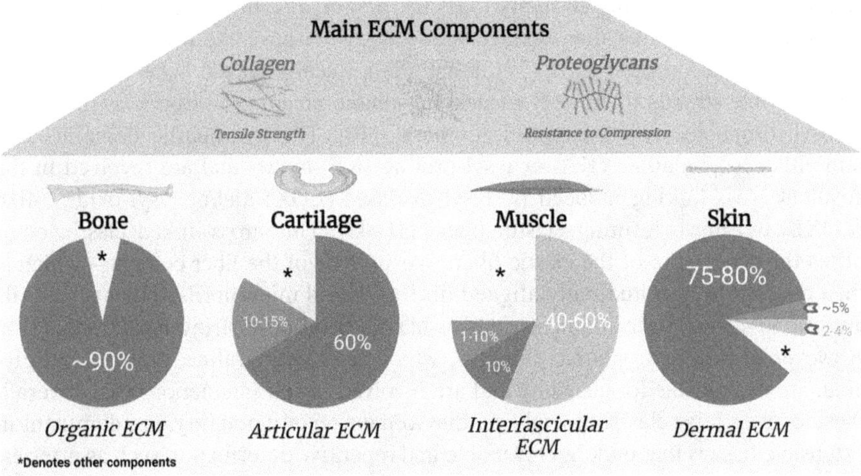

FIGURE 6.1 Ratio of the primary components in different tissues' ECM.

follicles or sweat glands, the skin's mechanical responsiveness, structural integrity, and tensegrity are maintained by the composition of its dermal ECM [53,54]. Here, collagen binds to elastic fibers, which although in a low amount (2%–4%) provide the tissue with the ability to recover from stretching, while the native structure of collagen fibers avoids the over-deformation of the skin [7].

In other tissues subjected to a higher degree of deformation, such as muscle, the major component elastin (40%–60%) confers springiness, while collagen (10%) and PGs (1%–10%) maintain their tensegrity and hydration [55–57]. Most of the muscle's ECM is located in the region limiting its fascicles – the interfascicular region – that divides skeletal muscle fiber subdivisions [58,59]. This ECM bears the majority of the passive load (e.g., supporting the contraction of muscle fibers) and is therefore a key player in the maintenance of overall tissue mechanical functionality [55]. Large muscles comprise a multi-compartment of fibers whose intrafascicular terminations have no direct tendinous attachments. Therefore, the contractile force produced in these fibers must be transmitted between adjacent muscle fibers via the endomysial connective tissue ECM that separates them [59,60].

6.3 DECELLULARIZATION METHODS

Decellularization has been defined as the process by which tissues are subjected to eliminate their cellular content, which are major immunogenic factors [61]. Ideally, this process should ultimately yield compounds completely deprived of those elements, while maintaining most of the acellular components of any tissue's ECM. Decellularization procedures generally begin with the lysis of the cellular and nuclear membranes, followed by the breakdown and rinsing of any cellular debris from the tissue. As previously mentioned, living tissues have distinct mechanical properties arising from distinct structures; therefore, their resistance to any decellularization method significantly varies among them [61,62]. As such, several methods have been developed and applied, singly or in combination, according to the target tissue to maximize the decellularization yield, while preserving their effect on the ECM composition (Table 6.1).

6.3.1 Chemical Methods

Chemical decellularization methodologies rely on either alkaline solutions such as ammonium hydroxide or acidic solutions such as acetic acid, peracetic acid, hydrochloric acid, and sulfuric acid to disrupt and dissolve the cellular membrane [49,63]. The length of exposure toward these chemicals is directly related to the tissue type and dimensions, since these features influence the diffusion of any given solution [64]. Prolonged exposure to those chemicals may raise potentially harmful effects on the ECM, such as the hydrolysis of structural proteins of interest or of decorating components such as GAGs [49,61,63,65]. Alternatively, cellular membrane dissolution may be achieved with the use of detergents, whose micellar structure successfully interacts with the phospholipid layer found on the cell's surface. There are three major types of detergents – ionic, nonionic, and zwitterionic – classified according to their molecular charges, which consequently have distinct degrees of

TABLE 6.1
Decellularization Methodologies

Method	Agent	Overall Outcome	Ref.
Chemical	Acid–base	Loss of collagen and GAG content Disrupted ECM via hydrolysis Lack of GFs Altered ECM mechanical properties	[49,61,63,65]
	Nonionic detergents	Loss of proteins and GAG content Disrupted ECM	[64,68,69]
	Ionic detergents	Loss of collagen and GAG content Lack of GFs	[61,69,70]
	Zwitterionic detergents	Denatured protein content	[72,73]
Physical	Freeze–thawing	Altered ECM ultrastructure Presence of cellular residues	[98–101]
	Mechanical force	Damaged and/or fragmented ECM	[61,115]
	Supercritical exposure	Damaged ECM	[16,108,109]
Biological	Enzymatic	Disrupted collagen Loss of laminin, fibronectin, elastin, and GAGs	[19,116]

interaction with the ECM components [66,67]. Nonionic detergents, such as Triton X-100, have been extensively used in decellularization protocols because of their relatively mild effects on ECM structure. These detergents disrupt lipid–lipid and lipid–protein interactions while leaving intact protein–protein interactions and maintaining their functional conformation [64,68,69]. Ionic detergents, however, are more effective for solubilizing both cytoplasmic and nuclear cellular membranes than nonionic, with the caveat of having a deleterious effect on native ECM structure. Exposure to the most used ionic detergents, such as sodium dodecyl sulfate (SDS), sodium deoxycholate, and Triton X-200, was shown to denatured proteins with loss of overall integrity and lead to a significant decrease in the GAG content [61,69,70]. Zwitterionic detergents, exhibiting both charges in their molecular structure, have the properties of both nonionic (milder effect on ECM) and ionic (efficiency at breaking protein–protein interactions) ones, while possessing an inferior micellization capability [71]. Consequently, this type of detergent, such as 3-[(3-cholamidopropyl) dimethylammonio]-1-propanesulfonate (CHAPS), sulfobetaine-10 (SB-10), and sulfobetaine-16 (SB-16), is not as frequently used as its ionic and nonionic counterparts [72,73]. Detergent-based approaches, however, still required extensive posttreatment rinsing with water or PBS, to eliminate any residual micellar agent within the decellularized tissue.

Overall, chemically driven decellularization is associated with the successful maintenance of the macrostructure and mechanical compliance of the retained ECM, with the caveat of a significant decrease in the overall contents of several components of functional interest, such as GAGs, fibronectin, and laminin. As these methodologies rely on the perfusion of solutions throughout the tissue samples, they are more commonly used in softer tissues and organs, such as the heart [70,74,75], liver [62,76], skin [67,77–79], adipose tissue [80,81], and muscle [82,83].

6.3.2 Enzymatic Methods

Methodologies based on treating native tissue with biological agents resort exclusively to enzymes, such as proteases, to dissociate cells from ECM and nucleases to break down nucleic acid chains [84–87]. Within proteases, trypsin and dispase II are the most used. Trypsin is a particular enzyme that cleaves the peptide bonds on the carbon side of arginine and lysine when the following residue is not proline [88]. Prolonged exposure to trypsin results in ECM structure disruption and loss of laminin, fibronectin, elastin, and GAG content [85,86,89,90]. Regarding dispase, it has a high affinity for specific ECM proteins such as fibronectin and collagen IV [84,91], and for this reason, it is less used in tissue decellularization. Nucleases such as endonucleases catalyze the hydrolysis of the internal bonds of the ribonucleotide or deoxyribonucleotide chains, whereas exonucleases catalyze the hydrolysis of their terminal bonds, ultimately leading to the degradation of ribonucleic acid (RNA) or deoxyribonucleic acid (DNA) [92]. Among them, deoxyribonuclease (DNase) I/II and ribonuclease (RNase) are the most commonly used endonucleases and are usually added to a decellularization protocol after cell membrane lysis to increase the efficiency of rinsing the nucleic acid content [93–95].

6.3.3 Physical Methods

Physical methods lack the capacity to break down or rinse the unwanted nuclear components; as such, they are used to facilitate the decellularization process coupled with other protocols. These approaches deal with the exertion of external stimuli or shocks, such as freeze–thawing, pressure, sonication, or agitation. The freezing of the tissue leads to the formation of ice crystals, which cause disruption of the cellular membranes aiding in cell lysis [96,97]. This approach is frequently applied to tough and robust tissues such as bone [98–101] and tendons [102,103], as a pretreatment to facilitate the perfusion of any solution during decellularization. However, in softer tissues, the perfusion of decellularization agents can be accomplished by mechanical agitation [104]. Mechanical pressure has also been used in these soft tissues to aid in the removal of cellular components after exposure to the decellularization agent [61]. Exposing tissue samples to high-frequency sound waves and/or vibrations, e.g., sonication, is also useful in breaking down or releasing cellular components from tissues of any kind [105–107].

Another physical approach that has been explored is the use of supercritical carbon dioxide ($scCO_2$) [16,108,109], taking advantage of two of the most important traits of a supercritical fluid (SCF): (i) gas-like diffusion/liquid-like mass transfer and (ii) variable density controlled by temperature and pressure. This technology also allows for the combination of the SCF with mild detergents, enhancing its efficacy since the polar entrainer/detergent fosters the interaction of CO_2 with other polar molecules, such as phospholipids and DNA molecules [110,111]. So far, the combination of supercritical CO_2 with other methodologies has been used to successfully remove DNA from tissues such as the aorta [112,113], skin [78], and bone [100].

Overall, the most robust and effective extraction protocols include a combination of physical, chemical, and enzymatic approaches, since each methodology excels at distinct aspects throughout the process [114].

6.4 PROCESSING OF EXTRACELLULAR MATRIX EXTRACTS

Originally, decellularization methodologies were developed to obtain ECM-based scaffolds that retain the composition, and biological and mechanical properties of the 3D ECM. Such templates, representative of the native microenvironment, would provide the necessary cues for cells to lead to neotissue formation. More recently, researchers have been looking past the traditional scaffolding and are adopting new procedures to utilize these ECM components in developing other biomaterials such as hydrogels [117,118].

After decellularization, the decellularized ECM (dECM) extracts require further processing (Figure 6.2) to be converted into hydrogels, since most of the retrieved components are not intrinsically gelling agents. At first, the proteins retained in the dECM are subjected to pepsin-mediated solubilization under acidic conditions [119]. Pepsin, an enzyme derived from porcine gastric juices that has long been used to solubilize acid-insoluble collagen, cleaves the telopeptide bonds of the collagen triple-helix structure to untangle collagen fibril aggregates [120]. Thus, this enzymatic solubilization process must be carefully tailored for each dECM extract, as its composition and morphology dictate the extent of the process. Overexposure of the dECM to these conditions may irreversibly alter the collagen's molecular structure, hindering the subsequent steps in the processing. The "solubilized dECM" – sol-dECM – becomes highly viscous when neutralized to physiologic pH and forms a hydrogel upon temperature increase in a process driven by the entropy associated with collagen fibrillogenesis [121–124]. This change in collagen conformation is partly modulated by the presence of GAGs, PGs, and other ECM proteins since these large macromolecules may spatially constrain the overall organization of the polymeric network [125,126]. Thus, it is influenced by the native biochemical profile of the source tissue and the content of the decellularized extract.

The gelation of this dECM/sol-dECM may also be triggered by the addition of a gelling agent [16,127–130]. The most common approach is the combination of dECM with cross-linkable polymers, due to their inherent rheological features and chemistry of their functional groups sensitive to various factors allowing for a multitude of different cross-linking reactions [131–137]. For instance, some polymers such as alginate and gellan gum are polyelectrolytes that carry a net negative charge on their carboxyl group, and are cross-linked by the addition of positive ions [134–137]. Others, containing light-sensitive elements, are cross-linked by exposure to a light source [131–133]. By triggering a swift and controlled cross-linking of these materials, researchers are able to retain the ECM components within the developed 3D mesh.

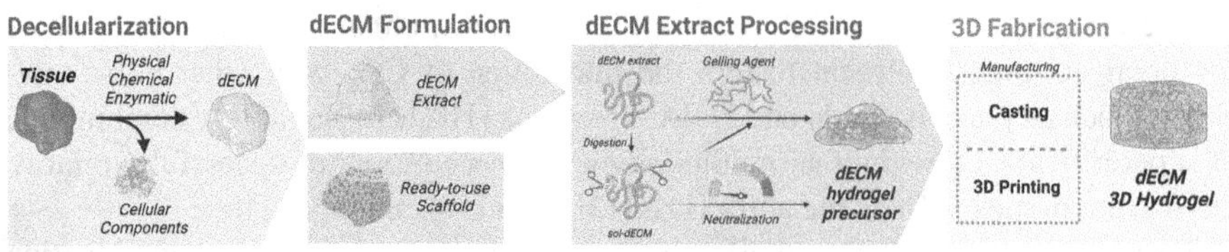

FIGURE 6.2 Pipeline for the development of dECM-based hydrogels. Decellularized extracellular matrix (dECM), solubilized dECM (sol-dECM).

6.5 DECELLULARIZED MATRICES FOR BIOPRINTING

6.5.1 Extracellular Matrix-Based Bioinks

Hydrogel precursors, including extract-based ECMs, have been combined with a wide range of cells to generate 3D constructs that, by having key tissue elements, hold great potential for tissue replacement/regeneration. If these hydrogel precursors are processed using 3D printing technologies, this potential further expands to the generation of tissue-like structures in which both material (ink) and cells can be three-dimensionally placed in a complex organization as in native tissues [138,139]. However, any ink candidate should address two main concerns: (i) its extrudability and (ii) the shape fidelity of the printed constructs, both of which can be partially determined by their rheological behavior [13,23,140,141]. Extrudability refers to the capability of a bioink to continuously flow through a printer's nozzle within a pressure range that also does not compromise cellular integrity. In turn, shape fidelity guarantees the resemblance of the final printed construct to the initial design of the desired structure. ECM-based inks typically have a viscosity that increases with protein concentration, and a shear-thinning behavior that is characterized by a decrease in the viscosity of the ink with increasing shear rate [21,138]. This characteristic translates into a lower pressure needed to print an object, allowing a reduction in the overall shear stress felt by cells during extrusion, positively impacting viability [142,143]. While this shear-thinning nature also contributes to the overall higher shape fidelity of the printed construct, there is another major factor influencing this aspect: the control of the ink's cross-linking [141,143,144]. Bioinks comprised exclusively of sol-dECM are normally cross-linked by increasing temperature to 37°C, where their solubilized collagen molecules rearrange to form a stable network, as previously described, entrapping the loaded cells. Although this thermal cross-linking has no adverse effects on the cell's viability, it limits the overall size of any printed construct, since fabricating large 3D constructs using dECM with weak mechanical properties and slow gelation time is an arduous task [145–147]. For this reason, dECM extracts have been combined with other materials such as alginate [130,148,149] or gellan gum [150,151] yielding inks with improved printability, since these materials readily cross-link when in contact with ions.

6.5.2 Extracellular Matrix-Based 3D-Printed Constructs

The numerous combinations of ECM sources and extraction and processing methodologies pose a wide range of possibilities to generate constructs decorated with the characteristic biological features of native tissues. Nonetheless, analysis of current dECM-based bioprinting approaches highlights that variations in the *modus operandi* are sparse and heavily focused on the chemically based ECM extraction from tissues of nonhuman source, followed by solubilization with acidic pepsin digestion (Table 6.2).

As previously mentioned, every step in the development of an ECM-based bioink should be adjusted to the selected ECM source. When bone is considered to fabricate osteogenic constructs, tissue demineralization is required to separate the organic and inorganic ECM fractions before decellularization [165,166]. So far, bone sol-dECM

TABLE 6.2
Extracellular Matrix-Based 3D-Printed Approaches

Decellularization		ECM Source	dECM Processing	Bioink Composition	Outcome	Ref.
Chemical	Triton	Porcine liver	dECM or dECM acid digested by pepsin	dECM/gelatin/HA or sol-dECM HUVECs or mouse hepatocytes	Increased albumin secretion when compared to collagen control	[152]
			dECM acid digested by pepsin	Sol-dECM hBMMSCs	Induced hepatic-associated gene expression	[153]
		Porcine skin		Sol-dECM hDFBs	Increased deposition of collagen I and thicker epidermal layer when compared to collagen control	[154]
				Sol-dECM hBMMSCs	Induced dermal-associated gene expression	[153]
		Porcine tendon		Sol-dECM hBMMSCs	Increased expression of tenogenic markers when compared to collagen control	[155]
		Porcine kidney		Sol-dECM/alginate HUVECs or RPTECs	Increased expression of renal phenotype markers by RPTECs, and CD31 and VE-cadherin by HUVECs, when compared to collagen control	[156]
		Porcine cornea		Sol-dECM hBMMSCs	Induced cornea-associated gene expression	[153]
		Bovine cornea		Sol-dECM hTMSCs	Increased expression of keratocan when compared to collagen controls	[157]
		Goat articular cartilage		Sol-dECM/SF hBMMSCs	Increased expression of chondrogenic markers when compared to SF control	[158]

(*Continued*)

TABLE 6.2 (*Continued*)
Extracellular Matrix-Based 3D-Printed Approaches

Decellularization	ECM Source	dECM Processing	Bioink Composition	Outcome	Ref.
SDS	Porcine heart		Sol-dECM/GelMA hCPC	Improved differentiation and angiogenic potential when compared to GelMA control	[159]
Triton SDS			Sol-dECM hBMMSCs	Induced cardio-associated gene expression	[153]
	Porcine aorta		Sol-dECM/alginate/ PLGA microspheres EPCs	Increased proliferation rate and expression of endothelial markers when compared to collagen and alginate control	[149]
	Porcine liver		Sol-dECM/GelMA iPSC-derived hepatocytes	Higher albumin secretion when compared to GelMA control	[160]
			Sol-dECM HepG2	Enhanced albumin secretion when compared to collagen controls	[161]
	Porcine pancreas		Sol-dECM human pancreatic islets or iPSC-derived insulin-producing cells	Islets showed higher levels of insulin and glucose-stimulated index when compared to alginate and collagen control Insulin-producing cells showed higher levels of insulin and increased expression of nuclear transcription factors when compared to collagen control	[162]

(*Continued*)

TABLE 6.2 (*Continued*)
Extracellular Matrix-Based 3D-Printed Approaches

Decellularization		ECM Source	dECM Processing	Bioink Composition	Outcome	Ref.
Enzymatic	Trypsin	Porcine bone		Sol-dECM hBMMSCs	Increased expression of osteogenic markers when compared to collagen controls	[155]
				Methacrylated sol-dECM/alginate hASCs	Increased matrix mineralization and expression of osteogenic markers when compared to alginate controls	[163]
	DNase	Porcine articular cartilage		Sol-dECM/alginate human or porcine BMMSCs	Increased expression of chondrogenic markers and ECM secretion when compared to alginate controls	[130]
Combinations	Freeze-thaw Detergent	Porcine heart ventricle		Sol-dECM/GelMA iPSC-derived cardiomyocytes	Increased expression of early and mature cardiac transcription factors when compared to collagen/GelMA controls	[164]
		Porcine liver		Sol-dECM/GelMA iPSC-derived hepatocytes	Increased expression of hepatocyte maturation markers when compared to collagen/GelMA control	
		Porcine ear cartilage		Methacrylated sol-dECM/gelatin/HA Rabbit auricular chondrocytes	Enhanced chondrocyte maturation and ECM secretion when compared to GelMA control	[128]

List of acronyms: *EPCs, endothelial progenitor cells; HA, hyaluronic acid; hASCs, human adipose-derived stem cells; hBMMSCs, human bone marrow-derived mesenchymal stem cells; hCPC, human cardiac progenitor cells; hDFBs, human dermal fibroblasts; hDMECs, human dermal microvascular endothelial cells; HepG2, human hepatocellular carcinoma; hMSCs, human mesenchymal stem cells; hSKMCs, human skeletal muscle cells; hTMSCs, human turbinate-derived mesenchymal stem cells; iPSC, human-induced pluripotent stem cell; RPTECs, renal proximal tubular epithelial cells; SF, silk fibroin.*

has been combined with bone marrow stromal [155] or adipose-derived stem [163] cells to develop bone-mimicking constructs using 3D printing. Independent of the type of cells composing the bioink, the dECM-containing constructs had enhanced the expression of osteogenic markers, such as osteocalcin, and alkaline phosphatase [155,163]. In constructs that attempt at mimicking the bone–tendon interface, respectively, using bone and tendon sol-dECM bioinks, the latter also lead to enhanced expression of tenogenic markers [155]. Furthermore, bone sol-dECM was methacrylated and combined with alginate, yielding a construct with not only enhanced mechanical properties post-printing but also an increased ability to support matrix mineralization along the culture [163].

The 3D printing of constructs with chondrogenic potential has resorted to the use of sol-dECM obtained from cartilage with materials such as silk fibroin [158], alginate [130], and bone marrow stromal cells. The incorporation of sol-dECM further triggered the expression of chondrogenic markers such as Transcription factor (SOX-9) and Aggrecan (ACAN) [130,158] and promoted the secretion of collagens and GAGs [130]. Similarly, a higher degree of maturation of auricular chondrocytes and enhanced secretion of collagen and GAGs were observed in constructs printed from methacrylated cartilage sol-dECM/gelatin/hyaluronic acid ink when compared to gelatin methacryloyl (GelMA)-based ones [128]. While skin is a multilayer tissue combining different independent appendages, which would highly benefit from 3D printing, this technology has been mostly used to generate the dermal component [167,168]. In agreement, dermal ECM has been shown to induce the expression of genes involved in biological processes of skin development, such as "positive regulation of keratinocyte migration – (GO:0051549)" in bone marrow stromal cells [153]. When combined with human dermal fibroblasts (hDFBs), sol-dECM allowed to fabricate stable dermal constructs with increased deposition of collagen I, while avoiding the deformation usually observed with typical skin collagen-based organotypic models. Moreover, it supported the development of a thicker and more stratified upper epidermal layer [154].

To replicate constituents of the circulatory system, researchers have developed heart sol-dECM-based bioinks with inherent cardiovascular [153,159,164] and angiogenic [159] potential. Cardiac progenitor cells loaded within sol-dECM/GelMA bioinks showed enhanced cardiac differentiation through increased expression of Myocyte-specific enhancer factor 2C (MEF2C), Connexin 43 (Cx43), and myosin heavy chain 7 (MYH7) and decreased expression of GATA Binding Protein 4 (GATA4), when compared to GelMA [159]. Interestingly, collecting the conditioned media from cells cultured in the sol-dECM/GelMA or GelMA constructs and supplementing human umbilical vein endothelial cells showed an increase in the angiogenic effect in the sol-dECM-enriched condition. Additionally, the influence of sol-dECM/GelMA composite in the differentiation of induced pluripotent stem cell (iPSC)-derived cardiomyocytes was assessed, with the authors stating an upregulation of the early cardiac transcription factor Tachykinin receptor 2 (NK2) homeobox 5 and a significantly higher expression of both mature markers such as myosin regulatory light chain 2 and troponin T when compared to collagen control [164]. Mimicking the aortic vessel has also been sought out by encapsulating endothelial progenitor cells in an amalgam of alginate, poly(lactic-co-glycolic acid) (PLGA) microspheres, and aortic sol-dECM [149]. Herein, it was possible to increase both the proliferation rate and the expression of endothelial markers, such as platelet/endothelial cell adhesion molecule 1 (CD31), vascular endothelial (VE)-cadherin, and von Willebrand factor, in sol-dECM-containing constructs.

In more specialized tissues, such as cornea, most of its functionality relies on specific structural requirements such as its transparency [169,170]. This was indeed achieved when cornea sol-dECM was combined with turbinate-derived mesenchymal stem cells to fabricate a cornea substitute [157]. Moreover, in the presence of cornea sol-dECM increased expression of representative markers of the cornea stromal layer, such as keratocan, was achieved when compared to collagen controls. Interestingly, an upregulation of the expression of genes associated with biological processes involved in both the development and function of the eye was reported in bone marrow-derived stem cells within cornea sol-dECM-based constructs [153].

Although the direct link between ECM and the secretory functions of certain organs is not straightforward, sol-dECM has been used to fabricate constructs supporting that ability in hepatic [153,160,161,164] and pancreatic [162] cells. Sol-dECM obtained from liver tissue was able to enhance the secretion of albumin from iPSC-derived hepatocytes [160], mouse primary hepatocytes [152], and hepatoma G2 (HepG2) cells [161], while pancreas-extracted sol-dECM supported the secretory function of pancreatic islets and iPSC-derived insulin-producing cells [162]. In addition to the secretion of insulin, the pancreatic islets showed significantly higher levels of glucose-stimulated index, and the iPSC-derived cells had an increased expression of nuclear transcription factors that are characteristic of adult human beta cells and secreting genes [162].

In other organs, the replication of their complexity or the multiple tissues that comprise them have not been the focus. In turn, the whole organ ECM has been used to fabricate specific compartments/tissues assuming the role of the neighboring ECM in any resident cells. For instance, kidney-derived dECM/alginate was combined with human umbilical vein endothelial cells or renal proximal tubular epithelial cells, respectively, to fabricate the vascular and tubular components of the renal parenchyma, using coaxial deposition [156]. When compared to collagen structures, these cells overexpressed their specific markers, such as CD31/VE-cadherin and aquaporin-1/organic cation transporter 2 (OCT2), respectively.

In summary, despite being originated from virtually every tissue, currently available dECM-based bioinks are relatively elementary in their ultimate composition: a gelatinized, collagenous mesh loaded with site-specific cells. This straightforward conjugate of sol-dECM with resident cells still does not represent the level of complexity found in tissues and organs. Moreover, the reported results for these methodologies only describe basic cellular responses and are focused on a few biological outcomes, with minimal assessment of more complex native tissue functions or overall level of maturation.

REFERENCES

1. Rosso F, Giordano A, Barbarisi M, Barbarisi A. From cell-ECM interactions to tissue engineering. *J Cell Physiol.* 2004;199(2):174–80.
2. Garreta E, Oria R, Tarantino C, Pla-Roca M, Prado P, Fernández-Avilés F, et al. Tissue engineering by decellularization and 3D bioprinting. *Mater Today.* 2017;20(4):166–78.

3. Hussey GS, Dziki JL, Badylak SF. Extracellular matrix-based materials for regenerative medicine. *Nat Rev Mater.* 2018;3(7):159–73.
4. Bosman FT, Stamenkovic I. Functional structure and composition of the extracellular matrix. *J Pathol.* 2003;200(4):423–8. Available from: https://onlinelibrary.wiley.com/doi/full/10.1002/path.1437
5. Mecham RP, Engel J, Chiquet M. The Extracellular Matrix: An Overview. In: Mecham RP, editor. *Biology of Extracellular Matrix* . Heidelberg: Springer Berlin 2011, pp. XIV, 426.
6. Mckee J, Perlman G, Morris M, Komarova S V. Extracellular matrix composition of connective tissues: A systematic review and meta-analysis. *Sci Rep.* 2019;9(1):10542. Available from: https://doi.org/10.1038/s41598-019-46896-0
7. Huang AH, Balestrini JL, Udelsman B V., Zhou KC, Zhao L, Ferruzzi J, et al. Biaxial stretch improves elastic fiber maturation, collagen arrangement, and mechanical properties in engineered arteries. *Tissue Eng Part C Methods.* 2016;22(6):524–33. Available from: http://online.liebertpub.com/doi/10.1089/ten.tec.2015.0309
8. O'brien FJ. Biomaterials & scaffolds for tissue engineering. *Mater Today.* 2011;14(3):88–95.
9. Place ES, Evans ND, Stevens MM. Complexity in biomaterials for tissue engineering. *Nat Mater.* 2009;8(6):457–70. Available from: http://dx.doi.org/10.1038/nmat2441
10. Kokkinis D, Bouville F, Studart AR. 3D printing of materials with tunable failure via bioinspired mechanical gradients. *Adv Mater.* 2018;30(19):1–9.
11. Wei TS, Ahn BY, Grotto J, Lewis JA. 3D printing of customized li-ion batteries with thick electrodes. *Adv Mater.* 2018;30(16):1–7.
12. Kirchmajer DM, Gorkin R, In Het Panhuis M. An overview of the suitability of hydrogel-forming polymers for extrusion-based 3D-printing. *J Mater Chem B.* 2015;3(20):4105–17.
13. Mobaraki M, Ghaffari M, Yazdanpanah A, Luo Y, Mills DK. Bioinks and bioprinting: A focused review. *Bioprinting.* 2020;18(August 2019):e00080. Available from: https://doi.org/10.1016/j.bprint.2020.e00080
14. Xu ZY, Huang JJ, Liu Y, Chen CW, Qu GW, Wang GF, et al. Extracellular matrix bioink boosts stemness and facilitates transplantation of intestinal organoids as a biosafe Matrigel alternative. *Bioeng Transl Med.* 2022;8(1):e10327. Available from: https://onlinelibrary.wiley.com/doi/full/10.1002/btm2.10327
15. Rao Y, Zhu C, Suen HC, Huang S, Liao J, Fei D, et al. Tenogenic induction of human adipose-derived stem cells by soluble tendon extracellular matrix: Composition and transcriptomic analyses. *Stem Cell Res Ther.* 2022;13(1):1–21. Available from: https://stemcellres.biomedcentral.com/articles/10.1186/s13287-022-03038-0
16. Reis DP, Domingues B, Fidalgo C, Reis RL, Gasperini L, Marques AP. Bioinks enriched with ECM components obtained by supercritical extraction. *Biomolecules.* 2022;12(3):1–15.
17. Chouhan D, Lohe T, Samudrala PK, Mandal BB. In situ forming injectable silk fibroin hydrogel promotes skin regeneration in full thickness burn wounds. *Adv Healthc Mater.* 2018;1801092:1–15.
18. Pati F, Ha DH, Jang J, Han HH, Rhie JW, Cho DW. Biomimetic 3D tissue printing for soft tissue regeneration. *Biomaterials.* 2015;62:164–75.
19. Choi Y-J, Jun Y-J, Kim DY, Yi HG, Chae SH, Kang J, et al. A 3D cell printed muscle construct with tissue-derived bioink for the treatment of volumetric muscle loss. *Biomaterials.* 2019;206(February):160–9. Available from: https://linkinghub.elsevier.com/retrieve/pii/S0142961219301863
20. Wainwright JM, Czajka CA, Patel UB, Freytes DO, Tobita K, Gilbert TW, et al. Preparation of cardiac extracellular matrix from an intact porcine heart. *Tissue Eng Part C Methods.* 2010;16(3):525–32. Available from: http://www.liebertonline.com/doi/abs/10.1089/ten.tec.2009.0392

21. Kim BS, Das S, Jang J, Cho DW. Decellularized extracellular matrix-based bioinks for engineering tissue- and organ-specific microenvironments. *Chem Rev.* 2020;120(19):10608–61.
22. Gorroñogoitia I, Urtaza U, Zubiarrain-laserna A, Alonso-varona A, Zaldua AM. A study of the printability of alginate-based bioinks by 3D bioprinting for articular cartilage tissue engineering. *Polymers (Basel).* 2022;14(2):354.
23. Lee SC, Gillispie G, Prim P, Lee SJ. Physical and chemical factors influencing the printability of hydrogel-based extrusion bioinks. *Chem Rev.* 2020;120(19):10834–86.
24. Nyström A, Bruckner-Tuderman L. Matrix molecules and skin biology. *Semin Cell Dev Biol.* 2018;89:136–46. Available from: https://www.sciencedirect.com/science/article/pii/S1084952118301046
25. Sorushanova A, Delgado LM, Wu Z, Shologu N, Kshirsagar A, Raghunath R, et al. The collagen suprafamily: From biosynthesis to advanced biomaterial development. *Adv Mater.* 2018;31(1):1801651. Available from: https://doi.org/10.1002/adma.201801651
26. Bell JS, Hayes S, Whitford C, Sanchez-weatherby J, Shebanova O, Terrill NJ, et al. Tropocollagen springs allow collagen fibrils to stretch elastically. *Acta Biomater.* 2022;141:185–93. Available from: https://doi.org/10.1016/j.actbio.2022.01.041
27. Karsdal MA, Leeming DJ, Henriksen K, Bay-Jensen AC. Biochemistry of Collagens, Laminins and Elastin. In: Morten A. Karsdal, editor. *Structure, Function and Biomarkers*; Nordic Bioscience, Herlev, Denmark and Southern Danish University, Odense, Denmark: Elsevier Inc; 2016. pp. 1–238.
28. Raghunath M, Bruckner P, Steinmann B. Delayed triple helix formation of mutant collagen from patients with osteogenesis imperfecta. *J Mol Biol.* 1994 Feb;236(3):940–9.
29. Engel J, Prockop DJ. The zipper-like folding of collagen triple helices and the effects of mutations that disrupt the zipper. *Annu Rev Biophys Biophys Chem.* 1991;20:137–52.
30. Sebastiano V, Zhen HH, Derafshi BH, Bashkirova E, Melo SP, Wang P, et al. Human COL7A1-corrected induced pluripotent stem cells for the treatment of recessive dystrophic epidermolysis bullosa. *Sci Transl Med.* 2014;6(264):264ra163.
31. D'hondt S, Guillemyn B, Syx D, Symoens S, De Rycke R, Vanhoutte L, et al. Type III collagen affects dermal and vascular collagen fibrillogenesis and tissue integrity in a mutant Col3a1 transgenic mouse model. *Matrix Biol.* 2018 Sep;70(C):72–83.
32. Varki R, Sadowski S, Uitto J, Pfendner E. Epidermolysis bullosa. II. Type VII collagen mutations and phenotype–genotype correlations in the dystrophic subtypes. *J Med Genet.* 2007 Mar;44(3):181.
33. Rodén L. Structure and Metabolism of Connective Tissue Proteoglycans. In: Lennarz WJ, editor. *The Biochemistry of Glycoproteins and Proteoglycans.* Boston, MA: Springer US; 1980. pp. 267–371. Available from: https://doi.org/10.1007/978-1-4684-1006-8_7
34. Lindahl U, Hook M. Glycosaminoglycans and their binding to biological macromolecules. *Annu Rev Biochem.* 1978 Jun 1;47(1):385–417. Available from: https://doi.org/10.1146/annurev.bi.47.070178.002125
35. Malmström A, Bartolini B, Thelin MA, Pacheco B, Maccarana M. Iduronic acid in chondroitin/dermatan sulfate: Biosynthesis and biological function. *J Histochem Cytochem.* 2012 Aug;60(12):916–25.
36. Iozzo R. Matrix proteoglycans: From molecular design to cellular function. *Annu Rev Biochem.* 1998;67(1):609–52. Available from: https://www.researchgate.net/publication/13525551
37. Couchman JR, Pataki CA. An introduction to proteoglycans and their localization. *J Histochem Cytochem.* 2012;60(12):885–97. Available from: https://journals.sagepub.com/doi/full/10.1369/0022155412464638

38. Schaefer L, Tredup C, Gubbiotti MA, Iozzo R V. Proteoglycan neofunctions: Regulation of inflammation and autophagy in cancer biology. *FEBS J*; 2017;284:10–26. Available from: https://febs.onlinelibrary.wiley.com/doi/10.1111/febs.13963
39. Frey H, Schroeder N, Manon-Jensen T, Iozzo R V, Schaefer L. Biological interplay between proteoglycans and their innate immune receptors in inflammation Helena. *FEBS J.* 2013;280(10):10–26. Available from: https://febs.onlinelibrary.wiley.com/doi/10.1111/febs.12145
40. Urry DW, Hugel T, Seitz M, Gaub HE, Sheiba L, Dea J, et al. Elastin: A representative ideal protein elastomer. *Philos Trans R Soc B Biol Sci.* 2002;357(1418):169–84.
41. Kagan HM, Li W. Lysyl oxidase: Properties, specificity, and biological roles inside and outside of the cell. *J Cell Biochem.* 2003;88(4):660–72.
42. Liu X, Zhao Y, Gao J, Pawlyk B, Starcher B, Spencer JA, et al. Elastic fiber homeostasis requires lysyl oxidase-like 1 protein. *Nat Genet.* 2004;36(2):178–82.
43. Urry DW, Pattanaik A, Xu J, Woods TC, Mc Pherson DT, Parker TM. Elastic protein-based polymers in soft tissue augmentation and generation. *J Biomater Sci Polym Ed.* 1998;9(10):1015–48.
44. Sato F, Wachi H, Starcher BC, Seyama Y. Biochemical analysis of elastic fiber formation with a frameshift-mutated tropoelastin (fmTE) at the C-terminus of tropoelastin. *J Heal Sci.* 2006 May;52(3):259–67.
45. Li B, Daggett V. Molecular basis for the extensibility of elastin. *J Muscle Res Cell Motil.* 2002;23(5):561–73. Available from: https://doi.org/10.1023/A:1023474909980
46. Karamanos NK, Theocharis AD, Piperigkou Z, Manou D, Passi A, Skandalis SS, et al. A guide to the composition and functions of the extracellular matrix. *FEBS J.* 2021;288(24):6850–912.
47. Andrew K. Baldwin, Simpson A, Steer R, Cain SA, Kielty CM. Elastic fibres in health and disease. *Expert Rev Mol Med.* 2006;8(19):1–23.
48. Vogel V. Unraveling the mechanobiology of extracellular matrix. *Ann Rev Physiol.* 2018;80:353–87. Available from: https://www.annualreviews.org/doi/abs/10.1146/annurev-physiol-021317-121312
49. Mansour A, Mezour MA, Badran Z, Tamimi F. Extracellular matrices for bone regeneration: A literature review. *Tissue Eng Part A.* 2017;23(23–24):1436–51. Available from: https://www.liebertpub.com/doi/10.1089/ten.tea.2017.0026
50. Mow VC, Holmes MH, Michael Lai W. Fluid transport and mechanical properties of articular cartilage: A review. *J Biomech.* 1984;17(5):377–94.
51. Sophia Fox AJ, Bedi A, Rodeo SA. The basic science of articular cartilage: Structure, composition, and function. *Sports Health.* 2009 Nov 1;1(6):461–8. Available from: https://doi.org/10.1177/1941738109350438
52. Gentili/snm C, Cancedda R. Cartilage and bone extracellular matrix. *Curr Pharm Des.* 2009 Mar 31;15(12):1334–48.
53. Cerqueira MT, Pirraco RP, Santos TC, Rodrigues DB, Frias AM, Martins AR, et al. Human Adipose Stem Cells Cell Sheet Constructs impact epidermal morphogenesis in full-thickness excisional wounds. *Biomacromolecules.* 2013;14:3997–4008. Available from: http://pubs.acs.org/doi/abs/10.1021/bm4011062
54. Malta MD, Cerqueira MT, Marques AP. Extracellular matrix in skin diseases: The road to new therapies. *J Adv Res.* 2022; Available from: http://www.ncbi.nlm.nih.gov/pubmed/36481476
55. Gillies AR, Lieber RL. Structure and function of the skeletal muscle extracellular matrix. *Muscle Nerve.* 2011;44:318–31. Available from: https://onlinelibrary.wiley.com/doi/10.1002/mus.22094
56. Bendall JR. The elastin content of various muscles of beef animals. *J Sci Food Agric.* 1967;18(12):553–8. Available from: https://sci-hub.se/10.1002/jsfa.2740181201

57. Dransfield E. Intramuscular composition and texture of beef muscles. *J Sci Food Agric.* 1977;28(9):833–42. Available from: https://onlinelibrary.wiley.com/doi/full/10.1002/jsfa.2740280910
58. Järvinen TAH, Józsa L, Kannus P, Järvinen TLN, Järvinen M. Organization and distribution of intramuscular connective tissue in normal and immobilized skeletal muscles. An immunohistochemical, polarization and scanning electron microscopic study. *J Muscle Res Cell Motil.* 2002;23(3):245–54. Available from: https://pubmed.ncbi.nlm.nih.gov/12500904/
59. Turrina A, Martínez-González MA, Stecco C. The muscular force transmission system: Role of the intramuscular connective tissue. *J Bodyw Mov Ther.* 2013 Jan;17(1):95–102.
60. Purslow PP, Trotter JA. The morphology and mechanical properties endomysium in series-fibred muscles: variations with muscle length. *J Muscle Res Cell Motil.* 1994;15(3):299–308.
61. Gilbert TW, Sellaro TL, Badylak SF. Decellularization of tissues and organs. *Biomaterials.* 2006;27(19):3675–83.
62. Arenas-Herrera JE, Ko IK, Atala A, Yoo JJ. Decellularization for whole organ bioengineering. *Biomed Mater.* 2013;8(1):014106.
63. Schneider C, Lehmann J, Van Osch GJVM, Hildner F, Teuschl A, Monforte X, et al. Systematic comparison of protocols for the preparation of human articular cartilage for use as scaffold material in cartilage tissue engineering. *Tissue Eng Part C Methods.* 2016;22(12):1095–107. Available from: https://www.liebertpub.com/doi/10.1089/ten.tec.2016.0380
64. Willemse J, Verstegen MMA, Vermeulen A, Schurink IJ, Roest HP, van der Laan LJW, et al. Fast, robust and effective decellularization of whole human livers using mild detergents and pressure controlled perfusion. *Mater Sci Eng C.* 2020 Mar 1;108: 110200.
65. Crapo PM, Gilbert TW, Badylak DVM. An overview of tissue and whole organ decellularization processes. *Biomaterials.* 2011;32(12):3233–43.
66. Farrokhi A, Pakyari M, Nabai L, Pourghadiri A, Hartwell R, Jalili RB, et al. Evaluation of detergent-free and detergent-based methods for decellularization of murine skin. *Tissue Eng Part A.* 2018;24(11–12):955–67. Available from: http://www.ncbi.nlm.nih.gov/pubmed/29303417%0Ahttp://online.liebertpub.com/doi/10.1089/ten.TEA.2017.0273
67. Moore MA, Samsell B, Wallis G, Triplett S, Chen S, Jones AL, et al. Decellularization of human dermis using non-denaturing anionic detergent and endonuclease: A review. *Cell Tissue Bank.* 2015;16(2):249–59. Available from: https://link.springer.com/article/10.1007/s10561-014-9467-4
68. Arechabala B, Coiffard C, Rivalland P, Coiffard LJM, De Roeck-Holtzhauer Y. Comparison of cytotoxicity of various surfactants tested on normal human fibroblast cultures using the neutral red test, MTT assay and LDH release. *J Appl Toxicol.* 1999;19(3):163–5.
69. Fernández-Pérez J, Ahearne M. The impact of decellularization methods on extracellular matrix derived hydrogels. *Sci Rep* [Internet]. 2019;9(1):1–12. Available from: https://www.nature.com/articles/s41598-019-49575-2
70. Seo Y, Jung Y, Kim SH. Decellularized heart ECM hydrogel using supercritical carbon dioxide for improved angiogenesis. *Acta Biomater.* 2018;67:270–81. Available from: https://doi.org/10.1016/j.actbio.2017.11.046
71. Sikorska E, Wyrzykowski D, Szutkowski K, Greber K, Lubecka EA, Zhukov I. Thermodynamics, size, and dynamics of zwitterionic dodecylphosphocholine and anionic sodium dodecyl sulfate mixed micelles. *J Therm Anal Calorim.* 2016;123(1):511–23. Available from: https://link.springer.com/article/10.1007/s10973-015-4918-0
72. Hudson TW, Zawko S, Deister C, Lundy S, Hu CY, Lee K, et al. Optimized acellular nerve graft is immunologically tolerated and supports regeneration. *Tissue Eng.*

2004;10(11–12):1641–51. Available from: https://www.liebertpub.com/doi/10.1089/ten.2004.10.1641

73. Hudson TW, Zawko S, Deister C, Lundy S, Hu CY, Lee K, et al. Engineering an improved acellular nerve graft via optimized chemical processing. *Tissue Eng.* 2004;10(9–10):1641–51. Available from: https://pubmed.ncbi.nlm.nih.gov/15588395/
74. Al-Hejailan R, Weigel T, Schürlein S, Berger C, Al-Mohanna F, Hansmann J. Decellularization of full heart – Optimizing the classical sodium-dodecyl-sulfate-based decellularization protocol. *Bioengineering.* 2022;9(4):147. Available from: https://www.mdpi.com/2306-5354/9/4/147/htm
75. Sánchez PL, Fernández-Santos ME, Costanza S, Climent AM, Moscoso I, Gonzalez-Nicolas MA, et al. Acellular human heart matrix: A critical step toward whole heart grafts. *Biomaterials.* 2015 Aug 1;61:279–89.
76. Daneshgar A, Klein O, Nebrich G, Weinhart M, Tang P, Arnold A, et al. The human liver matrisome – Proteomic analysis of native and fibrotic human liver extracellular matrices for organ engineering approaches. *Biomaterials.* 2020 Oct 1;257: 120247.
77. Jorgensen AM, Chou Z, Gillispie G, Lee SJ, Yoo JJ, Soker S, et al. Decellularized skin extracellular matrix (dsECM) improves the physical and biological properties of fibrinogen hydrogel for skin bioprinting applications. *Nanomaterials.* 2020;10(8):1484.
78. Antons J, Marascio MGM, Aeberhard P, Weissenberger G, Hirt-Burri N, Applegate LA, et al. Decellularised tissues obtained by a CO_2-Philic detergent and supercritical CO_2. *Eur Cells Mater.* 2018;36:81–95.
79. Brouki Milan P, Pazouki A, Joghataei MT, Mozafari M, Amini N, Kargozar S, et al. Decellularization and preservation of human skin: A platform for tissue engineering and reconstructive surgery. *Methods.* 2020 Jan 15;171: 62–7.
80. Turner AEB, Yu C, Bianco J, Watkins JF, Flynn LE. The performance of decellularized adipose tissue microcarriers as an inductive substrate for human adipose-derived stem cells. *Biomaterials.* 2012 Jun 1;33(18):4490–9.
81. Omidi E, Fuetterer L, Reza Mousavi S, Armstrong RC, Flynn LE, Samani A. Characterization and assessment of hyperelastic and elastic properties of decellularized human adipose tissues. *J Biomech.* 2014 Nov 28;47(15):3657–63.
82. Reyna WE, Pichika R, Ludvig D, Perreault EJ. Efficiency of skeletal muscle decellularization methods and their effects on the extracellular matrix. *J Biomech.* 2020;110:109961. Available from: https://doi.org/10.1016/j.jbiomech.2020.109961
83. Naik A, Griffin MF, Szarko M, Butler PE. Optimizing the decellularization process of human maxillofacial muscles for facial reconstruction using a detergent-only approach. *J Tissue Eng Regen Med.* 2019;13(9):1571–80. Available from: https://onlinelibrary.wiley.com/doi/full/10.1002/term.2910
84. Takami Y, Matsuda T, Yoshitake M, Hanumadass M, Walter RJ. Dispase/detergent treated dermal matrix as a dermal substitute. *Burns.* 1996;22(3):182–90.
85. Dziki JL, Wang DS, Pineda C, Sicari BM, Rausch T, Badylak SF. Solubilized extracellular matrix bioscaffolds derived from diverse source tissues differentially influence macrophage phenotype. *J Biomed Mater Res Part A.* 2017 Jan 1;105(1):138–47.
86. Nowocin AK, Southgate A, Gabe SM, Ansari T. Biocompatibility and potential of decellularized porcine small intestine to support cellular attachment and growth. *J Tissue Eng Regen Med.* 2016 Jan 1;10(1):E23–33.
87. Cui H, Chai Y, Yu Y. Progress in developing decellularized bioscaffolds for enhancing skin construction. *J Biomed Mater Res Part A.* 2019 Aug 1;107(8):1849–59.
88. Al-Qurayshi Z, Wafa EI, Meyer MKR, Owen S, Salem AK. Tissue engineering the pinna: Comparison and characterization of human decellularized auricular biological scaffolds. *ACS Appl Bio Mater.* 2021;4(9):7234–42. Available from: https://doi.org/10.1021/acsabm.1c00766

89. McFetridge PS, Daniel JW, Bodamyali T, Horrocks M, Chaudhuri JB. Preparation of porcine carotid arteries for vascular tissue engineering applications. *J Biomed Mater Res Part A.* 2004;70A(2):224–34. Available from: https://onlinelibrary.wiley.com/doi/full/10.1002/jbm.a.30060
90. Schenke-Layland K, Vasilevski O, Opitz F, König K, Riemann I, Halbhuber KJ, et al. Impact of decellularization of xenogeneic tissue on extracellular matrix integrity for tissue engineering of heart valves. *J Struct Biol.* 2003 Sep 1;143(3):201–8.
91. Stenn KS, Link R, Moellmann G, Madri J, Kuklinska E. Dispase, a neutral protease from *Bacillus polymyxa*, is a powerful fibronectinase and type IV collagenase. *J Invest Dermatol.* 1989;93(2):287–90.
92. Shiokawa D, Tanuma SI. Characterization of human DNase I family endonucleases and activation of DNase γ during apoptosis. *Biochemistry.* 2001;40(1):143–52. Available from: https://pubs.acs.org/sharingguidelines
93. Wang Z, Sun F, Lu Y, Pan S, Yang W, Zhang G, et al. Rapid preparation of decellularized trachea as a 3D scaffold for organ engineering. *Int J Artif Organs.* 2021;44(1):55–64.
94. Wang Z, Sun F, Lu Y, Zhang B, Zhang G, Shi H. Rapid preparation method for preparing tracheal Decellularized scaffolds: Vacuum assistance and optimization of DNase I. *ACS Omega.* 2021;6(16):10637–44.
95. Shirakigawa N, Ijima H, Takei T. Decellularized liver as a practical scaffold with a vascular network template for liver tissue engineering. *J Biosci Bioeng.* 2012;114(5):546–51.
96. Balasubramanian SK, Bischof JC, Hubel A. Water transport and IIF parameters for a connective tissue equivalent. *Cryobiology.* 2006;52(1):62–73.
97. Mazur P. Freezing of living cells: Mechanisms and implications. *Am J Physiol Physiol.* 1984;247(3):C125–42. Available from: http://www.physiology.org/doi/10.1152/ajpcell.1984.247.3.C125
98. Smith CA, Board TN, Rooney P, Eagle MJ, Richardson SM, Hoyland JA. Human decellularized bone scaffolds from aged donors show improved osteoinductive capacity compared to young donor bone. *PLoS One.* 2017 May 1;12(5):e0187783.
99. Smith CA, Richardson SM, Eagle MJ, Rooney P, Board T, Hoyland JA. The use of a novel bone allograft wash process to generate a biocompatible, mechanically stable and osteoinductive biological scaffold for use in bone tissue engineering. *J Tissue Eng Regen Med.* 2015;9(5):595–604. Available from: https://onlinelibrary.wiley.com/doi/full/10.1002/term.1934
100. Ling Y, Xu W, Yang L, Liang C, Xu B. Improved the biocompatibility of cancellous bone with compound physicochemical decellularization process. *Regen Biomater.* 2020;7(5):443–51. Available from: https://academic.oup.com/rb/article/7/5/443/5899252
101. Gardin C, Ricci S, Ferroni L, Guazzo R, Sbricoli L, De Benedictis G, et al. Decellularization and delipidation protocols of bovine bone and pericardium for bone grafting and guided bone regeneration procedures. *PLoS One.* 2015;10(7):e0132344.
102. Tao M, Liang F, He J, Ye W, Javed R, Wang W, et al. Decellularized tendon matrix membranes prevent post-surgical tendon adhesion and promote functional repair. *Acta Biomater.* 2021;134:160–76. Available from: https://doi.org/10.1016/j.actbio.2021.07.038
103. Burk J, Erbe I, Berner D, Kacza J, Kasper C, Pfeiffer B, et al. Freeze-thaw cycles enhance decellularization of large tendons. *Tissue Eng Part C Methods.* 2014;20(4):276–84. Available from: http://online.liebertpub.com/doi/abs/10.1089/ten.tec.2012.0760
104. Daryabari SS, Fendereski K, Ghorbani F, Dehnavi M, Shafikhani Y, Omranipour A, et al. Whole-organ decellularization of the human uterus and in vivo application of the bio-scaffolds in animal models. *J Assist Reprod Genet.* 2022;39(6):1237–47. Available from: https://link.springer.com/article/10.1007/s10815-022-02492-2

105. Lin CH, Hsia K, Su CK, Chen CC, Yeh CC, Ma H, et al. Sonication-assisted method for decellularization of human umbilical artery for small-caliber vascular tissue engineering. *Polymers (Basel).* 2021 May;13(11):1699.
106. Syazwani N, Azhim A, Morimoto Y, Furukawa KS, Ushida T. Decellularization of aorta tissue using sonication treatment as potential scaffold for vascular tissue engineering. *J Med Biol Eng.* 2015;35(2):258–69. Available from: https://doi.org/10.1007/s40846-015-0028-5
107. Koo MA, Jeong H, Hong SH, Seon GM, Lee MH, Park JC. Preconditioning process for dermal tissue decellularization using electroporation with sonication. *Regen Biomater.* 2022 Jan 1;9:rbab071. Available from: https://doi.org/10.1093/rb/rbab071
108. Guler S, Aslan B, Hosseinian P, Aydin HM. Supercritical carbon dioxide-assisted decellularization of aorta and cornea. *Tissue Eng Part C Methods.* 2017;23(9):540–7. Available from: http://online.liebertpub.com/doi/10.1089/ten.tec.2017.0090
109. Halfwerk FR, Rouwkema J, Gossen JA, Grandjean JG. Supercritical carbon dioxide decellularised pericardium: Mechanical and structural characterisation for applications in cardio-thoracic surgery. *J Mech Behav Biomed Mater.* 2018;77(September 2017):400–7. Available from: http://dx.doi.org/10.1016/j.jmbbm.2017.10.002
110. Kankala RK, Zhang YS, Wang S Bin, Lee CH, Chen AZ. Supercritical fluid technology: An emphasis on drug delivery and related biomedical applications. *Adv Healthc Mater.* 2017;6(16):1700433.
111. Teoh WH, Mammucari R, Foster NR. Solubility of organometallic complexes in supercritical carbon dioxide: A review. *J Organomet Chem.* 2013;724:102–16. Available from: http://dx.doi.org/10.1016/j.jorganchem.2012.10.005
112. Sawada K, Terada D, Yamaoka T, Kitamura S, Fujisato T. Cell removal with supercritical carbon dioxide for acellular artificial tissue. *J Chem Technol Biotechnol.* 2008;83(May):1163–9.
113. Casali DM, Handleton RM, Shazly T, Matthews MA. A novel supercritical CO_2-based decellularization method for maintaining scaffold hydration and mechanical properties. *J Supercrit Fluids.* 2018 Jan 1;131:72–81.
114. Kawecki M, Łabuś W, Klama-Baryla A, Kitala D, Kraut M, Glik J, et al. A review of decellurization methods caused by an urgent need for quality control of cell-free extracellular matrix' scaffolds and their role in regenerative medicine. *J Biomed Mater Res Part B Appl Biomater.* 2018;106(2):909–23.
115. Hsiong S, Huber A, Kullas KE, Tottey S, Badylak SF. The effects of processing methods upon mechanical and biologic properties of porcine dermal extracellular matrix scaffolds. *Biomaterials.* 2011;31(33):8626–33.
116. Remlinger NT, Czajka CA, Juhas ME, Vorp DA, Stolz DB, Badylak SF, et al. Hydrated xenogeneic decellularized tracheal matrix as a scaffold for tracheal reconstruction. *Biomaterials.* 2010;31(13):3520–6. Available from: http://dx.doi.org/10.1016/j.biomaterials.2010.01.067
117. Poon CJ, Cotta MVPE, Sinha S, Palmer JA, Woods AA, Morrison WA, et al. Preparation of an adipogenic hydrogel from subcutaneous adipose tissue. *Acta Biomater.* 2013;9(3):5609–20.
118. Uriel S, Huang JJ, Moya ML, Francis ME, Wang R, Chang S, et al. The role of adipose protein derived hydrogels in adipogenesis. *Biomaterials.* 2008;29(27):3712–9.
119. Freytes DO, Martin J, Velankar SS, Lee AS, Badylak SF. Preparation and rheological characterization of a gel form of the porcine urinary bladder matrix. *Biomaterials.* 2008;29(11):1630–7.
120. Qian J, Okada Y, Ogura T, Tanaka K, Hattori S, Ito S, et al. Kinetic analysis of the digestion of bovine type I collagen telopeptides with porcine pepsin. *J Food Sci.* 2016;81(1):C27–34. Available from: https://ift.onlinelibrary.wiley.com/doi/10.1111/1750-3841.13179

121. Parkinson J, Kadler KE, Brass A. Simple physical model of collagen fibrillogenesis based on diffusion limited aggregation. *J Mol Biol.* 1995 Apr 7;247(4):823–31.
122. Hulmes DJS. Collagen Diversity, Synthesis and Assembly. In: Fratzl P, editor. *Collagen: Structure and Mechanics.* Boston, MA: Springer US; 2008. pp. 15–47. Available from: https://doi.org/10.1007/978-0-387-73906-9_2
123. Koide T, Nagata K. Collagen Biosynthesis BT – Collagen: Primer in Structure, Processing and Assembly. In: Brinckmann J, Notbohm H, Müller PK, editors. *Collagen.* Berlin, Heidelberg: Springer Berlin Heidelberg; 2005. pp. 85–114. Available from: https://doi.org/10.1007/b103820
124. Jonker AM, Löwik DWPM, Van Hest JCM. Peptide-and protein-based hydrogels. *Chem Mater.* 2012;24(5):759–73.
125. Brightman AO, Rajwa BP, Sturgis JE, McCallister ME, Robinson JP, Voytik-Harbin SL. Time-lapse confocal reflection microscopy of collagen fibrillogenesis and extracellular matrix assembly in vitro. *Biopolymers.* 2000 Sep;54(3):222–34.
126. Saldin LT, Cramer MC, Velankar SS, White LJ, Badylak SF. Extracellular matrix hydrogels from decellularized tissues: Structure and function. *Acta Biomater.* 2017;49:1–15.
127. Kesti M, Eberhardt C, Pagliccia G, Kenkel D, Grande D, Boss A, et al. Bioprinting complex cartilaginous structures with clinically compliant biomaterials. *Adv Funct Mater.* 2015;25(48):7406–17.
128. Visscher DO, Lee H, van Zuijlen PPM, Helder MN, Atala A, Yoo JJ, et al. A photo-crosslinkable cartilage-derived extracellular matrix bioink for auricular cartilage tissue engineering. *Acta Biomater.* 2021 Feb 1;121: 193–203.
129. Ooi HW, Mota C, Cate AT, Calore A, Moroni L, Baker MB. Thiol – Ene alginate hydrogels as versatile bioinks for bioprinting. *Biomacromolecules.* 2018;19(8):3390–400.
130. Rathan S, Dejob L, Schipani R, Haffner B, Möbius ME, Kelly DJ. Fiber reinforced cartilage ECM functionalized bioinks for functional cartilage tissue engineering. *Adv Healthc Mater.* 2019;8(7):1–11.
131. Lim KS, Klotz BJ, Lindberg GCJ, Melchels FPW, Hooper GJ, Malda J, et al. Visible light cross-linking of gelatin hydrogels offers an enhanced cell microenvironment with improved light penetration depth. *Macromol Biosci.* 2019;19(6):1900098.
132. Noshadi I, Hong S, Sullivan KE, Sani ES, Portillo-Lara R, Tamayol A, et al. In vitro and in vivo analysis of visible light crosslinkable gelatin methacryloyl (GelMA) hydrogels. *Biomater Sci.* 2017;5(10):2093–105.
133. Liu Y, Wong CW, Chang SW, Hsu S. An injectable, self-healing phenol-functionalized chitosan hydrogel with fast gelling property and visible light-crosslinking capability for 3D printing. *Acta Biomater.* 2021;122:211–9.
134. Saini K. Preparation method, properties and crosslinking of hydrogel: A review. *PharmaTutor.* 2017;5(1):27–36.
135. Coutinho DF, Sant S V, Shin H, Oliveira JT, Gomes ME, Neves NM, et al. Modified Gellan Gum hydrogels with tunable physical and mechanical properties. *Biomaterials.* 2010;31(29):7494–502.
136. Ostrowska-Czubenko J, Gierszewska-Drużyńska M. Effect of ionic crosslinking on the water state in hydrogel chitosan membranes. *Carbohydr Polym.* 2009;77(3):590–8.
137. Wen C, Lu L, Li X. Mechanically robust gelatin–A lginate IPN hydrogels by a combination of enzymatic and ionic crosslinking approaches. *Macromol Mater Eng.* 2014;299(4):504–13.
138. Kabirian F, Mozafari M. Decellularized ECM-derived bioinks: Prospects for the future. *Methods.* 2020;171(April):108–18.
139. Dzobo K, Motaung KSCM, Adesida A. Recent trends in decellularized extracellular matrix bioinks for 3D printing: An updated review. *Int J Mol Sci.* 2019;20(18:4628.
140. Mironov V, Prestwich G, Forgacs G. Bioprinting living structures. *J Mater Chem.* 2007;17(20):2054–60.

141. Schwab A, Levato R, Este MD, Piluso S, Eglin D, Malda J. Printability and shape fidelity of bioinks in 3D bioprinting. *Chem Rev.* 2020;120(19):10850–77.
142. Derakhshanfar S, Mbeleck R, Xu K, Zhang X, Zhong W, Xing M. 3D bioprinting for biomedical devices and tissue engineering: A review of recent trends and advances. *Bioact Mater.* 2018;3(2):144–56. Available from: https://doi.org/10.1016/j.bioactmat.2017.11.008
143. Paxton N, Smolan W, Böck T, Melchels F, Groll J, Jungst T. Proposal to assess printability of bioinks for extrusion-based bioprinting and evaluation of rheological properties governing bioprintability. *Biofabrication.* 2017;9(4):044107.
144. He Y, Yang F, Zhao H, Gao Q, Xia B, Fu J. Research on the printability of hydrogels in 3D bioprinting. *Sci Rep.* 2016;6:1–13. Available from: http://dx.doi.org/10.1038/srep29977
145. Hölzl K, Lin S, Tytgat L, Van Vlierberghe S, Gu L, Ovsianikov A. Bioink properties before, during and after 3D bioprinting. *Biofabrication.* 2016;8(3):032002.
146. Murphy SV, Skardal A, Atala A. Evaluation of hydrogels for bio-printing applications. *J Biomed Mater Res Part A.* 2013;101A(1):272–84.
147. Wilson SA, Cross LM, Peak CW, Gaharwar AK. Shear-thinning and thermo-reversible nanoengineered inks for 3D bioprinting. *ACS Appl Mater Interfaces.* 2017;9(50):43449–58.
148. Curley CJ, Dolan EB, Otten M, Hinderer S, Duffy GP, Murphy BP. An injectable alginate/extra cellular matrix (ECM) hydrogel towards acellular treatment of heart failure. *Drug Deliv Transl Res.* 2019;9(1):1–13. Available from: https://doi.org/10.1007/s13346-018-00601-2.
149. Gao G, Lee JH, Jang J, Lee DH, Kong JS, Kim BS, et al. Tissue engineered bio-blood-vessels constructed using a tissue-specific bioink and 3D coaxial cell printing technique: A novel therapy for ischemic disease. *Adv Funct Mater.* 2017;27(33):1700798.
150. Mouser VHM, Melchels FPW, Visser J, Dhert WJA, Gawlitta D, Malda J. Yield stress determines bioprintability of hydrogels based on gelatin-methacryloyl and gellan gum for cartilage bioprinting. *Biofabrication.* 2016;8(3):1–24.
151. Akkineni AR, Ahlfeld T, Lode A, Gelinsky M. A versatile method for combining different biopolymers in a core/shell fashion by 3D plotting to achieve mechanically robust constructs. *Biofabrication.* 2016;8(4):1–15. Available from: http://dx.doi.org/10.1088/1758-5090/8/4/045001
152. Kim MK, Jeong W, Lee SM, Kim JB, Jin S, Kang HW. Decellularized extracellular matrix-based bio-ink with enhanced 3D printability and mechanical properties. *Biofabrication.* 2020;12(2):025003.
153. Han W, Singh NK, Kim JJ, Kim H, Kim BS, Park JY, et al. Directed differential behaviors of multipotent adult stem cells from decellularized tissue/organ extracellular matrix bioinks. *Biomaterials.* 2019;224(February):119496. Available from: https://doi.org/10.1016/j.biomaterials.2019.119496
154. Kim BS, Kwon YW, Kong J, Park GT, Gao G, Kim BS. 3D cell printing of in vitro stabilized skin model and in vivo pre-vascularized skin patch using tissue-specific extracellular matrix bioink: A step towards advanced skin tissue engineering. *Biomaterials.* 2018;168:38–53. Available from: https://doi.org/10.1016/j.biomaterials.2018.03.040
155. Chae S, Sun Y, Choi YJ, Ha DH, Jeon I, Cho DW. 3D cell-printing of tendon-bone interface using tissue-derived extracellular matrix bioinks for chronic rotator cuff repair. *Biofabrication.* 2021;13(3):10. Published 2021 Apr 2. Available from: https://doi.org/10.1088/1758-5090/abd159.
156. Singh NK, Han W, Nam SA, Kim JW, Kim JY, Kim YK, et al. Three-dimensional cell-printing of advanced renal tubular tissue analogue. *Biomaterials.* 2020;232(June 2019):119734. Available from: https://doi.org/10.1016/j.biomaterials.2019.119734

157. Kim H, Park MN, Kim J, Jang J, Kim HK, Cho DW. Characterization of cornea-specific bioink: High transparency, improved in vivo safety. J Tissue Eng. 2019;10: 2041731418823382. Published 2019 Jan 25. Available from: https://doi.org/10.1177/2041731418823382.
158. Zhang X, Liu Y, Luo C, Zhai C, Li Z, Zhang Y, et al. Crosslinker-free silk/decellularized extracellular matrix porous bioink for 3D bioprinting-based cartilage tissue engineering. *Mater Sci Eng C*. 2021;118(August 2020):111388. Available from: https://doi.org/10.1016/j.msec.2020.111388
159. Bejleri D, Streeter BW, Nachlas ALY, Brown ME, Gaetani R, Christman KL, et al. A bioprinted cardiac patch composed of cardiac-specific extracellular matrix and progenitor cells for heart repair. *Adv Healthc Mater*. 2018;7(23):1–13.
160. Mao Q, Wang Y, Li Y, Juengpanich S, Li W. Fabrication of liver microtissue with liver decellularized extracellular matrix (dECM) bioink by digital light processing (DLP) bioprinting. *Mater Sci Eng C*. 2020;109(August 2019):110625. Available from: https://doi.org/10.1016/j.msec.2020.110625
161. Lee H, Han W, Kim H, Ha DH, Jang J, Kim BS, et al. Development of liver decellularized extracellular matrix bioink for three-dimensional cell printing-based liver tissue engineering. *Biomacromolecules*. 2017;18(4):1229–37.
162. Kim J, Shim IK, Hwang DG, Lee YN, Kim M, Kim H, et al. 3D cell printing of islet-laden pancreatic tissue-derived extracellular matrix bioink constructs for enhancing pancreatic functions. *J Mater Chem B*. 2019;7(10):1773–81.
163. Lee J, Hong J, Kim WJ, Kim GH. Bone-derived dECM/alginate bioink for fabricating a 3D cell-laden mesh structure for bone tissue engineering. *Carbohydr Polym*. 2020;250:116914. Available from: https://doi.org/10.1016/j.carbpol.2020.116914
164. Yu C, Ma X, Zhu W, Wang P, Miller KL, Stupin J, et al. Scanningless and continuous 3D bioprinting of human tissues with decellularized extracellular matrix. *Biomaterials*. 2019;194(December 2018):1–13. Available from: https://doi.org/10.1016/j.biomaterials.2018.12.009
165. Piattelli A, Scarano A, Corigliano M, Piattelli M. Comparison of bone regeneration with the use of mineralized and demineralized freeze-dried bone allografts: A histological and histochemical study in man. *Biomaterials*. 1996 Jun 1;17(11):1127–31.
166. Castro-Ceseña AB, Novitskaya EE, Chen PY, Hirata GA, McKittrick J. Kinetic studies of bone demineralization at different HCl concentrations and temperatures. *Mater Sci Eng C*. 2011 Apr 8;31(3):523–30.
167. Kang MS, Kwon M, Lee SY, Lee SH, Jo HJ, Kim B, et al. In situ crosslinkable collagen-based hydrogels for 3D printing of dermis-mimetic constructs. *ECS J Solid State Sci Technol*. 2022;11(4):045014. Available from: https://iopscience.iop.org/article/10.1149/2162-8777/ac6897
168. Ng WL, Qi JTZ, Yeong WY, Naing MW. Proof-of-concept: 3D bioprinting of pigmented human skin constructs. *Biofabrication*. 2018;10(2):025005. Available from: http://stacks.iop.org/1758-5090/10/i=2/a=025005?key=crossref.7902e79941ef0af1941e16958babce0e
169. Hazra S, Nandi S, Naskar D, Guha R, Chowdhury S, Pradhan N, et al. Non-mulberry silk fibroin biomaterial for corneal regeneration. *Sci Rep*. 2016;6(1):1–13. Available from: https://www.nature.com/articles/srep21840
170. Gil ES, Mandal BB, Park SH, Marchant JK, Omenetto FG, Kaplan DL. Helicoidal multi-lamellar features of RGD-functionalized silk biomaterials for corneal tissue engineering. *Biomaterials*. 2010;31(34):8953–63. Available from: http://dx.doi.org/10.1016/j.biomaterials.2010.08.017

7 3D Bioprinting for Musculoskeletal Applications

Sandra Ruiz-Alonso, Fátima García-Villén, Ilia Villate-Beitia, Fouad Alhakim-Khalak, Jorge Ordoyo-Pascual, Lucía Enriquez-Rodríguez, Jon Zarate Sesma, Gustavo Puras Ochoa, Laura Saenz Del Burgo Martínez, and Jose Luis Pedraz Muñoz
University of the Basque Country (UPV/EHU)
Institute of Health Carlos III

CONTENTS

7.1 INTRODUCTION: BACKGROUND AND DRIVING FORCES

The anatomy of the musculoskeletal system includes bones, cartilages, ligaments, tendons, and muscles, which form the main architecture of the body and are necessary to provide stability and movement, with tendons connecting muscle to bone and ligaments binding bone to bone [1]. Therefore, the musculoskeletal system is essential for allowing locomotion and maintaining posture, as well as for other vital functions including the protection of organs and the regulation of many homeostatic functions such as the storage of minerals and hematopoiesis [2].

DOI: 10.1201/9781003274568-7

Nowadays, musculoskeletal disorders are the most important health problems worldwide. In fact, approximately 1.71 billion people globally are affected by them [3]. This prevalence has an enormous impact on direct healthcare costs (primary care, specialist care, emergency department care, day surgery, inpatient hospitalizations, and compensation payments, among others) and indirect costs (i.e., replacement employees, work absenteeism, or productivity loss). For example, it is estimated that Germany accounted for 17.2 billion € of production loss (production loss costs based on labor costs) in 2016 and 30.4 billion € in loss of gross value added (loss of labor productivity) [4]. The treatment to be carried out is not always clear and is highly conditioned by the type of injury. Severe injuries may require surgery in order to restore the structure and function of this tissue [5]. In this regard, the implant of grafts to defective sites is currently the most used therapeutic method to recover the functionality of damaged or diseased musculoskeletal tissue. Among the different grafting options, autografts are normally preferred due to the avoidance of immune rejection; allografts and xenografts have also been used, but they present many limitations related to the risk of rejection and the shortage of suitable donors [6].

In order to overcome these issues, tissue engineering strategies have been proposed for the biofabrication of tissue constructs with regenerative potential. In this regard, three-dimensional (3D) bioprinting has emerged as one of the most promising technologies to that end. This technique allows the production of living tissue-engineered constructs with precise positioning of a wide variety of biomaterials and cells [7]. The distribution of biological materials with high spatial control enables the recapitulation of the desired tissue heterogeneity; however, the biofabrication of a complete functional organ integrated with other systems, such as the vascular or nervous systems, remains a challenge [5]. Compared to standard 3D printing, 3D bioprinting needs to address other issues related to the sensitivities of living cells, the choice of suitable biomaterials, and the intricate structure and functionality of different tissues. In particular, in the case of the musculoskeletal system, the combination of different constructs, including tendon/muscle, bone/muscle, or bone/tendon, represents an additional challenge.

The choice of the most suitable bioink composition constitutes a key factor for 3D bioprinting. Bioinks are formed by the mixture of cells and natural and/or synthetic biomaterials and allow for high versatility due to their ability to incorporate a wide range of different components and cell types. An ideal bioink should present a suitable balance between both biological and mechanical properties, which is often difficult to achieve. First, the bioink should guarantee cell viability and dispersion within the bioprinted scaffold, as well as cell adhesion, proliferation, and differentiation. In addition, the scaffold should also simulate the native extracellular environment and present a moderate biodegradation rate with nontoxic degradation products [8]. Regarding mechanical features, an adequate printability of the material and viscosity, flexibility, and strength similar to the native tissue is pivotal. In general, the biomaterials used to prepare bioinks are classified into naturally derived biomaterials and synthetic polymers. Examples of naturally derived polymers include collagen (COL), gelatin (GEL), fibrin, hyaluronic acid (HA), chitosan (CHIT), or alginate (ALG), among others, and their high similarity with native extracellular matrix offers a propitious environment for cell adhesion, proliferation, and migration as well as for maintaining good cell viability. However, they usually show weak mechanical properties and poor printability [2]. Therefore, a combination with synthetic polymers is often necessary in order to overcome this issue and the most used ones for 3D bioprinting of the musculoskeletal system include the following: polyethylene glycol (PEG), PEG diacrylate (PEGDA), polycaprolactone (PCL), polylactic acid (PLA), and poly(lactic-co-glycolic) acid (PLGA) [2,5,9]. The printability and controllability of these polymers normally exceed those of natural materials and, additionally, they offer the possibility to specifically tune their rheological and mechanical properties for each application by changing their molecular weight or grade of chemical polymerization [10]. Bioinks are also composed of specific cell types depending on the target tissue and the degree of complexity of the construct. Most common cell sources include cell lineages, primary cells harvested from native tissues, and cells differentiated from mesenchymal stem cells (MSC) and induced pluripotent stem cells (iPSC) [11,12]. Moreover, bioinks also offer the possibility to incorporate other biochemical compounds, such as growth factors, to promote cell growth and/or differentiation within the scaffold [5]. Figure 7.1 summarizes the main 3D bioprinting techniques used for the musculoskeletal system, as well as the most relevant cell types and biomaterials used to prepare the bioinks for the biofabrication of that tissue, which are further described throughout this chapter.

In this chapter, the main studies involving 3D bioprinting of the musculoskeletal system, and the current limitations and future perspectives of these methods will be discussed.

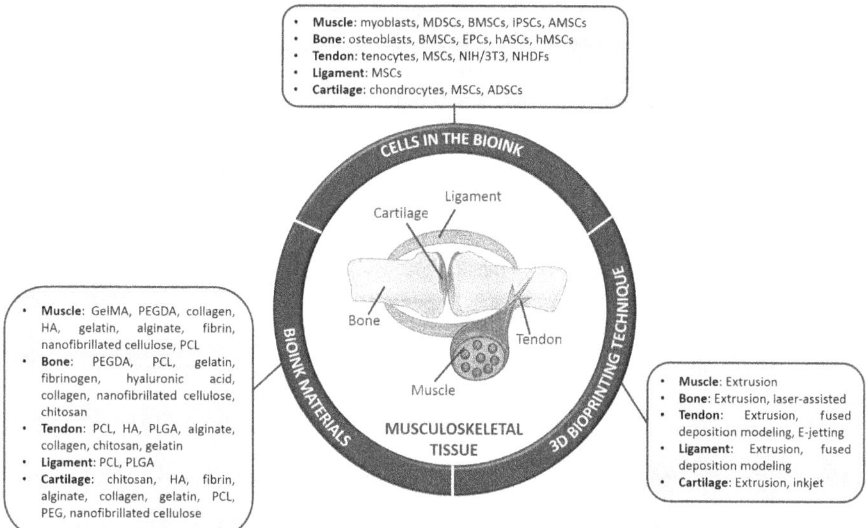

FIGURE 7.1 Schematic representation of the main components of the musculoskeletal system, the principal 3D bioprinting techniques and the cell types and biomaterials used to prepare the bioinks for biofabrication of the musculoskeletal tissue. Acronyms. MDSC: myeloid-derived suppressor cell, BMSC: bone mesenchymal cell, IPSC: induced pluripotent stem cell, AMSC: autologous marrow stem cell, EPC: endothelial progenitor cell, hASC: human adipose-derived stem cell, hMSC: human mesenchymal cell, MSC: mesenchymal cell, NHDF: normal human diploid fibroblast, ADSC: adipose-derived stem cell, GelMA: gelatin methacryloyl, PEGDA: poly(ethylene glycol) diacrylate, HA: hyaluronic acid, PCL: polycaprolactone, PLGA: poly(lactic-co-glycolic)acid, PEG: polyethylene glycol.

7.2 3D BIOPRINTING FOR BONE TISSUE REGENERATION

Traumas, fractures, and congenital and osteodegenerative diseases such as osteoporosis are some of the disorders and diseases that affect bones. Their natural regeneration is not always adequate, particularly in large injuries, since the intrinsic capacity of bone regeneration can be exceeded [13,14]. Current treatments primarily utilize auto-, allo-, xeno- and synthetic grafts, but they carry the risk of producing immune rejection and increased morbidity [14,15]. For this reason, promising techniques such as 3D bioprinting are currently being used for the development of scaffolds that promote bone regeneration [13,16].

To develop scaffolds that support a high mechanical load such as bone's, synthetic polymers such as PCL, polyurethane (PU), PLA, and PLGA are the essential candidates [14]. Bioceramics are used to restore hard tissues such as bone, being hydroxyapatite and beta-tricalcium phosphate the best known, usually combined with other materials [17]. Apart from these materials, currently, the use of native tissue-derived decellularized extracellular matrix (dECM) has emerged as a potential biomaterial as it contains tissue-specific composition [18].

Regarding the cell types laden in the bioinks, in most cases, cells that are part of the "Basic Multicellular Unit (BMU)" are used. BMU is responsible for bone formation and regeneration. Therefore, the cells that are most used are MSCs, preosteoblasts, and human adipose-derived stem cells (hASCs). In addition, iPSCs can be used as long as their tumorigenic potential is evaluated [19].

The interaction between the biomaterials used and the cells is important in bone tissue engineering; therefore, the structure of the scaffold has been modified by adding pores, adhesion proteins, or functional groups [16]. In most cases, the developed structures for bone regeneration are porous cylinders, disks, and cubic structures [20–24]. More complex structures may contain bone osteon-like structures which can include Haversian, medullary, and Volkmann's canals, as shown in Figure 7.2a.I [21].

For bone 3D bioprinting, techniques such as inkjet, extrusion, and light-based printers are used. Since the macrostructure and geometry of the scaffold directly affect the result, it is necessary to optimize the printing parameters. For instance, porosity and pore size directly affect osteo- and angiogenesis [14]. Also, pore size, pore geometry, and porosity of the bone scaffold directly affect the compressive and flexural strength, thus affecting the mechanical properties, as shown in Figure 7.2a.II–IV [17].

One of the frequently used strategies for the development of more complex and effective scaffolds is the incorporation of bioactive molecules into the inks and bioinks. In the case of bone regeneration, the most used ones are vascular endothelial growth factor (VEGF), bone morphogenetic protein (BMP), and transforming growth factor-β (TGF-β) [25]. BMPs, especially BMP-2, are frequently used because they promote osteogenic action and thus, bone formation [16,26]. The addition of genetically modified cells to express BMP-2 has also been studied [27]. Since the greatest challenge in the regeneration of large fractures is to develop the vasculature [25], factors such as VEGF, platelet-derived growth factor (PDGF)-BB, and TGF-β1 [28] are used to stimulate angiogenesis, along with the addition of endothelial cells such as human umbilical vein endothelial cells (HUVEC) [14]. Furthermore, BMPs, TFG-β1, VEGF, and placental growth factor are considered to be the most important bone growth factors [13,16,26,28]. To improve the properties of bioinks, growth factors can also be added in the form of nanoparticles (NPs) [28]. There are also

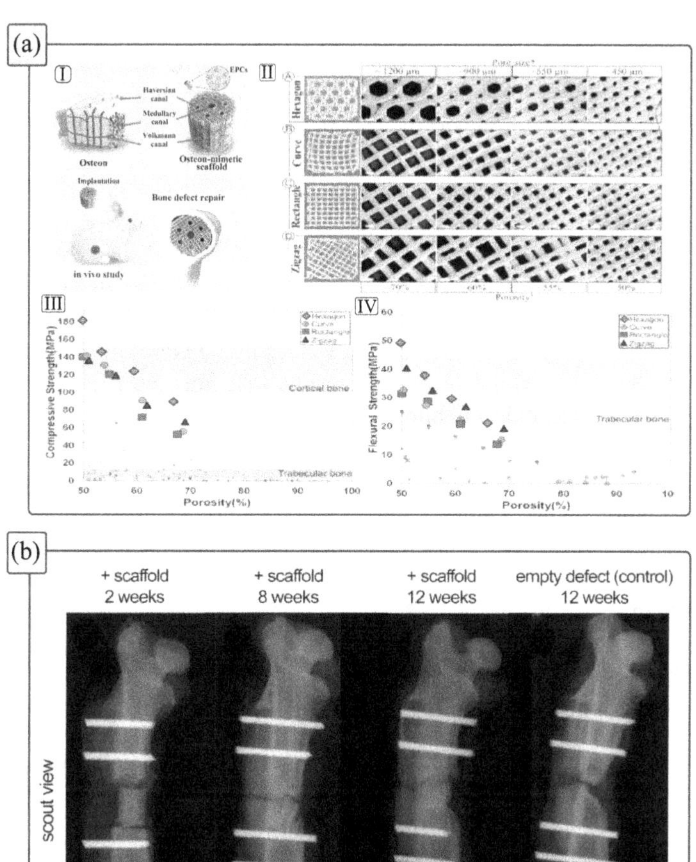

FIGURE 7.2 (a) I: 3D-bioprinted osteon-mimetic scaffolds integrated with medullary, Haversian, and Volkmann's canal structures. Adapted from *3D Bioprinting Of Osteon-Mimetic Scaffolds With Hierarchical Microchannels for Vascularized Bone Tissue Regeneration* by Xin Sun et al. (2022) [21]. II: Models (left column) and scanning electron microscopy (SEM) images of inspected scaffolds; Hexagonal (table top), curved, rectangular, and zigzag shape (table bottom). The microstructure of scaffolds with distinct pore geometries vs porosity, (III) compressive strength, and (IV) flexural strength of the scaffolds. Adapted from *3D Printing of Bioceramics for Bone Tissue Engineering* by Muhammad Jamshaid Zafar et al. (2019) licensed under CC BY 4.0 [17]. (b) Scout views and micro-computed X-ray tomography (μCT) axial cuts of the rat femur at 2, 8, and 12 weeks post-surgery, with and without bone scaffold. Adapted from *3D Bioprinted Bacteriostatic Hyperelastic Bone Scaffold for Damage-Specific Bone Regeneration* by Mohammadreza Shokouhimehr et al. (2021) licensed under CC BY 4.0 [24].

bioactive ions that are added to promote bone regeneration, such as strontium and magnesium, or to reduce the risk of infections, such as silver [29]. *In vitro* maturation of the scaffold is normally achieved through the addition of an osteogenic medium (dexamethasone, B-glycerophosphate, and ascorbic acid) to stimulate the differentiation of the added cells [20,22,23].

Most of the *in vivo* tests have been performed with small animals such as rats, mice, and rabbits. They focus on the regeneration of critical-size defects where the bone cannot regenerate on its own. The most studied defects *in vivo* are femoral and calvarial defects. In addition to the foregoing, these animals are also widely used for biocompatibility tests like the subcutaneous implantation of the scaffold [21,22,24]. As shown in Figure 7.2b [24], the latest advances in 3D bioprinting for bone regeneration in most cases exhibit promising results that must be further investigated, especially in larger animals and humans.

7.3 3D BIOPRINTING FOR MUSCLE TISSUE REGENERATION

The muscular tissue is responsible for all the movements of an organism, both conscious and unconscious. Although all of them share common features and histology, three different types of muscle tissues can be found: skeletal, cardiac, and smooth muscle. The differential histological and hierarchical architecture of each muscle type makes muscle tissue engineering (MTE) rather challenging.

Unlike other tissues (such as bone or tendon) for which replication of the native mechanical properties is of crucial importance, for muscle 3D bioprinting, the main challenges are related to the cellular density, organization, alignment, and connections together with synchronized contraction, proper circulation of nutrients, and neurovascular integration. Therefore, the vast majority of MTE bioink formulations are based on highly biocompatible and biosimilar ingredients (i.e., dECM, COL, fibrinogen, etc.). Since the printability of these bioinks is often jeopardized due to low mechanical strength, different strategies such as the inclusion of printing supports [PCL, polyvinyl alcohol (PVA), and PEG], the use of sacrificial inks [32–36] and/or photo-polymerizable materials [i.e., gelatin methacryloyl (GelMA), collagen methacryloyl (ColMA), poly(ethyleneglycol)dimethacrylate (PEGDMA), and glycidyl methacrylate-hyaluronic acid (GM-HA)] [30,31,35,37–48] have been implemented. Bioink resorption is likewise desirable since it drives additional space for cells and nutrients, further enhancing the maturation and integration of the muscular 3D implant.

The cell type laden in the MTE bioinks depends on the type of muscle tissue to be reproduced (cardiac or skeletal tissue) [43,49–51], but in most cases, undifferentiated cells, such as human iPSCs, are used. Although differentiated cells are less used, some, such as mouse myoblast cells (C2C12), have been frequently selected for their incorporation in the inks for MTE regeneration. Some studies have proven the usefulness of combining different cell types within the same scaffold as a successful strategy to better mimic the hierarchical architecture of the muscle, such as neural stem cells, fibroblasts, endothelial cells, and/or adipose cells [30,34,36,39,40,43,44,51,52]. This cellular combination results in better cell-to-cell interactions, the formation of junctions, as well as synergistic effects during differentiation and myoblast alignment. For instance, HUVEC's cytokines have proven to induce C2C12 myogenic-specific gene expression [39].

Topographical cues (typically contour-like staircases) are generally undesirable for 3D-bioprinted scaffolds, except for MTE, since they induce proper alignment of muscular cells [36,41,44,53–56]. Therefore, linear or rectilinear motions and mesh-line scaffolds are common in 3D-bioprinted MTE. The importance of this feature is such that some studies have focused on the optimization of the printing parameters to maximize cellular alignment and differentiation [34,40,41,53]. Fibrous-like bioink ingredients such as COL or fibrin (among others) can also provide an additional degree of topographical cue to the final scaffold. Regarding 3D CAD designs, the most recent studies attempt to reproduce the hierarchical structure of the skeletal muscle (fibrous multilayer bundles parallel to each other) [32,34,45,57]. For the cardiac muscle, more complex structures have been attempted, like the curved scaffold to reproduce the cardiac topology [40], the Purkinje network developed by Tracy and co-workers [58], or the murine heart from a magnetic resonance imaging scanning by Kupfer and co-workers [37].

As previously highlighted, cellular viability takes precedence over mechanical properties in MTE. Effective nutrients and oxygen diffusion and adequate waste elimination (Figure 7.3a) are of crucial importance for proper scaffold maturation (cellular migration, proliferation, and differentiation) [31–34,38,49]. When it comes to maintaining cellular viability, pneumatic extrusion 3D bioprinting has been established as the most convenient and versatile strategy. Moreover, this technique enables the printing of highly porous, labile bioinks, like the foam-like proposed by Mostafavi and collaborators [32].

Maturation of the artificial 3D tissue *in vitro* is of great importance to discern the appropriateness of the formulation and the scaffolds for *in vivo* implantation. Nonetheless, only a minority of the most recent studies exert external stimulation on the 3D scaffolds. Electric stimulation of artificial muscle tissue is known to induce and accelerate scaffold maturation, promoting cell communication, alignment (Figure 7.3b), proliferation, synapse formation, muscular contraction, etc. [33,40,43,45–47]. Graphene [40], polyethylene dioxythiophene [47], gold NPs, and two-dimensional transition metal carbide [46] can improve the electrical conductivity of MTE bioinks, yielding positive results. In this regard, electric-based 3D printing processes, such as electrically assisted cell printing [45] or electrohydrodynamic direct writing [39], have proven to be a useful strategy. Magnetic fields are also able to induce muscle maturation by mediating a mechanical stretch stimulation of a cell-laden hydrogel containing Fe_3O_4 [59]. Stretching devices can also be used to mechanically stimulate muscle 3D scaffolds, though the bioink should have minimum mechanical properties to withstand this kind of maturation [60].

Rats and mice are the most common platforms for *in vivo* MTE tests. Only a few studies have been recently dedicated to *in vivo* MTE of cardiac tissue [51,52], yielding improved cardiac tissue regeneration and minimum scar tissue formation. The vast majority of recent studies are focused on skeletal muscle, particularly in the treatment of volumetric muscle loss (VML, muscle losses of more than 20%), since in these conditions, the tissue is unable to regenerate through self-healing. The *in vivo* tests herein reported revealed that 3D bioprinting is an effective and promising strategy to address VML by achieving neural and vascular integration, more than 80% of functional recovery within 8 weeks, and preventing muscle atrophy, functional impairment, and physical deformities [32,33,38,44,54].

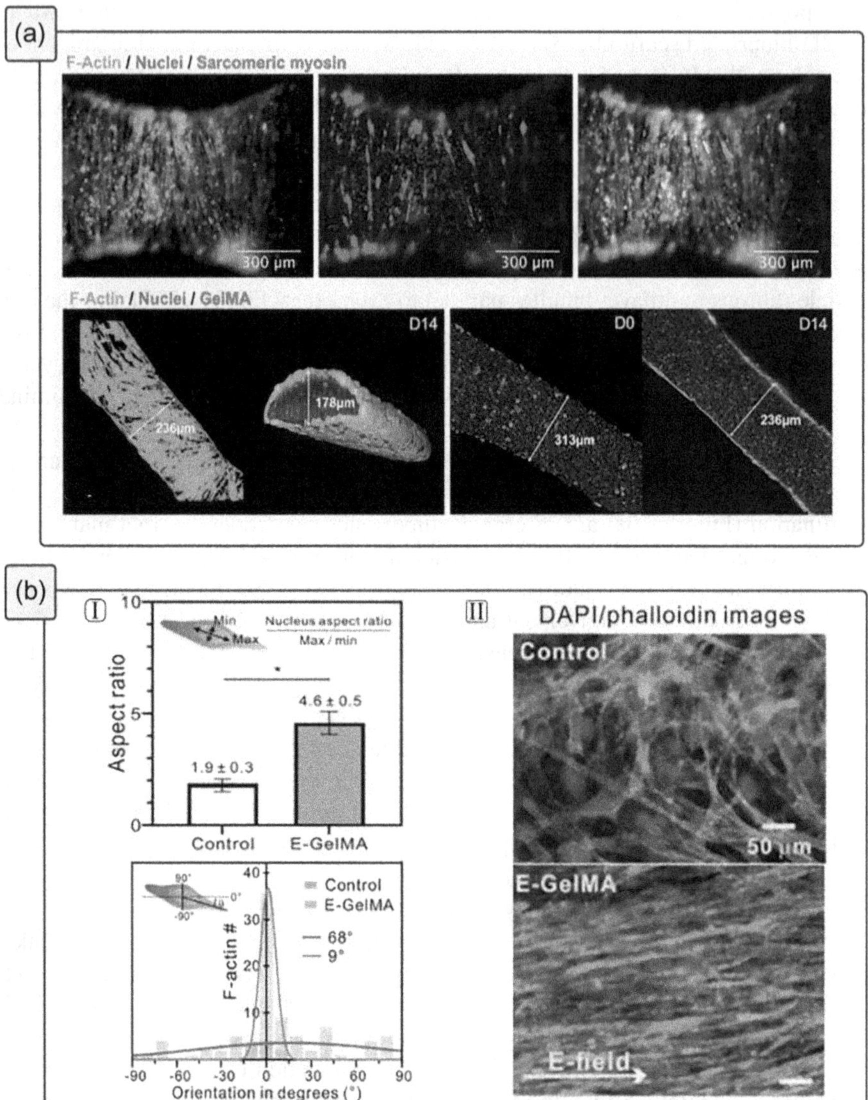

FIGURE 7.3 (a) Up: Myoblasts stained for F-actin, sarcomeric myosin, and DNA. The presence of myosin-positive fibers indicates maturing contractile mechanisms. Down: confocal imaging of cells migrating to the boundaries of the material, where they fused into multinucleated myotubes on the material surface. This migration toward the edges of the scaffold is believed to be induced by the lack of nutrients and/or oxygen diffusion within the scaffold. Adapted from *A Skeleton Muscle Model Using Gelma-Based Cell-Aligned Bioink Processed With An Electric-Field Assisted 3D/4D Bioprinting* by Gi Hoon Yang et al. (2021) licensed under CC BY 4.0 [30]. (b) I: aspect ratio of cell nuclei and orientation (degrees) of actin filaments (F-actin). II: fluorescence images of the control and gelatin methacryloyl (GelMA)-based muscle bioink (white arrows indicate the electric field direction during stimulation). Extracted from *Matured Myofibers in Bioprinted Constructs with In Vivo Vascularization and Innervation* by Catherine G Y Ngan et al. (2021) licensed under CC BY 4.0 [31].

7.4 3D BIOPRINTING FOR TENDON AND LIGAMENT REGENERATION

Tendons and ligaments are tissues responsible for withstanding and transmitting forces, a function that is closely related to their high tensile strength (ranging from 50 to 150MPa) and their high elastic modulus (ranging from 1 to 2GPa) [61].

The materials used in 3D printing applied to tendon and ligament regeneration have been very varied. Initially, there was a strong case for the use of organic materials. However, in recent years, the vast majority of the research has been carried out with the use of synthetic materials. Among these synthetic materials are PCL [62–67], PLA [68], and PLGA [64,69–71]. They allowed for achieving highly defined structures with good mechanical properties. Although they showed hardly any cytotoxicity effect, in none of the approaches were the cells included in the ink or printed on the structure, but rather they were seeded onto the obtained construct after being printed. As an alternative, different biological materials have also been used. The most widespread approach has been the use of tendon and ligament dECM to obtain bioinks with good biocompatibility and reduced cytotoxicity [72–74]. The results in terms of mechanical properties were low, which showed the need for subsequent maturation of the structures. Other materials of biological origin used have been nanofibrillar cellulose [75], ALG [75], and HA [76,77]. Unlike inorganic materials, with natural materials, cells were incorporated into the inks before being printed.

As is the case for the major part of tissue engineering approaches, tendon and ligament studies often resort to undifferentiated cells. In this particular case, human bone marrow-derived -MSCs [62,63,69,71,73], human umbilical cord blood-MSCs [64,76], human ASCs [70,75], human dermal fibroblasts, tendon stem/progenitor cells, and NIH 3T3 fibroblasts [72,74] can be mentioned. Generally, differentiation mediums are used for the differentiation of these cells (example in Figure 7.4a.V). In some cases, the use of already differentiated cells such as human tenocytes was preferred [67,77].

So far, the structures developed for the regeneration of tendons and ligaments have been very simple. In most cases, they do not attempt to mimic the morphology of the damaged tissues. Instead, they are limited to mesh-like structures [66,67,74,76], meshed cubes and cylinders, [64,69,71,75] or more or less solid rectangular prisms [62,63,65,70,72,73,77]. Two of the developed structures for tendon and ligament tissue regeneration can be observed in Figure 7.4a and b, respectively. The developed structures were simple and not similar to the natural tendons and ligaments; nevertheless, it served to determine the printability of inorganic materials in combination with hydrogels, in the case of the tendon scaffold, and the printability of GelMa, in the case of the ligament scaffold. There are a few cases where an attempt has been made to mimic the structure of tendons or ligaments [79]. It is reasonable to believe that these tissue-like structures will have better results in tissue regeneration.

As for the 3D printing techniques used to obtain the scaffolds, they are highly influenced by the type of ink or bioink used. As previously mentioned, the vast majority of materials used in recent years have been thermoplastic inorganic materials. Therefore, the most widely used technique has been fused deposition modeling. Another most used technique is extrusion. In this case, materials of natural origin are usually used. The remaining 3D printing techniques have hardly been used in recent years for the regeneration of tendons and ligaments.

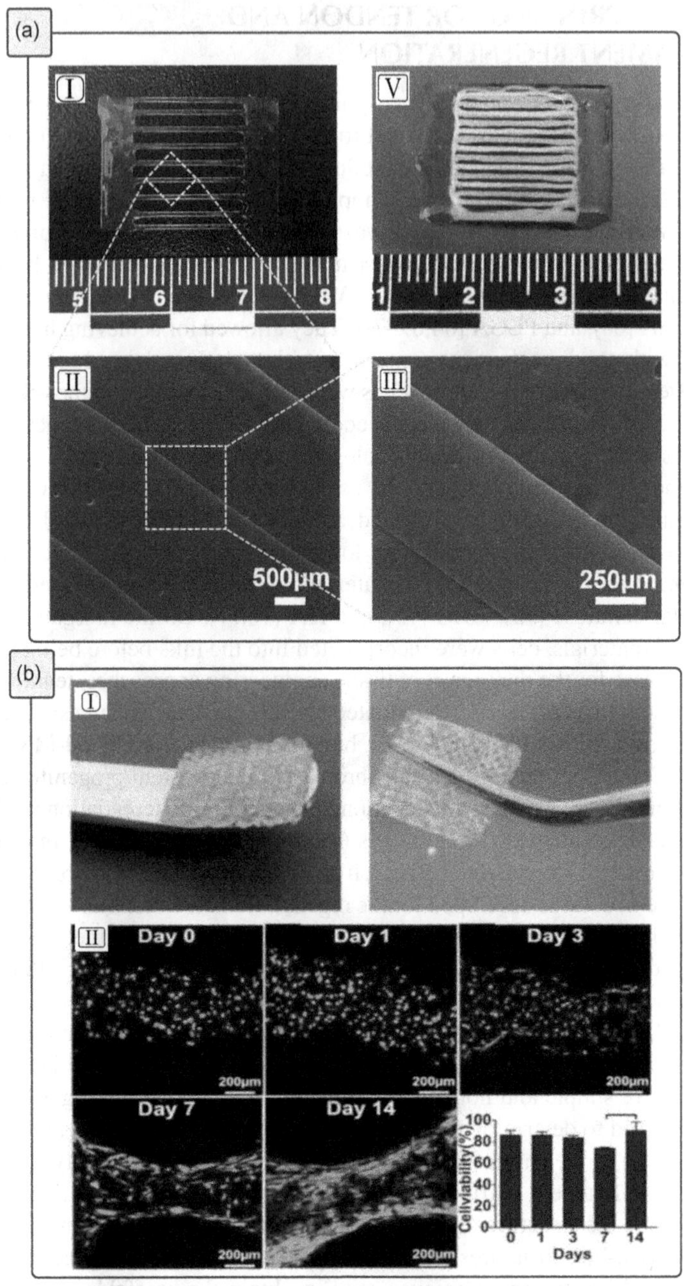

FIGURE 7.4 (a) I: 3D-printed one-layer PLGA scaffold for tendon regeneration. II y III: SEM images of one-layer PLGA scaffold. V: 3D-printed tri-layered scaffold model. Excerpt from *3D Printing of Multilayered Scaffolds for Rotator Cuff Tendon Regeneration* by Xiping Jiang et al. (2020) licensed under CC BY-NC-ND 4.0 [70]. (b) I: Thermally cross-linked 3D-bioprinted GelMA hydrogel scaffolds. II: viability of ligament stem cells embedded in the 3D-bioprinted constructs during 14 days. (*, $p < 0.05$, **, $p < 0.05$). Adapted from *Optimization of 3D Bioprinting of Periodontal Ligament Cells* by Nimal Thattaruparambil Raveendran et al. (2018) [78].

Maturation of the structures obtained is very important to increase their complexity and achieve better results both *in vitro* and *in vivo*. Maturation of the scaffolds for tendon and ligament regeneration has been carried out using different strategies: gene editing (use of NPs loaded with a plasmid to silence the expression of TGF-β1) [65], uniaxial static tension [73,80], or culture with a tissue-specific dECM cue [73,77]. In recent years, there are only a few examples of *in vitro* maturation. However, it is worth highlighting the good results that have been obtained with them. By means of these techniques, it is possible to prevent adhesion in tendons, achieve differentiation of cells into tenocytes, or increase the mechanical properties of the structures.

There are many tests that have been performed *in vivo*, mainly using rabbits, rats, and mice. In the case of mice, being much smaller, they have been used mainly for subcutaneous implantation of scaffolds (biocompatibility analysis). In the case of tests involving the analysis of the regeneration capacity of tendons and ligaments, the use of slightly larger animals is preferred. In this sense, most *in vivo* studies have been carried out using rabbits as model animals.

7.5 3D BIOPRINTING FOR CARTILAGE REGENERATION

Cartilage is one of the connective tissues that are widely distributed throughout the body, constituting one of the main components of joints, spine, ribs, outer ears, nose… Cartilage tissue is difficult to repair because it is avascular and aneural and the cell density is very low. For all these reasons, spontaneous tissue repair is very limited [81]. Furthermore, when cartilage is injured, the joint slowly and irrevocably deteriorates if left untreated. This entails a serious problem for society since about 6% of disabled people over 30 years of age have defects and diseases related to cartilage tissues [82]. Current strategies to treat these cartilage defects include mosaicplasties, some cell-based techniques, and remodeling through microfractures. Despite their use in clinical practice, they have a number of limitations, such as short-term resolution, the high cost of the procedures, and the impossibility of recreating the native cartilage structure [83]. In this context, tissue engineering is highlighted as the most promising option.

In 3D printing of cartilage tissues, inkjet-based bioprinting, laser-assisted bioprinting, extrusion-based bioprinting, and stereolithography (SLA) bioprinting have been used. Nevertheless, the most used ones are extrusion and SLA bioprinting since they have great biocompatibility and are very easy to combine with different cross-linking mechanisms [84]. A different example of extrusion 3D bioprinting is shown in Figure 7.5b, which consists of using a handheld coaxial 3D printer.

Some of the most commonly used natural polymers in the preparation of bioinks for cartilage bioprinting include GEL [85], COL, fibrin [86], ALG [87], and HA [88]. In contrast, the most widely used synthetic polymers for cartilage bioprinting include PCL [89], PEG [90], and methacrylated hyaluronic acid [90]. Natural polymers have hydrophilic properties and high cytocompatibility and biocompatibility, making them suitable candidates for the production of cartilage bioinks. Despite this, the mechanical properties they possess are insufficient to reproduce native tissue performance. Therefore, the combination of these ingredients with synthetic polymers, with better mechanical properties, is essential [91]. In these cases, the proportion of synthetic ingredients can be higher than normal since the cellular density is not the key point. One example of the combination of synthetic polymers and natural

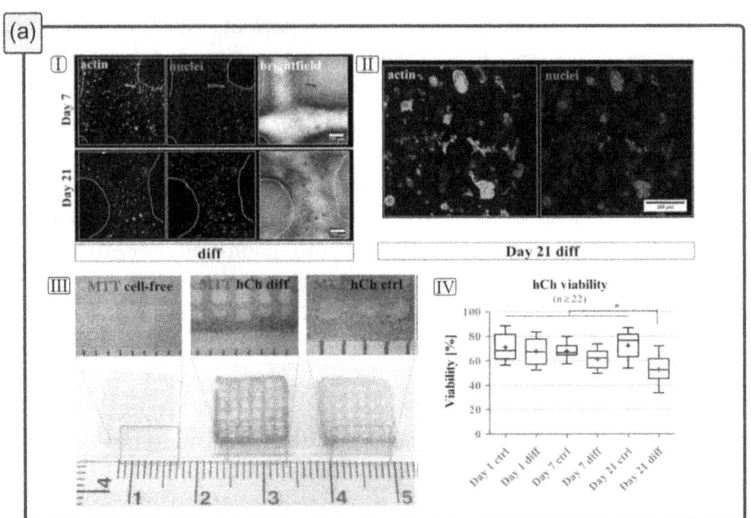

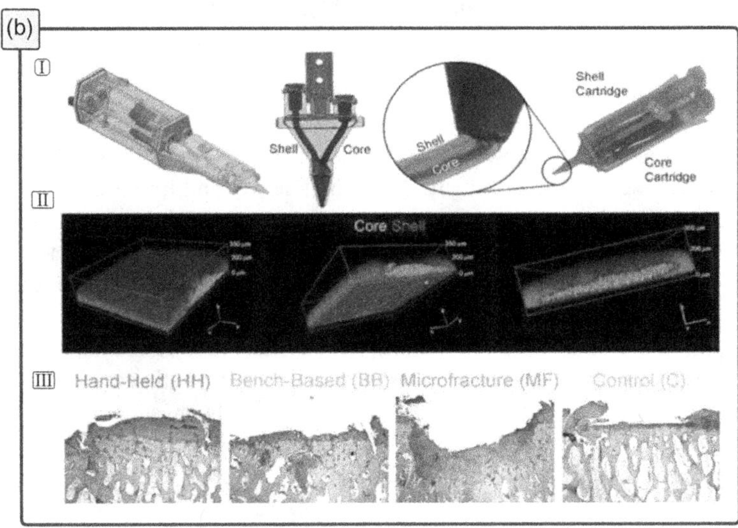

FIGURE 7.5 (a) I, II: Distribution and morphology of the cytoskeleton of chondrocytes within the bioprinted scaffolds. 4′,6-Diamidino-2-phenylindole (DAPI) staining (cell nuclei) and phalloidin (actin filaments of the cytoskeleton). III: Use of 2,5-diphenyl-2H-tetrazolium bromide (MTT) staining to observe metabolically active cells on day 21 of cell culture. A scaffold without cells (left), a scaffold in control conditions (right), and another in differentiation conditions (center) were used. IV: Viability of human chondrocytes on algMC scaffolds obtained with 3D bioprinting. Proportion of viable cells and the total number of cells after 1, 7, and 21 days under control (ctrl) and differentiation (diff) conditions, $n \geq 22$, * $p < 0.05$. Adapted from *3D Bioprinting of Osteochondral Tissue Substitutes – In Vitro-Chondrogenesis in Multi-Layered Mineralized Constructs* by David Kilian et al. (2020) licensed under CC BY 4.0 [97]. (b) Core/Shell 3D printing by extrusion with a handheld coaxial 3D printer. I: Schematic representation II: 3D-rendered confocal images of scaffolds III: Histology with safranin/fast green staining showing better new cartilage formation in the hand-held (HH) group than in the others. Adapted from *Cartilage Tissue Engineering Using Stem Cells and Bioprinting Technology-Barriers to Clinical Translation* by Sam L Francis et al. (2018) licensed under CC BY [93].

polymers is shown in Figure 7.4b, where the intercalation of PCL layers and COL1/fibrinogen layers with chondrocytes embedded can be observed.

Regarding cell components, the combination of different cell types in the same bioink can increase the performance of the bioprinted cartilage. Chondrocyte- or mesenchymal cell-laden bioinks are the most commonly reported [92]. In relation to the use of chondrocytes, the main benefit is their low immunogenicity, although they may have limited availability. On the other hand, MSCs constitute an important approximation in the 3D bioprinting of cartilage tissue since they show high chondrogenic potential. MSCs derived from the adipose tissues have superior chondrogenic differentiation capacity than those derived from the bone marrow [93]. It is worth mentioning the ability of MSCs to self-renew, release active factors that modify the microenvironment, and differentiate into multiple cell lines, including chondrocytes [94].

The incorporation of particles carrying bioactive molecules, such as growth factors and hormones, in scaffolds is a promising strategy to improve bioinks and tissue regeneration. In this way, the release of growth factors can be controlled to promote cell differentiation of stem cells, vascularization of the surrounding tissues, cell growth, and proliferation [95]. Among the growth factors and hormones most used in bioinks for printing cartilage tissue are TGFs, insulin-like growth factors (IGFs), BMPs, and PDGFs. The growth factor TGF-β3 is capable of maintaining the chondrogenic phenotype of MSCs for the regeneration of cartilage tissue and induces chondrogenic differentiation of stem cells. IGF-1 is used in cartilage repair due to its effects on cartilage homeostasis. BMPs are capable of inducing cartilage formation. BMP-2 and BMP-7 induce chondrogenic differentiation generating cartilage formation. The use of PDGF-AB or PDGF-BB is useful for the proliferation, migration, and growth of endothelial cells, as well as for increasing the synthesis of type I COL [92,96].

7.6 3D BIOPRINTING FOR "INTER" TISSUE REGENERATION

When trying to replicate natural tissues from the human body, it is important to note that they are generally constituted by different layers or sub-tissues, each of them with a different composition, function, and properties. 3D bioprinting has postulated itself to be an incredible technology with endless possibilities, but it has been facing some challenges when it comes to bioprinting different tissue types under the same print run [98].

As previously stated, the musculoskeletal system is composed of different tissues coexisting and working together to present a wide range of different mechanical, structural, and biological properties. Preserving these properties is crucial when properly replicating what happens in the human body [5]. For instance, taking a look at a kneecap, it is important to have the mechanic resistance that the bone provides, but it is also needed the elasticity of the ligaments and the dim action of the cartilage, as well as a good transition from tissue to tissue to ensure the stability of the structure [99]. Generally, the solution that is being used to approach this issue is the formation of a fibrovascular scar between two different tissues, that is, bone and tendon. Even though this physically links both tissues, the biomechanics of the interface are not preserved, and therefore, the functional properties *in vivo* are not properly restored [100,101].

With the intention of overcoming this downside and acknowledging the characteristics of the junction between tissues, the concept of interface tissue bioprinting was born. Even though there are still limited studies, interface bioprinting has proven to be crucial in restoring musculoskeletal damage, thus being in the vanguard of the tissue regeneration field [102].

When bioprinting an interface tissue, three different parts can be distinguished: tissue A, the interface, and tissue B. In order to have a continuous but stratified scaffold, the transitions from tissue A to B must be gradual, not only in the bioink but also in the cellular and molecular microenvironment, avoiding the boundaries between phases [103]. When it comes to the bioink, there are two approaches to achieve this task, either by using a mixture of both bioinks in a gradient manner or using a bioink that presents intermediate characteristics [104–106].

Another critical aspect of 3D interface bioprinting is the cell type used in the scaffold. In this regard, there are several possibilities: (i) the use of stem cells and their subsequent differentiation by means of different stimuli, (ii) the use of differentiated cells, or (iii) a combination of both, this being the most promising approach [64,101,103,107].

7.6.1 Tendon-to-Muscle Interface

Due to its ability to contract and transmit the nervous impulse for this contraction, muscle recreation is one of the major challenges in this field [13], and the interface is not different at all since it has to present a high resistance to mechanic forces but also a great elastic capacity to return to a relaxed state without the risk of tearing [11,39,108]. One of the complex developed interfaces can be observed in Figure 7.6a. Therein, the combination of different materials (PU and PCL) and cell lines (C2C12 cells NIH/3T3 cells) was analyzed obtaining very promising results [11].

7.6.2 Bone-to-Cartilage Interface

This is especially important to treat osteochondral damages derived from osteoarthritis, trauma, or inflammation. The importance of cartilage in protecting the bone from wearing away is crucial for a good articular function, and to achieve this, the cartilage must be blended into the bone structure. This takes place through a calcified cartilage layer that not only unifies both tissues but also presents intermediate characteristics between both [106]. An interesting calcified cartilage layer was developed by Wang and co-workers [109] as can be observed in Figure 7.6b.

7.6.3 Bone-to-Tendon Interface

This interface has shown to be a key point when treating rotator cuff injuries, for example. The restoration of the elasticity and the rest of the mechanical properties in this fibrocartilaginous insertion are crucial to prevent re-tears in the tissue and these rely on the proper repair of the tendon-to-bone interface [107]. This interface includes four structural areas that present themselves in a continuous manner—tendon, non-mineralized fibrocartilage, mineralized fibrocartilage, and bone—therefore increasing its rigidity and decreasing its elasticity from tendon to bone [103]. An example of this type of interface can be seen in Figure 7.7, where different materials (PCL and PCL/tricalcium phosphate) were alternated to achieve a good interface between the two tissues.

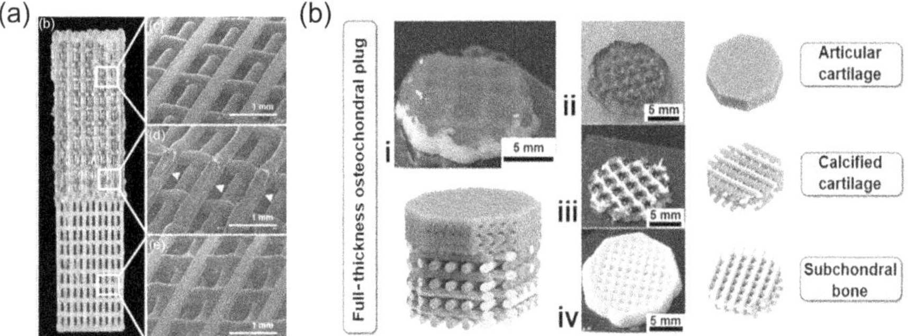

FIGURE 7.6 (a) Tendon-to-muscle interface. The topside (ii) is printed with polyurethane (PU) and C2C12 cells, and the bottom side (iv) is composed of polycaprolactone (PCL) with NIH/3T3 cells. The structure presents a 10% overlap as shown in picture (iii). Adapted from *A 3D Bioprinted Complex Structure for Engineering The Muscle–Tendon Unit* by Tyler K Merceron et al. (2015) [11] (b) Bone to cartilage. Adapted from *Nanotechnologies And Nanomaterials in 3D (Bio)Printing Toward Bone Regeneration* by Zongliang Wang et al. (2021) licensed under CC BY 4.0 [109].

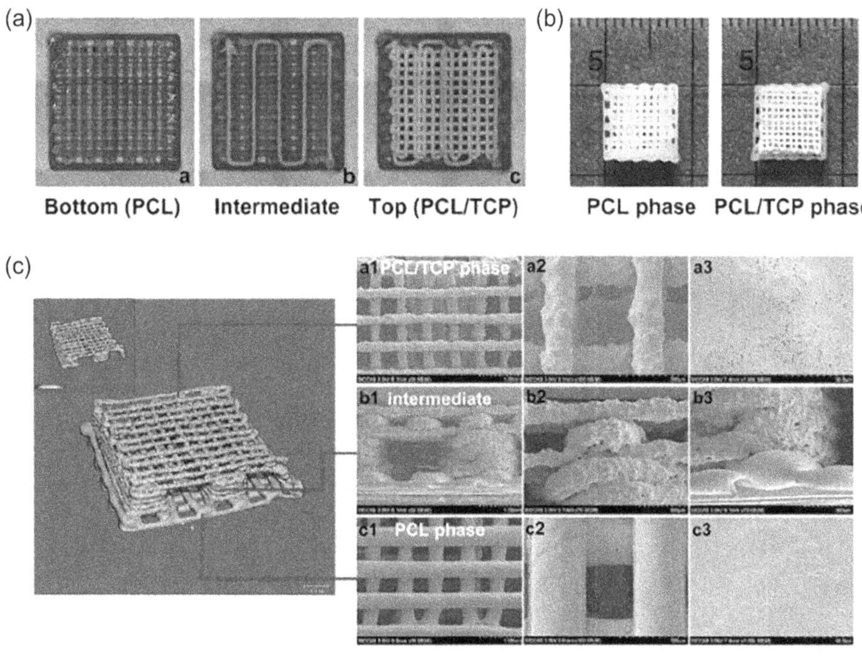

FIGURE 7.7 Bone-to-tendon interface. (a) Real-time images of the 3D printed patterns. (b) Morphology and size of the 3D-printed scaffold. (c) MicroCT (left) demonstrated print quality and the predesigned structure. SEM micrographs (right) displaying surface microstructures of the PCL/TCP phase (a1~a3), intermediate ducts (b1~b3), and PCL phase (c1~c3). Excerpt from *Three-Dimensional Printed Multiphasic Scaffolds With Stratified Cell-Laden Gelatin Methacrylate Hydrogels for Biomimetic Tendon-To-Bone Interface Engineering* by Yi Cao et al. (2020) licensed under CC BY-NC-ND 4.0 [107]. PCL: polycaprolactone, TCP: tricalcium phosphate.

7.7 FUTURE PERSPECTIVES AND GOALS OF THE APPLICATION OF 3D BIOPRINTING TO MUSCULOSKELETAL REGENERATION

Tissue engineering and, specifically, 3D bioprinting have made great progress in the development of structures that could help musculoskeletal system regeneration. Nevertheless, there are still a number of limitations that make it difficult to lead the obtained products straight to the clinic. Ultimately, these limitations constitute the future challenges that 3D bioprinting applied to the regeneration of the musculoskeletal system has to face. First, there is a fine balance between the mechanical properties of the constructs and the viability of the cells embedded in them. A large number of materials and combinations of them have been studied to achieve mechanical properties similar to those of the original tissue; however, to date, no combination has been found that achieves these mechanical properties without hindering the integrity of the cells or without causing an unwanted immune response. Second, the use of bioactive molecules in the bioprinted scaffold has also been very limited mainly due to three reasons: (i) the molecules that participate in the regeneration processes of the musculoskeletal system are still being clarified, (ii) they are molecules that generally have a low half-life at 37°C (limits their use when they are needed in the late phases of the regeneration process), and (iii) it is necessary to ensure that the biomolecules will remain in the target area without diffusing to other areas. Third, the studies carried out so far are generally simple and limited to the analysis of one or two specific factors (the combination of materials, the printability of the material, the orientation of the fibers, the viability of the cells…). In this regard, still, very preliminary studies have been performed. It is expected that in the coming years, the proposed approaches will be more complex: the combination of different materials and cells, the incorporation of circulatory and nervous systems to the scaffolds, their maturation through mechanical and nervous stimulation, the incorporation of active biomolecules with a controlled release during the phases of interest (for example, through the use of NPs), and the development of interfaces between tissues that are better defined and similar to the original tissues, among others. Being able to develop 3D-bioprinted scaffolds that allow the regeneration of musculoskeletal tissues requires overcoming these aforementioned limitations.

It should also be noted that there is currently no standard or unified legislation on this type of biomedical products (the materials, the cells, the technology used,… are affected by different legislation). This lack of unification is compromising the transfer to the clinic. Significant progress in this area is expected in the coming years, thus defining the minimum criteria that the 3D-printed scaffolds must meet in order to reach patients.

Overcoming the aforementioned challenges and limitations is crucial to allow the regeneration of musculoskeletal tissues. Despite the difficulties, the combined efforts of research groups and institutions all over the world make the musculoskeletal bioprinting to be closer to the real clinical practice.

ACKNOWLEDGMENTS

This project was supported by the Basque Country Government (Consolidated Groups, IT1448-22, and predoctoral grants PRE_2021_2_0153 and PRE_2021_2_0181), by the University of Basque Country UPV/EHU (postdoctoral fellowship ESPDOC19/47) and by the TriAnkle European project (Horizon 2020 TriAnkle

952981-2). This research was also supported by CIBER-Consorcio Centro de Investigación Biomédica en Red- CB06/01/1028, Instituto de Salud Carlos III, Ministerio de Ciencia e Innovación. The authors wish to thank the intellectual and technical assistance from the ICTS "NANBIOSIS," more specifically by the Drug Formulation Unit (U10) of the CIBER in Bioengineering, Biomaterials, and Nanomedicine (CIBER-BBN) at the University of the Basque Country (UPV/EHU).

REFERENCES

1. Walker J. Skeletal system 2: Structure and function of the musculoskeletal system. *Nursing Times*. 2020;116(3):52–6.
2. Park W, Gao G, Cho DW. Tissue-specific decellularized extracellular matrix bioinks for musculoskeletal tissue regeneration and modeling using 3D bioprinting technology. *Int J Mol Sci*. 2021;22(15):7837.
3. Cieza A, Causey K, Kamenov K, Hanson SW, Chatterji S, Vos T. Global estimates of the need for rehabilitation based on the Global Burden of Disease study 2019: A systematic analysis for the Global Burden of Disease Study 2019. *Lancet*. 2021;396(10267):2006–17.
4. de Kok J, Vroonhof P, Snijders J, Roullis G, Clarke M, Peereboom K, et al. *Work-Related MSDs: Prevalence, Costs and Demographics in the EU*. Luxembourg: European Agency for Safety and Health at Work; 2019.
5. Potyondy T, Uquillas JA, Tebon PJ, Byambaa B, Hasan A, Tavafoghi M, et al. Recent advances in 3D bioprinting of musculoskeletal tissues. *Biofabrication*. 2021;13(2):10.1088/1758-5090/abc8de. Published 2021 Mar 10. doi:10.1088/1758-5090/abc8de.
6. Li Z, Xiang S, Li EN, Fritch MR, Alexander PG, Lin H, et al. Tissue engineering for musculoskeletal regeneration and disease modeling. *Handb Exp Pharmacol*. 2021;265:235–68.
7. Murphy SV, Atala A. 3D bioprinting of tissues and organs. *Nat Biotechnol*. 2014;32(8):773–85.
8. Weng T, Zhang W, Xia Y, Wu P, Yang M, Jin R, et al. 3D bioprinting for skin tissue engineering: Current status and perspectives. *J Tissue Eng*. 2021;12:20417314211028574.
9. Ostrovidov S, Salehi S, Costantini M, Suthiwanich K, Ebrahimi M, Sadeghian RB, et al. 3D bioprinting in skeletal muscle tissue engineering. *Small*. 2019;15(24):e1805530.
10. Gungor-Ozkerim PS, Inci I, Zhang YS, Khademhosseini A, Dokmeci MR. Bioinks for 3D bioprinting: An overview. *Biomater Sci*. 2018;6(5):915–46.
11. Merceron TK, Burt M, Seol YJ, Kang HW, Lee SJ, Yoo JJ, et al. A 3D bioprinted complex structure for engineering the muscle-tendon unit. *Biofabrication*. 2015;7(3):035003.
12. Ashammakhi N, Ahadian S, Xu C, Montazerian H, Ko H, Nasiri R, et al. Bioinks and bioprinting technologies to make heterogeneous and biomimetic tissue constructs. *Mater Today Bio*. 2019;1:100008.
13. Lin X, Patil S, Gao YG, Qian A. The bone extracellular matrix in bone formation and regeneration. *Front Pharmacol*. 2020;11:757.
14. Genova T, Roato I, Carossa M, Motta C, Cavagnetto D, Mussano F. Advances on bone substitutes through 3D bioprinting. *Int J Mol Sci*. 2020;21(19):7012.
15. Elalouf A. Immune response against the biomaterials used in 3D bioprinting of organs. *Transpl Immunol*. 2021;69:101446.
16. Ansari M. Bone tissue regeneration: Biology, strategies and interface studies. *Prog Biomater*. 2019;8(4):223–37.
17. Zafar MJ, Zhu D, Zhang Z. 3D printing of bioceramics for bone tissue engineering. *Materials (Basel)*. 2019;12(20):3361.
18. De Santis MM, Alsafadi HN, Tas S, Bölükbas DA, Prithiviraj S, Da Silva IAN, et al. Extracellular-matrix-reinforced bioinks for 3D bioprinting human tissue. *Adv Mater*. 2021;33(3):e2005476.

19. Yang WS, Kim WJ, Ahn JY, Lee J, Ko DW, Park S, et al. New bioink derived from neonatal chicken bone marrow cells and its 3D-bioprinted niche for osteogenic stimulators. *ACS Appl Mater Interfaces*. 2020;12(44):49386–97.
20. Lee J, Hong J, Kim W, Kim GH. Bone-derived dECM/alginate bioink for fabricating a 3D cell-laden mesh structure for bone tissue engineering. *Carbohydr Polym*. 2020;250:116914.
21. Sun X, Jiao X, Yang X, Ma J, Wang T, Jin W, et al. 3D bioprinting of osteon-mimetic scaffolds with hierarchical microchannels for vascularized bone tissue regeneration. *Biofabrication*. 2022;14(3):10.1088/1758-5090/ac6700.
22. Touya N, Devun M, Handschin C, Casenave S, Ahmed Omar N, Gaubert A, et al. *In vitro* and *in vivo* characterization of a novel tricalcium silicate-based ink for bone regeneration using laser-assisted bioprinting. *Biofabrication*. 2022;14(2):10.1088/1758-5090/ac584b. Published 2022 Mar 9. doi:10.1088/1758-5090/ac584b.
23. Maturavongsadit P, Narayanan LK, Chansoria P, Shirwaiker R, Benhabbour SR. Cell-laden nanocellulose/chitosan-based bioinks for 3D bioprinting and enhanced osteogenic cell differentiation. *ACS Appl Bio Mater*. 2021;4(3):2342–53.
24. Shokouhimehr M, Theus AS, Kamalakar A, Ning L, Cao C, Tomov ML, et al. 3D bioprinted bacteriostatic hyperelastic bone scaffold for damage-specific bone regeneration. *Polymers (Basel)*. 2021;13(7):1099.
25. Midha S, Dalela M, Sybil D, Patra P, Mohanty S. Advances in three-dimensional bioprinting of bone: Progress and challenges. *J Tissue Eng Regen Med*. 2019;13(6):925–45.
26. Gresham RCH, Bahney CS, Leach JK. Growth factor delivery using extracellular matrix-mimicking substrates for musculoskeletal tissue engineering and repair. *Bioact Mater*. 2021;6(7):1945–56.
27. Wang M, Li H, Yang Y, Yuan K, Zhou F, Liu H, et al. A 3D-bioprinted scaffold with doxycycline-controlled BMP2-expressing cells for inducing bone regeneration and inhibiting bacterial infection. *Bioact Mater*. 2021;6(5):1318–29.
28. Gomez-Florit M, Pardo A, Domingues RMA, Graça AL, Babo PS, Reis RL, et al. Natural-based hydrogels for tissue engineering applications. *Molecules*. 2020;25(24):5858.
29. Jiang S, Wang M, He J. A review of biomimetic scaffolds for bone regeneration: Toward a cell-free strategy. *Bioeng Transl Med*. 2021;6(2):e10206.
30. Yang GH, Kim W, Kim J, Kim G. A skeleton muscle model using GelMA-based cell-aligned bioink processed with an electric-field assisted 3D/4D bioprinting. *Theranostics*. 2021;11(1):48–63.
31. Ngan CGY, Quigley A, Williams RJ, O'Connell CD, Blanchard R, Boyd-Moss M, et al. Matured myofibers in bioprinted constructs with in vivo vascularization and innervation. *Gels*. 2021;7(4):171.
32. Kim JH, Ko IK, Jeon MJ, Kim I, Vanschaayk MM, Atala A, et al. Pelvic floor muscle function recovery using biofabricated tissue constructs with neuromuscular junctions. *Acta Biomater*. 2021;121:237–49.
33. Kim JH, Seol YJ, Ko IK, Kang HW, Lee YK, Yoo JJ, et al. 3D bioprinted human skeletal muscle constructs for muscle function restoration. *Sci Rep*. 2018;8(1):12307.
34. Kim JH, Kim I, Seol YJ, Ko IK, Yoo JJ, Atala A, et al. Neural cell integration into 3D bioprinted skeletal muscle constructs accelerates restoration of muscle function. *Nat Commun*. 2020;11(1):1025.
35. Constante G, Apsite I, Alkhamis H, Dulle M, Schwarzer M, Caspari A, et al. 4D biofabrication using a combination of 3d printing and melt-electrowriting of shape-morphing polymers. *ACS Appl Mater Interfaces*. 2021;13(11):12767–76.
36. Yeo M, Kim G. Micro/nano-hierarchical scaffold fabricated using a cell electrospinning/3D printing process for co-culturing myoblasts and HUVECs to induce myoblast alignment and differentiation. *Acta Biomater*. 2020;107:102–14.

37. Kupfer ME, Lin WH, Ravikumar V, Qiu K, Wang L, Gao L, et al. In situ expansion, differentiation, and electromechanical coupling of human cardiac muscle in a 3D bioprinted, chambered organoid. *Circ Res.* 2020;127(2):207–24.
38. Xu L, Varkey M, Jorgensen A, Ju J, Jin Q, Park JH, et al. Bioprinting small diameter blood vessel constructs with an endothelial and smooth muscle cell bilayer in a single step. *Biofabrication.* 2020;12(4):045012.
39. Laternser S, Keller H, Leupin O, Rausch M, Graf-Hausner U, Rimann M. A novel microplate 3D bioprinting platform for the engineering of muscle and tendon tissues. *SLAS Technol.* 2018;23(6):599–613.
40. Ronzoni FL, Aliberti F, Scocozza F, Benedetti L, Auricchio F, Sampaolesi M, et al. Myoblast 3D bioprinting to burst in vitro skeletal muscle differentiation. *J Tissue Eng Regen Med.* 2022;16(5):484–95.
41. Urciuolo A, Poli I, Brandolino L, Raffa P, Scattolini V, Laterza C, et al. Intravital three-dimensional bioprinting. *Nat Biomed Eng.* 2020;4(9):901–15.
42. Boularaoui S, Shanti A, Lanotte M, Luo S, Bawazir S, Lee S, et al. Nanocomposite conductive bioinks based on low-concentration GelMA and MXene nanosheets/gold nanoparticles providing enhanced printability of functional skeletal muscle tissues. *ACS Biomater Sci Eng.* 2021;7(12):5810–22.
43. Wang Y, Wang Q, Luo S, Chen Z, Zheng X, Kankala RK, et al. 3D bioprinting of conductive hydrogel for enhanced myogenic differentiation. *Regen Biomater.* 2021;8(5):rbab035.
44. Mostafavi A, Samandari M, Karvar M, Ghovvati M, Endo Y, Sinha I, et al. Colloidal multiscale porous adhesive (bio)inks facilitate scaffold integration. *Appl Phys Rev.* 2021;8(4):041415.
45. Yeo M, Kim G. Electrohydrodynamic-direct-printed cell-laden microfibrous structure using alginate-based bioink for effective myotube formation. *Carbohydr Polym.* 2021;272:118444.
46. Wang Y, Cui H, Xu C, Esworthy TJ, Hann SY, Boehm M, et al. 4D printed cardiac construct with aligned myofibers and adjustable curvature for myocardial regeneration. *ACS Appl Mater Interfaces.* 2021;13(11):12746–58.
47. Kim W, Lee H, Lee J, Atala A, Yoo JJ, Lee SJ, et al. Efficient myotube formation in 3D bioprinted tissue construct by biochemical and topographical cues. *Biomaterials.* 2020;230:119632.
48. Hwangbo H, Lee H, Jin EJ, Lee J, Jo Y, Ryu D, et al. Bio-printing of aligned GelMa-based cell-laden structure for muscle tissue regeneration. *Bioact Mater.* 2022;8:57–70.
49. Choi YJ, Jun YJ, Kim DY, Yi HG, Chae SH, Kang J, et al. A 3D cell printed muscle construct with tissue-derived bioink for the treatment of volumetric muscle loss. *Biomaterials.* 2019;206:160–9.
50. Liu J, Miller K, Ma X, Dewan S, Lawrence N, Whang G, et al. Direct 3D bioprinting of cardiac micro-tissues mimicking native myocardium. *Biomaterials.* 2020;256:120204.
51. Ong CS, Fukunishi T, Zhang H, Huang CY, Nashed A, Blazeski A, et al. Biomaterial-free three-dimensional bioprinting of cardiac tissue using human induced pluripotent stem cell derived cardiomyocytes. *Sci Rep.* 2017;7(1):4566.
52. Yeung E, Fukunishi T, Bai Y, Bedja D, Pitaktong I, Mattson G, et al. Cardiac regeneration using human-induced pluripotent stem cell-derived biomaterial-free 3D-bioprinted cardiac patch in vivo. *J Tissue Eng Regen Med.* 2019;13(11):2031–9.
53. Fan T, Wang S, Jiang Z, Ji S, Cao W, Liu W, et al. Controllable assembly of skeletal muscle-like bundles through 3D bioprinting. *Biofabrication.* 2021;14(1):10.1088/1758-5090/ac3aca. Published 2021 Dec 1. doi:10.1088/1758-5090/ac3aca.
54. Lee H, Kim W, Lee J, Park KS, Yoo JJ, Atala A, et al. Self-aligned myofibers in 3D bioprinted extracellular matrix-based construct accelerate skeletal muscle function restoration. *Appl Phys Rev.* 2021;8(2):021405.

55. Kim D, Hwangbo H, Kim G. Engineered myoblast-laden collagen filaments fabricated using a submerged bioprinting process to obtain efficient myogenic activities. *Biomacromolecules*. 2021;22(12):5042–51.
56. Miao S, Nowicki M, Cui H, Lee SJ, Zhou X, Mills DK, et al. 4D anisotropic skeletal muscle tissue constructs fabricated by staircase effect strategy. *Biofabrication*. 2019;11(3):035030.
57. Christensen KW, Turner J, Coughenour K, Maghdouri-White Y, Bulysheva AA, Sergeant O, et al. Assembled cell-decorated collagen (AC-DC) fiber bioprinted implants with musculoskeletal tissue properties promote functional recovery in volumetric muscle loss. *Adv Healthc Mater*. 2022;11(3):e2101357.
58. Tracy EP, Gettler BC, Zakhari JS, Schwartz RJ, Williams SK, Birla RK. 3D bioprinting the cardiac purkinje system using human adipogenic mesenchymal stem cell derived purkinje cells. *Cardiovasc Eng Technol*. 2020;11(5):587–604.
59. Li Y, Huang G, Gao B, Li M, Genin GM, Lu TJ, et al. Magnetically actuated cell-laden microscale hydrogels for probing strain-induced cell responses in three dimensions. *NPG Asia Materials*. 2016;8(1):e238.
60. Matsumoto T, Sasaki J, Alsberg E, Egusa H, Yatani H, Sohmura T. Three-dimensional cell and tissue patterning in a strained fibrin gel system. *PLoS One*. 2007;2(11):e1211.
61. Martin RB, Burr DB, Sharkey NA, Fyhrie DP. Mechanical Properties of Ligament and Tendon. In: Martin RB, Burr DB, Sharkey NA, Fyhrie DP, editors. *Skeletal Tissue Mechanics*. New York: Springer New York; 2015. p. 175–225.
62. Lui H, Vaquette C, Denbeigh JM, Bindra R, Kakar S, van Wijnen AJ. Multiphasic scaffold for scapholunate interosseous ligament reconstruction: A study in the rabbit knee. *J Orthop Res*. 2021;39(8):1811–24.
63. Lui H, Bindra R, Baldwin J, Ivanovski S, Vaquette C. Additively manufactured multiphasic bone-ligament-bone scaffold for scapholunate interosseous ligament reconstruction. *Adv Healthc Mater*. 2019;8(14):e1900133.
64. Park SH, Choi YJ, Moon SW, Lee BH, Shim JH, Cho DW, et al. Three-dimensional bio-printed scaffold sleeves with mesenchymal stem cells for enhancement of tendon-to-bone healing in anterior cruciate ligament reconstruction using soft-tissue tendon graft. *Arthroscopy*. 2018;34(1):166–79.
65. Wu G, Sun B, Zhao C, Wang Z, Teng S, Yang M, et al. Three-Dimensional Tendon Scaffold Loaded with TGF-β1 gene silencing plasmid prevents tendon adhesion and promotes tendon repair. *ACS Biomater Sci Eng*. 2021;7(12):5739–48.
66. Touré ABR, Mele E, Christie JK. Multi-layer scaffolds of poly(caprolactone), poly(glycerol sebacate) and bioactive glasses manufactured by combined 3D printing and electrospinning. *Nanomaterials (Basel)*. 2020;10(4):626.
67. Wu Y, Wong YS, Fuh JY. Degradation behaviors of geometric cues and mechanical properties in a 3D scaffold for tendon repair. *J Biomed Mater Res A*. 2017;105(4):1138–49.
68. Pitaru AA, Lacombe JG, Cooke ME, Beckman L, Steffen T, Weber MH, et al. Investigating commercial filaments for 3D printing of stiff and elastic constructs with ligament-like mechanics. *Micromachines (Basel)*. 2020;11(9):846.
69. Chen P, Cui L, Fu SC, Shen L, Zhang W, You T, et al. The 3D-printed PLGA scaffolds loaded with bone marrow-derived mesenchymal stem cells augment the healing of rotator cuff repair in the rabbits. *Cell Transplant*. 2020;29:963689720973647.
70. Jiang X, Wu S, Kuss M, Kong Y, Shi W, Streubel PN, et al. 3D printing of multilayered scaffolds for rotator cuff tendon regeneration. *Bioact Mater*. 2020;5(3):636–43.
71. Chen P, Cui L, Chen G, You T, Li W, Zuo J, et al. The application of BMP-12-overexpressing mesenchymal stem cells loaded 3D-printed PLGA scaffolds in rabbit rotator cuff repair. *Int J Biol Macromol*. 2019;138:79–88.
72. Nocera AD, Comín R, Salvatierra NA, Cid MP. Development of 3D printed fibrillar collagen scaffold for tissue engineering. *Biomed Microdevices*. 2018;20(2):26.

73. Chae S, Choi YJ, Cho DW. Mechanically and biologically promoted cell-laden constructs generated using tissue-specific bioinks for tendon/ligament tissue engineering applications. *Biofabrication.* 2022;14(2):025013.
74. Toprakhisar B, Nadernezhad A, Bakirci E, Khani N, Skvortsov GA, Koc B. Development of bioink from decellularized tendon extracellular matrix for 3D bioprinting. *Macromol Biosci.* 2018;18(10):e1800024.
75. Stanco D, Boffito M, Bogni A, Puricelli L, Barrero J, Soldati G, et al. 3D bioprinting of human adipose-derived stem cells and their tenogenic differentiation in clinical-grade medium. Int J Mol Sci. 2020;21(22):8694.
76. Rak Kwon D, Jung S, Jang J, Park GY, Suk Moon Y, Lee SC. A 3-dimensional bioprinted scaffold with human umbilical cord blood-mesenchymal stem cells improves regeneration of chronic full-thickness rotator cuff tear in a rabbit model. *Am J Sports Med.* 2020;48(4):947–58.
77. Zhang Y, Lei T, Tang C, Chen Y, Liao Y, Ju W, et al. 3D printing of chemical-empowered tendon stem/progenitor cells for functional tissue repair. *Biomaterials.* 2021;271:120722.
78. Thattaruparambil Raveendran N, Vaquette C, Meinert C, Samuel Ipe D, Ivanovski S. Optimization of 3D bioprinting of periodontal ligament cells. *Dent Mater.* 2019;35(12):1683–94.
79. Ruiz OG, Dhaher Y. Multi-color and multi-material 3D printing of knee joint models. *3D Print Med.* 2021;7(1):12.
80. Nakanishi Y, Okada T, Takeuchi N, Kozono N, Senju T, Nakayama K, et al. Histological evaluation of tendon formation using a scaffold-free three-dimensional-bioprinted construct of human dermal fibroblasts under. *Regen Ther.* 2019;11:47–55.
81. Zhang YS, Yue K, Aleman J, Moghaddam KM, Bakht SM, Yang J, et al. 3D bioprinting for tissue and organ fabrication. *Ann Biomed Eng.* 2017;45(1):148–63.
82. Yang J, Zhang YS, Yue K, Khademhosseini A. Cell-laden hydrogels for osteochondral and cartilage tissue engineering. *Acta Biomater.* 2017;57:1–25.
83. Di Piazza E, Pandolfi E, Cacciotti I, Del Fattore A, Tozzi AE, Secinaro A, et al. Bioprinting technology in skin, heart, pancreas and cartilage tissues: Progress and challenges in clinical practice. *Int J Environ Res Public Health.* 2021;18(20):10806.
84. Mei Q, Rao J, Bei HP, Liu Y, Zhao X. 3D bioprinting photo-crosslinkable hydrogels for bone and cartilage repair. *Int J Bioprint.* 2021;7(3):367.
85. Olate-Moya F, Arens L, Wilhelm M, Mateos-Timoneda MA, Engel E, Palza H. Chondroinductive alginate-based hydrogels having graphene oxide for 3D printed scaffold fabrication. *ACS Appl Mater Interfaces.* 2020;12(4):4343–57.
86. Dasargyri A, Reichmann E, Moehrlen U. Bio-engineering of fetal cartilage for in utero spina bifida repair. *Pediatr Surg Int.* 2020;36(1):25–31.
87. Trachsel L, Zenobi-Wong M, Benetti EM. The role of poly(2-alkyl-2-oxazoline)s in hydrogels and biofabrication. *Biomater Sci.* 2021;9(8):2874–86.
88. Schuurman W, Levett PA, Pot MW, van Weeren PR, Dhert WJ, Hutmacher DW, et al. Gelatin-methacrylamide hydrogels as potential biomaterials for fabrication of tissue-engineered cartilage constructs. *Macromol Biosci.* 2013;13(5):551–61.
89. Xu T, Binder KW, Albanna MZ, Dice D, Zhao W, Yoo JJ, et al. Hybrid printing of mechanically and biologically improved constructs for cartilage tissue engineering applications. *Biofabrication.* 2013;5(1):015001.
90. Mouser VH, Abbadessa A, Levato R, Hennink WE, Vermonden T, Gawlitta D, et al. Development of a thermosensitive HAMA-containing bio-ink for the fabrication of composite cartilage repair constructs. *Biofabrication.* 2017;9(1):015026.
91. Abdollahiyan P, Oroojalian F, Mokhtarzadeh A, de la Guardia M. Hydrogel-based 3D bioprinting for bone and cartilage tissue engineering. *Biotechnol J.* 2020;15(12):e2000095.
92. Murphy SV, De Coppi P, Atala A. Opportunities and challenges of translational 3D bioprinting. *Nat Biomed Eng.* 2020;4(4):370–80.

93. Francis SL, Di Bella C, Wallace GG, Choong PFM. Cartilage tissue engineering using stem cells and bioprinting technology-barriers to clinical translation. *Front Surg.* 2018;5:70.
94. Petretta M, Desando G, Grigolo B, Roseti L. Cartilage tissue engineering by extrusion bioprinting: Process analysis, risk evaluation, and mitigation strategies. *Materials (Basel).* 2021;14(13):3528.
95. Daly AC, Freeman FE, Gonzalez-Fernandez T, Critchley SE, Nulty J, Kelly DJ. 3D bioprinting for cartilage and osteochondral tissue engineering. *Adv Healthc Mater.* 2017;6(22).
96. Zhang J, Wehrle E, Rubert M, Müller R. 3D bioprinting of human tissues: Biofabrication, bioinks, and bioreactors. *Int J Mol Sci.* 2021;22(8):3971. Published 2021 Apr 12. doi:10.3390/ijms22083971.
97. Kilian D, Ahlfeld T, Akkineni AR, Bernhardt A, Gelinsky M, Lode A. 3D bioprinting of osteochondral tissue substitutes – in vitro-chondrogenesis in multi-layered mineralized constructs. *Sci Rep.* 2020;10(1):8277.
98. Choe R, Devoy E, Jabari E, Packer JD, Fisher JP. Biomechanical aspects of osteochondral regeneration: Implications and strategies for three-dimensional bioprinting. *Tissue Eng Part B Rev.* 2022;28(4):766–88.
99. Melrose J. The importance of the knee joint meniscal fibrocartilages as stabilizing weight bearing structures providing global protection to human knee-joint tissues. *Cells.* 2019;8(4):324.
100. Abdulghani S, Morouço PG. Biofabrication for osteochondral tissue regeneration: Bioink printability requirements. *J Mater Sci Mater Med.* 2019;30(2):20.
101. Pitta Kruize C, Panahkhahi S, Putra NE, Diaz-Payno P, van Osch G, Zadpoor AA, et al. Biomimetic approaches for the design and fabrication of bone-to-soft tissue interfaces. *ACS Biomater Sci Eng.* 2021;10.1021/acsbiomaterials.1c00620.
102. Luo W, Liu H, Wang C, Qin Y, Liu Q, Wang J. Bioprinting of human musculoskeletal interface. *Adv Eng Mater.* 2019;21:1900019.
103. Chae S, Sun Y, Choi YJ, Ha DH, Jeon I, Cho DW. 3D cell-printing of tendon-bone interface using tissue-derived extracellular matrix bioinks for chronic rotator cuff repair. *Biofabrication.* 2021;13(3): 10.1088/1758-5090/abd159. Published 2021 Apr 2. doi:10.1088/1758-5090/abd159.
104. Bittner SM, Guo JL, Melchiorri A, Mikos AG. Three-dimensional printing of multilayered tissue engineering scaffolds. *Mater Today (Kidlington).* 2018;21(8):861–74.
105. Choe R, Devoy E, Kuzemchak B, Sherry M, Jabari E, Packer JD, et al. Computational investigation of interface printing patterns within 3D printed multilayered scaffolds for osteochondral tissue engineering. *Biofabrication.* 2022;14(2):10.1088/1758-5090/ac5220 . Published 2022 Feb 23. doi:10.1088/1758-5090/ac5220
106. Xu J, Ji J, Jiao J, Zheng L, Hong Q, Tang H, et al. 3D printing for bone-cartilage interface regeneration. *Front Bioeng Biotechnol.* 2022;10:828921.
107. Cao Y, Yang S, Zhao D, Li Y, Cheong SS, Han D, et al. Three-dimensional printed multiphasic scaffolds with stratified cell-laden gelatin methacrylate hydrogels for biomimetic tendon-to-bone interface engineering. *J Orthop Translat.* 2020;23:89–100.
108. Volpi M, Paradiso A, Costantini M, Święszkowski W. Hydrogel-based fiber biofabrication techniques for skeletal muscle tissue engineering. *ACS Biomater Sci Eng.* 2022;8(2):379–405.
109. Wang Z, Agrawal P, Zhang YS. Nanotechnologies and nanomaterials in 3D (bio)printing toward bone regeneration. *Adv NanoBiomed Res.* 2021;1(11):2100035.

8 3D Bioprinting for Cardiovascular Applications

N. Matthews, S. Ly, D. West, and C. Gentile
University of Technology Sydney

CONTENTS

8.1 INTRODUCTION

Ischaemic heart disease is characterised by occlusion of the coronary circulation to the heart, leading to myocardial damage and death of cardiomyocytes in the impacted region [1]. This is common for myocardial infarction (MI), which may eventually lead to heart failure (HF) in more severe conditions [1]. End-stage HF is a serious condition with a poor survival rate, and the gold standard treatment option remains a heart transplant. Lack of donors, requirement for specialist surgical centres and high cost prevent access to the treatment for a vast majority of the 26 million HF patients globally [1].

More recently, there has been evidence for a potential alternative to replacing the whole heart by using donor transplant with a bioengineered heart tissue that combines

DOI: 10.1201/9781003274568-8

state-of-the-art 3D bioprinting technology and stem cell-derived cardiac cells [2,3]. 3D bioprinting technology is an adaptable method of biofabrication for the precise geometrical deposition of cells and biomaterials to create a viable and functional tissue [3]. The accuracy of the biofabricated tissue is limited by the technical specifications of the 3D bioprinting system used [4]. Being able to determine where in the engineered tissue-specific cell types or non-cellular material resides is a distinct benefit compared to seeding cells and fabricating tissue in a Petri dish [5]. Similarly, 3D bioprinting, as the abbreviation suggests, makes it possible to create tissue according to 3D geometry [4]. Compared to two-dimensional shapes fabricated in a cell culture or a well plate, 3D designs are more detailed allowing complexity in the design [4]. Stem cell technologies enable the use of a patient-specific biological blueprint [6]. The latest advancements in the field have led to the use of either human embryonic or induced pluripotent stem cells (iPSCs) into cell types found in myocardial tissue [2,6]. The benefits of using patient-derived iPSCs prevent the likely risk of transplant rejection [5].

Cardiac tissue engineering has proven to be challenging due to the complex anatomy and physiology of the human heart [3]. First, emulating the complexity of the myocardial tissue using 3D bioprinting requires a perfect balance of printability and biocompatibility of the chosen biomaterials [3]. Then, from a biomechanical perspective, a healthy human heart beats and contracts in a variety of directions and acts like a pump to circulate blood around the body, as well as it contracts [7]. When the heart contracts to circulate blood to the rest of the body, the top region twists clockwise while the bottom of the heart twists counter-clockwise [7]. This adds to the complexity of engineering cardiac tissue because correct mechanical properties such as rigidity and elasticity are required to accommodate this ventricular motion. For optimal myocardial tissue engineering, the engrafted cardiac tissue should contract synchronously with the native myocardium [8]. Finally, the engineered tissue should be able to engraft and ultimately improve the cardiac function of a failing heart [2].

The myocardium is composed of three major cell types: cardiac myocytes, endothelial cells and fibroblasts [5]. The adult myocardium cannot regenerate itself following an injury [2]. Angiogenesis and biocompatibility of biomaterials used are important aspects for the successful transplantation of a biofabricated myocardial tissue. This will ensure proper neovascularisation in the infarcted area for nutrient and oxygen supply, as well as the prevention of graft rejection and undesired immune response [2].

This book chapter aims at highlighting the requirements of optimal myocardial tissues, as well as the outcomes of recent studies using biofabricated tissues for myocardial regeneration, including considerations for the translation of patient-specific, 3D bioprinted cardiac patches from exploratory studies to the clinic.

8.2 ANATOMY OF THE HUMAN HEART

The heart acts as the muscular pump of the circulatory system [9]. It is located in the middle mediastinum and surrounded by a pericardial sac, consists of a left and a right side divided by a septum, and is formed by four distinct chambers [9]. The chamber walls have three layers: a thin internal layer of endocardium that lines the chamber walls; a thick, muscular myocardium in the middle responsible for contractions; and a thin external layer, epicardium [9]. The atrium and the ventricle on the right collect and distribute deoxygenated blood, while the same structures on the left circulate oxygenated blood [10]. The human heart has the following four exterior surfaces: anterior surface formed mainly by the right ventricle; diaphragmatic surface formed primarily by the left ventricle and partly by the right ventricle; right pulmonary surface comprising the right atrium; and left pulmonary surface encompassing the left ventricle [9]. The heart has its own systemic blood supply, coronary circulation, which is responsible for the delivery and return of the blood flow to and from the myocardium [9]. If the coronary arteries become occluded, the blood supply to the myocardial wall is compromised, which can ultimately lead to MI.

The biological function of the heart is divided into two phases, diastole and systole, which together complete the cardiac cycle as presented in Figure 8.1 [11]. During diastole, blood is returned to the right atrium via the inferior and superior vena cava, and via pulmonary veins to the left atrium. Returning blood flow increases the pressure within the atria, and when it exceeds ventricular pressure, atrioventricular valves open passively allowing blood flow into the ventricles [11]. At the start of systole, atrial walls contract filling the ventricles. During a brief period of isovolumetric contraction of the ventricular walls, the atrioventricular, pulmonary and aortic valves remain closed. As the pressure inside the ventricles increases and exceeds the systemic arterial pressure, pulmonary and aortic valves open ejecting the blood into the circulatory system. After contracting, the ventricular walls relax and the next cardiac cycle begins [11].

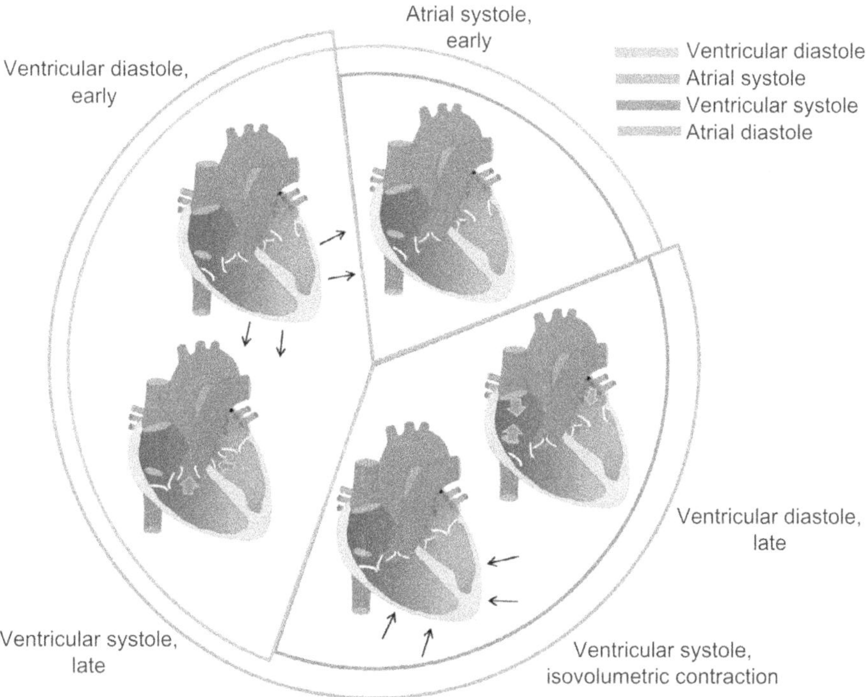

FIGURE 8.1 Phases of the cardiac cycle. Blood is collected in the atria during diastole, flows into the ventricles, and is ejected to the aorta and pulmonary trunk in systole. Source: Athanasiou et al. [12] used with permission.

8.3 IMPACT OF MI

The sudden occlusion of the blood flow to the myocardium causes MI in the impacted region, leading to pathological cell death or necrosis [13]. The impact of MI on the myocardial wall leads to the build-up of fibrous tissue in infarcted areas. This event is known as cardiac remodelling and results in alterations in the tissue composition, increased stiffness in the cardiac tissue, thinning of the walls, ischaemic mitral regurgitation and further death of cardiomyocytes [14]. The end result of cardiac remodelling is ventricular dysfunction, which leads to reduction in stroke volume and cardiac output [14,15]. Eventually, MI can lead to HF due to the death of cardiomyocytes and fibrosis that consequently forms on the myocardial wall [14]. Despite significant advances in preventative treatments for MI, end-stage HF does not have a successful cure yet [16].

8.4 3D BIOPRINTING AND BIOFABRICATION METHODS

3D bioprinting of cardiac cells in a hydrogel suspension may offer an alternative treatment option to individuals with myocardial damage. 3D bioprinting constitutes precise layering and positioning of cells, biomaterials and biochemicals in a defined 3D structure. This defined structure is known as a scaffold which is the structural basis for 3D bioprinting tissues. The scaffold provides a foundation for cells to adhere, proliferate and produce an extracellular matrix (ECM) to mimic living tissues [17].

The emergence of 3D bioprinting has generated widespread interest and continued growth of technological advancements in the field of regenerative medicine [18]. These advancements assist in further improvement of different techniques and methods required to successful fabricating of cardiovascular tissue structures.

Different 3D bioprinting systems operate on varying printing methods, and each has their own advantages and limitations. Common 3D bioprinting methods that have been explored for bioprinting constructs for cardiovascular regeneration include extrusion-based, inkjet-based and stereolithography modalities [19]. Classification of the bioprinting methods is presented in Table 8.1 and Figure 8.2.

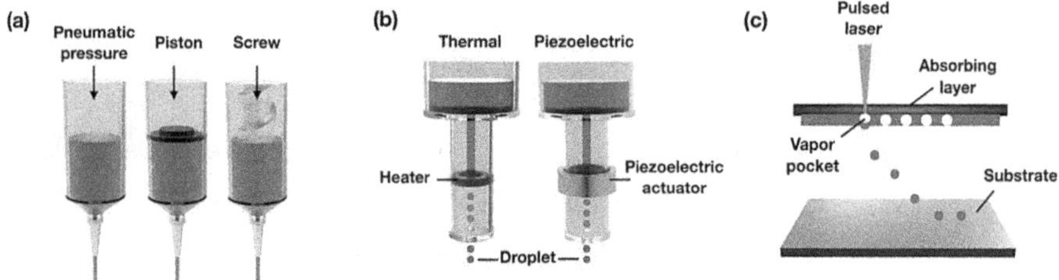

FIGURE 8.2 Major bioprinting methods. Schematic of (a) extrusion-based, (b) inkjet-based and (c) stereolithography bioprinting systems. Source: Fatimi et al. [27] used with permission.

TABLE 8.1
Classification of Bioprinting Methods, Their Applications, Advantages and Limitations

Bioprinting Method	Principle	Applications	Advantages	Limitations
Extrusion-based [20–22]	Semi-solid extrusion (SSE) and Pressure-assisted bioprinting (PAB) – rotating screw or pressurised air drives material through a loaded nozzle that deposits the material on a plane to form a desired 3D structure.	Biofabricate scaffolds that closely resemble tissue structures. Production of soft tissue models and bone structures for use as implants. Biofabrication of heart valves, blood vessels and myocardial constructs.	Capable of printing in the X, Y, Z axes. Temperature controlled printing environment. Able to use multiple nozzles to allow serial deposits.	Filament material used must transition to a stable state to preserve a three-dimensional structure.
	Fused deposition modelling(FDM)– a custom temperature environment is created to melt thermo-filament materials to extrude through a nozzle that deposits on a plane to form the 3D structure.			Filament materials that require high temperatures to extrude will be detrimental to cells during bioprinting
Inkjet-based [21,23,24]	Thermal inkjet bioprinting – electrical heat is applied to the print head which creates pressure that forces droplets to release from the nozzle.	Functional skin regeneration as this technique allows for direct deposits of biomaterials onto skin Production of layered cartilage constructs.	High speed allows for direct deposit and increased chances of cell viability.	Materials used to print must be in liquid state. Clogged nozzles droplet-based printing requires nozzles to have small diameter outlets.

(Continued)

TABLE 8.1 (*Continued*)
Classification of Bioprinting Methods, Their Applications, Advantages and Limitations

Bioprinting Method	Principle	Applications	Advantages	Limitations
	Acoustic inkjet bioprinting – a crystal is used to convert electrical energy into mechanical energy to break the liquid material into droplets which is then deposited via the nozzle. This is the result of a piezoelectric crystal which allows for a change in elemental bonds when a voltage is applied.		Avoids thermal stress on cells such as temperature increase while bioprinting.	Frequencies used may disrupt the cell membranes of bioprints. Technology is not widely available where most equipment is custom-made.
Stereolithography [20,25,26]	Freeform bioprinting method that does not use a nozzle to deposit materials. A computer-controlled laser, typically ultra-violet (UV), is pointed at a liquid material to solidify into a specified design. Micromirror arrays are used to adjust the light intensity of the beam to polymerise specific light-sensitive materials.	Production of tissue scaffolds and organs Fabrication of vascular networks. Biofabrication of personalised constructs for disease modelling to deliver patient-specific procedures. That is, modelling of plaque formed, calcified vessels.	Highest printing accuracy compared to the other methods. Relatively rapid printing speed. Able to produce large scaffolds. Able to fabricate complex and intricate geometrical designs.	Laser light source may affect DNA structure of autologous materials used to print.

8.5 BIOINKS

A bioink is commonly composed of a mixture of biomaterials and desired cell types for bioprinting tissue. Two dominant types of bioink structures are currently used: scaffold-based bioinks consist of encapsulated cells in biomaterials, while cell-free bioinks are used for cells to adhere to them in a second time [28]. Selection of biomaterials for formulating bioinks must demonstrate biocompatibility and printability, and exhibit desired rheological properties required for the intended 3D bioprinting technique and application [28]. These characteristics are important as the material used to 3D bioprint must facilitate cell adhesion, differentiation and proliferation [28]. These in turn determine cell viability and the ability of the biofabricated tissue to support living cells after transplantation.

A challenge in 3D bioprinting is the need to yield a robust structure where embedded cells can proliferate and adhere. A soft structure provides a softer matrix environment which is favourable for cell viability of soft tissues, while a stiffer structure may be suitable for other tissues and organs [29]. To bridge tissue-specific requirements, cross-linking strategies have been applied to polymers in low-viscosity bioinks for 3D bioprinting solid-like constructs. *In situ* and post-cross-linking approaches have both been explored, demonstrating high cell viability and improved printability *via* enhanced bioink viscosity [29].

8.6 HYDROGEL COMPOSITION

Hydrogels have been heavily explored in 3D bioprinting of cardiac patches as they are able to support cell growth and adhesion, and have tunable mechanical characteristics [30]. In addition, hydrogels provide mechanical support for cardiac cells and allow the deposition of cell-laden matrices to biofabricate a cardiac patch. Use of hydrogels formulated from natural polymers is common as they demonstrate good biocompatibility. However, synthetic hydrogels are easily produced compared to natural bioinks and often meet the required specifications of stability and reproducibility in 3D bioprinting [31]. Therefore, to meet mechanical properties and biocompatibility, a combination of natural and synthetic polymers is commonly used to form a hybrid hydrogel. Depending on the polymer properties, bioinks have been formulated to achieve optimal printability and cell-to-cell function. Commonly used natural bioinks are discussed below and presented in Figure 8.3.

8.6.1 ALGINATE

Derived from brown algae, alginate exhibits water-soluble properties that are suitable for preparing hydrogels [36]. An alginate solution can be cross-linked with calcium chloride to obtain a gelatinous structure (Figure 8.3a). Alginate is highly abundant and cost-effective resulting in its widespread use in regenerative medicine such as in 3D bioengineering tissue. Furthermore, it is non-toxic and has been shown to not cause an inflammatory response *in vivo* [36].

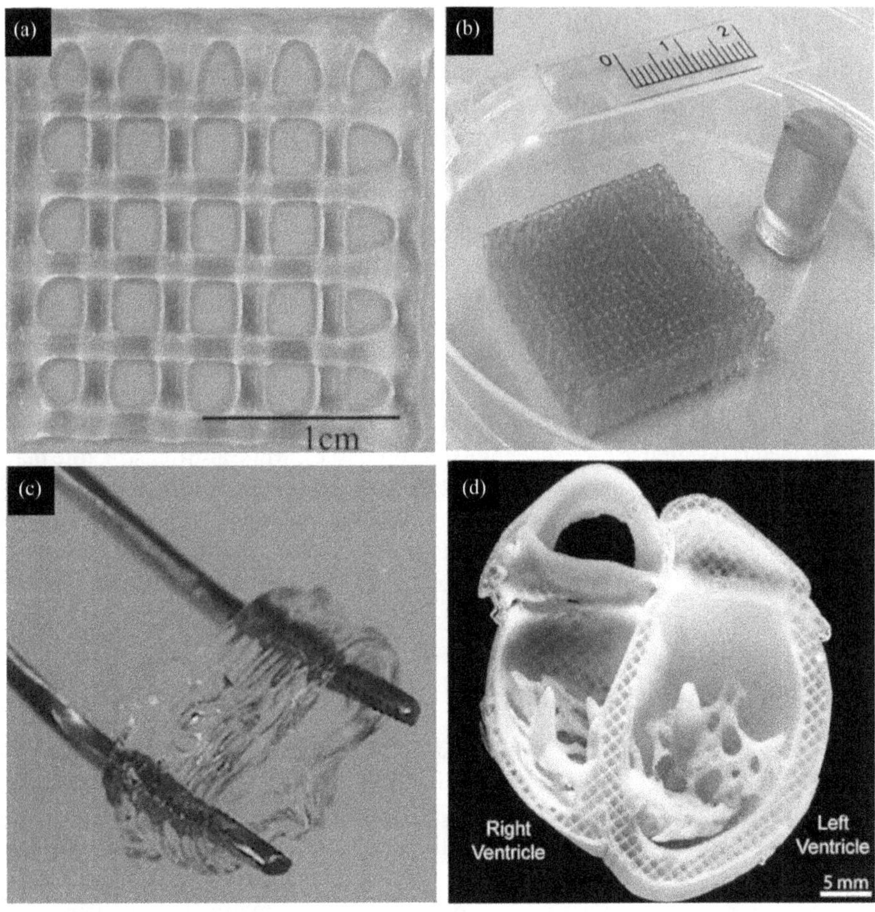

FIGURE 8.3 Examples of scaffolds containing hydrogels used to bioprint tissues. 3D bioprinted hydrogel scaffolds using (a) alginate, (b) gelatin, (c) gelatin methacrylate (GelMA) and (d) collagen. Adapted from Refs. [32–35].

8.6.2 Collagen

Collagen has been explored as a natural polymer for 3D bioprinting as it is a common protein that facilitates structural integrity and mechanical support in mammalian tissues (Figure 8.3b). Collagen for 3D bioprinting applications can be derived from a variety of sources, including bovine, porcine and fish skin [37]. The insoluble nature of collagen requires an acidic solvent to transform it into a hydrogel for use as a bio-ink [36]. A disadvantage of 3D bioprinting with collagen is the requirement for a long cross-linking process and the material's lack of stiffness. This limits the applications of collagen when 3D bioprinting of bulky or complex structures.

8.6.3 Gelatin

Gelatin is commonly used as a bioink in 3D bioprinting due to its gelation reversibility, processability and minimal immune response during surgical application. Gelatin is sourced from Type I collagen. While collagen is an insoluble protein, gelatin can dissolve in water in temperatures over 30°C due to its thermal denaturation. The process is reversible as gelatin can undergo gelation at 4°C and become a solution at 37°C [36]. Due to this gelation property, cross-linking of gelatin is required using chemicals such as aldehyde derivatives to ensure structural integrity during 3D bioprinting (Figure 8.3c) [38].

8.6.4 Gelatin Methacrylate

Gelatin methacrylate (GelMa) is a common fabricated gelatin-based ink used for 3D bioprinting complex structures (Figure 8.3d). It is also used as an additive in bioinks to enhance mechanical properties and printability. GelMa is a product of the reaction between gelatin and methacryclic anhydride. When photocured into a hydrogel with a photoinitiator, GelMa exhibits essential properties of an ECM to promote cell growth and proliferation, which allows cells to populate the scaffold [39].

8.7 CELL TYPES USED IN BIOINKS

Cardiac monocytes and non-myocytes, such as endothelial cells and fibroblasts, constitute approximately 70% of the cells in the human heart [40]. Along with vascular cells and blood cells in the heart, they are vital in providing structural integrity and electrical stimulation to the myocardium.

Cells used in 3D bioprinting can be autologous or allogeneic; to date, both have been investigated for use in cardiac regeneration. These cells are mixed with various polymers and structures to formulate a bioink used in 3D bioprinting. Multi-potent and pluripotent stem cells have been explored for 3D bioprinting cardiac patches to restore cardiomyocytes and vascular networks in myocardial infarcted areas. Multi-potent stem cells can be sourced from peripheral blood, bone marrow and living tissue. This cell type has been reported to possess cardiogenic differentiation capabilities, which improves the cardiac patch cell viability [41]. Pluripotent stem cells can be sourced from embryonic and induced pluripotent stem cells. This cell type is highly attractive for use in cardiac regeneration due to its ability to self-renew and multi-lineage differentiation. Embryonic stem cell-derived cardiomyocytes (ESC-CMs) have been reported to be able to electromechanically couple with the host cells [41]. This allows for simultaneous contraction between the host's heart and the implanted cardiomyocytes.

8.8 SPHEROIDS FOR 3D BIOPRINTING

For successful biomimicry and biocompatibility of forming complex engineered tissue, cell-to-cell contact is essential for intra-cellular functions. Surrounding the intra-cellular region is the ECM that supports cell differentiation, homeostasis and cell proliferation [42].

Cells in the heart are surrounded and subjected to physiological stimulations such as other mass components interfering spatial distributions of oxygen, nutrients and signalling molecules [43]. This is important to consider when 3D bioprinting engineered tissues as the vascular network is critical since the transplantation of the tissue to support healthy transportation of nutrient and oxygen supplies. To mimic these physiological conditions in 3D-bioprinted tissues and to achieve optimal biomimicry and biocompatibility, the use of spheroids has been explored as building blocks for tissue engineering [42].

Spheroids are generated to facilitate cell-to-cell interactions while maintaining cell-matrix adhesion. Spheroids harness unique properties which make them advantageous for tissue engineering applications. When compared to a 2D single cell approach, spheroids exhibit greater regenerative properties [42]. Complex tissues can be biofabricated with spheroids as incorporating multiple cell types in the same media is possible with co-culture spheroids. In addition, spheroids can be manipulated into macro-tissue constructs for the possibility of engineering large tissue constructs. Pairs of uniluminal vascular spheroids in cultured medium have been investigated and found to form larger spheroid structures *via* self-assembly [44]. This potentially allows for the use of vascular spheroids to be the building blocks to 3D bioprint blood vessels.

It is important to highlight that there are limitations with current *in vitro* models in 3D bioprinting and the methods of using a single layer of cells to 3D bioprint. A significant limitation of this is that the cell growth remains linear, known as "2D cultures", which impacts transplantation on the natural three-dimensional structure of the tissue [45]. It has been researched that 3D cultures have an advantage of having better biomimicry *in vivo. In vitro,* 3D cultures can better mimic the cardiac tissue microenvironment which assists in improving the accuracy of *in vitro* and *in vivo* testing. A major 3D culture type is spheroid. Spheroid cultures have been used to 3D bioprint tissue and organ models [46].

More specifically, cardiac spheroids have been investigated with human patient-derived cardiomyocytes in a range of culture and 3D bioprinting techniques. Using cardiac spheroids to biofabricate cardiac tissue offers increased potential for improved cell-cell interactions, vascularisation via co-culture of fibroblast-based cells and endothelial cells, and the production of ECM via the spheroid's nature of self-assembly [45].

Techniques when 3D bioprinting with spheroids include scaffold-free where spheroids are suspended in media and scaffold-based where spheroids are embedded in a hydrogel and then printed. A cardiac spheroid, alginate-gelatin-based hydrogel was reported to enable fusion of the spheroids which resulted in the cardiac spheroids exhibiting contractions when stimulated [46]. This highlights the long-term use of cardiac spheroids potentially being used to biofabricate cardiac tissues. Another study explored the biofabrication of myocardium layers with isolated, autologous cardiac progenitor cells (CPCs) to form cardiac spheroids. These CPCs-based spheroids found to 3D bioprint ideal gelatin and collagen scaffolds to regenerated damaged myocardium [47].

8.9 CONSIDERATIONS FOR TESTING OF REGENERATIVE PROPERTIES OF 3D BIOPRINTED TISSUES IN PRECLINICAL AND CLINICAL STUDIES

Several different small and large animal models have been used in cardiac research to date. Selecting an animal model that is the best fit for the study design depends on the scientific hypothesis of the experiment, availability of resources for managing the animals for the duration of the study, and how well the anatomical features under investigation match human anatomy [48].

Rats and mice are commonly used small animal models in cardiac studies as they exhibit similar coronary circulation architecture to humans [48,49]. Canine, ovine and porcine models have been used in large animal studies investigating the mechanism of MI [48,50]. It is important to highlight that the heart of a pig is anatomically and physiologically closest to its human counterpart. The anatomical position, shape, average rest heart rate, weight ratio to body weight, and thickness of the left ventricular (LV) wall in humans, pigs, rats and mice are presented for comparison in Figure 8.4.

The anatomical orientation and physiology of the heart in small and large animals differ to that of humans. In rodents, the heart is significantly smaller, has a more rounded shape and the apex of the heart points caudally. Residing in a pericardial sack in the mediastinum, the rodent heart does not have a ligament attachment to the diaphragm allowing it to maintain a spherical silhouette [49].

In large quadruped animals such as pigs, the size of the heart is similar to bipedal humans, but the anatomical positioning and overall shape of the organ are different [49,51,52]. The porcine heart is more elongated with a valentine shape compared to the human heart. In pigs, the heart rests on its apex with the anterior border near the sternum, while the flat inferior border of the human heart rests on the diaphragmatic surface giving the organ a trapezoidal shape. In both species, the heart is firmly attached to the central tendinous aponeurosis of the diaphragm.

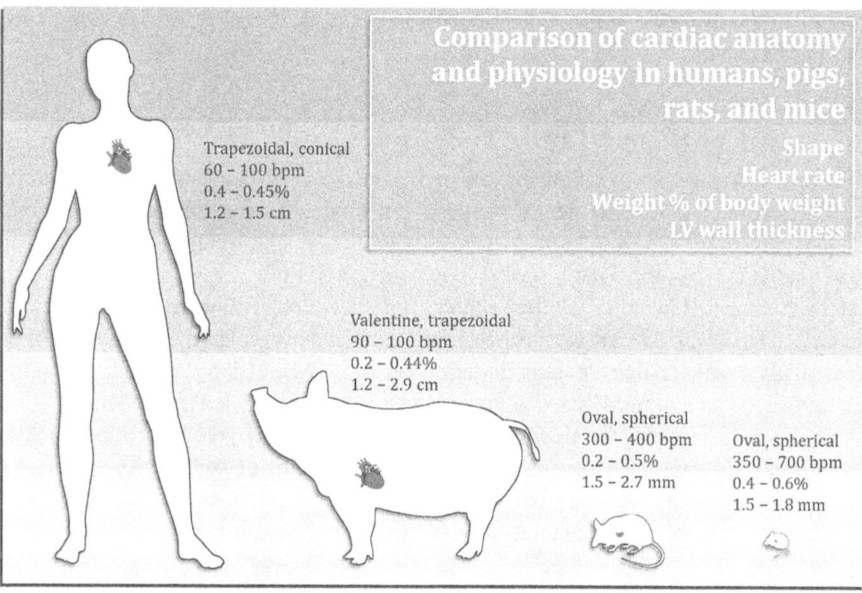

FIGURE 8.4 Comparison of cardiac anatomy and physiology between humans, pigs, rats and mice. The anatomical size and orientation of the heart are similar in humans and pigs but notably different when compared to rodents. In contrast, the comparative size of the heart to body weight and thickness of the LV wall are similar across all species.

A handful of clinical studies have so far been conducted where stem cell therapies were tested for the treatment of MI. As a comparison to other approaches, none of them are yet to use a 3D bioprinted cardiac patch in humans but have instead tested cell sheets [53–56] and injectable stem cell treatments [57–60]. Autologous cell sheets formed of skeletal myoblasts [54–56] and hESC-derived cardiovascular progenitors embedded in a fibrin patch [53] are the closest experimental methods to a 3D bioprinted cardiac patch tested clinically to date.

Although the clinical studies using a cell sheet approach recruited small cohorts between 1 and 7 patients, results showed promising trends in the areas of efficacy, feasibility and safety [53–56]. In terms of efficacy, all the clinical studies saw a trend in improvement of the LV ejection fraction (LVEF) with increases ranging between 7.1% and 20%; however, none of the results were statistically significant [53–56]. Two of the clinical studies measured local changes to the LV wall motion in the treated area [53,56]. Menasché et al. [53] used a scoring system for the LV wall motion measurement and reported a significant change from 4.2 ± 0.8 at baseline to 2.5 ± 0.4 at 1 year where a lower number indicates an improved outcome. Yoshikawa et al. [56] measured systolic wall motion in the region of transplanted cell sheets and recorded a change from 4.6 ± 1.0 to 5.0 ± 1.4 mm after the treatment; however, the change was not significant.

Two clinical studies discussed the better safety and feasibility of the cell sheet method over injectables [55,56]. Main benefits cited were improved cell delivery to the transplant site, increased cell survivability, reduced risk of inflammation in the myocardium and reduced myocardial damage. None of the clinical studies encountered major or severe adverse events such as severe arrhythmia, post-procedural MI, or patient death attributed to a cell sheet transplant, or reported on rejection of the cellular transplant [53–56].

8.9.1 Studies Using 3D Bioprinted Cardiac Patches in Animal Models

To date, a handful of *in vivo* studies investigating the use of 3D bioprinted cardiac patches for the treatment of MI have been conducted. Six small animal studies where a 3D bioprinted patch has been transplanted to the left ventricular wall were completed between 2011 and 2022 [61–66]. Findings of studies where a 3D bioprinted cardiac patch was used are presented in Table 8.2. Two of the studies were done on mice and four on rats; so far, studies of 3DBP cardiac patches have not been done on large animal models. In general, the results indicate a trend in improvement in the ejection fraction and fraction shortening, reduction in MI size and neovascularisation after patch implantation.

Four out of the six studies testing a bioprinted patch *in vivo* used a permanent left anterior descending artery (LAD) ligation model, one an ischaemic reperfusion (I/R) model, and in one study, MI was not induced. Engraftment to the epicardium ranged from freeform transplantation to the use of sutures, fibrin glue or a combination of both.

Duration of the studies ranged between 7 and 120 days, where available results of cardiac performance measurements are included at 28 days post-MI in Table 8.2. As the studies were designed and performed independently, measurement times and end points, size of control and treatment groups, as well as cardiac and patch performance indicators vary between the studies making them difficult to contrast and compare.

TABLE 8.2
Studies Testing 3D Bioprinted Cardiac Patches In Vivo

Study	Hydrogel Composition	Cells (Type, Ratio, #)	Patch Geometry (Layers, Thickness (mm), Diameter (mm))	Animal/MI Model	Suture /Glue	Measu-Rement Timing Post-MI (*d*)	EF% (*n*) (Sham, MI Only, Acellular Patch, Random Cell-Seed, Engineered Patch)	FS% (*n*) (Sham, MI Only, Acellular Patch, Random Cell-Seed, Engineered Patch)	MI Size (*n*) (Sham, MI Only, Acellular Patch, Random Cell-Seed, Engineered Patch)	Graft Presence (Macro / Micro Scale)	Vascularisation (*n*)
Jiang et al. [61]	ASP-A35m	CMs, neonatal mice N/A N/A	2 1 5	ICR mouse, permanent	None	28	55.58 ± 2.62 (7) 22.49 ± 1.67 (7) 23.33 ± 1.49 (7)- 29.31 ± 7.32# (7)	28.57 ± 1.37 (7) 10.27 ± 0.78 (7) 10.74 ± 0.78 (7)- 13.83 ± 3.75# (7)	- ns. (7) ns. (7) - Significant# (7)	Macro	ns. (-)
Cui et al. [62]	GelMA / PEGDA	hiPSC-CMs, hMSCs, hECs 1:1:1 N/A	2, 4, 8 0.6 4	NSG mouse, I/R	None	120	- 56.1 ± 1.5 (-) 64.1 ± 3.5 (-) 64.1 ± 3.5 (-) -	- - - - -	- 8.4 ± 1.1% (-) 3.8 ± 0.7% (-) 3.8 ± 0.7% (-) -	Macro, micro	Significant** (≥6)
Yang et al. [64]	PGS-PCL	CMs, H9c2 rat N/A 10 × 10^4/ well	4, 15 1.2, 4.5 2	Sprague-Dawley rat, permanent	Suture	28	ns. (8) ns. (8) ns.† (8) ns.‡ (8) Significant** (8)	ns. (8) ns. (8) ns.† (8) ns.‡ (8) Significant** (8)	- ns. (8) ns.† (8) ns.‡ (8) Significant** (8)	-	Significant** (8)

(Continued)

TABLE 8.2 (*Continued*)
Studies Testing 3D Bioprinted Cardiac Patches In Vivo

Study	Hydrogel Composition	Cells (Type, Ratio, #)	Patch Geometry (Layers, Thickness (mm), Diameter (mm))	Animal/MI Model	Suture /Glue	Measu-Rement Timing Post-MI (*d*)	EF% (*n*) (Sham, MI Only, Acellular Patch, Random Cell-Seed, Engineered Patch)	FS% (*n*) (Sham, MI Only, Acellular Patch, Random Cell-Seed, Engineered Patch)	MI Size (*n*) (Sham, MI Only, Acellular Patch, Random Cell-Seed, Engineered Patch)	Graft Presence (Macro / Micro Scale)	Vascularisation (*n*)
Yeung et al. [63]	Cardiac spheroid	hiPSC-CMs, FBs, HUVECs 70:15:15 3.3×10^4/ well	1 0.35–0.40 3.6	Lewis nude rat, permanent	Suture, glue	28	- - 40.1 ± 14.4 (6) 50.0 ± 18.9 (6) -	- - - - -	- - 19.39 ± 8.1% (6) 10.6 ± 5.1%* (6) -	-	Significant*** (6)
Ong et al. [65]	Cardiac spheroid	hiPSC-CMs, FBs, HUVECs 70:15:15 3.3×10^4/ CS	1 - -	Rowett nude rat, none	Suture, glue	7	- - - - -	- - - - -	- - - - -	Macro, micro	ns. (-)
Gaebel et al. [66]	Polyester urethane urea	HUVECs, hMSCs 3:1 18×10^4/ cm2	2 0.3 8	Rowett nude rat, permanent	Suture	56	ns. (4) ns. (3) ns. (6) ns. (6) Significant* (7)	- - - - -	ns. (3) ns. (3) ns. (3) ns. (3) ns. (3)	Macro, micro	Significant* (4)

All values mean ± SD, ns, non-significant; *$p<0.05$, **$p<0.01$, ***$p<0.001$, #$p<0.0001$. † cellular cardiac patch with a PCL scaffold, ‡ cellular cardiac patch with a PGS scaffold. ASP-A35m, leucine zipper-based protein bi-layer hydrogel; CM, cardiomyocyte; EF, ejection fraction; FB, fibroblast; FS, fraction shortening; GelMA, gelatin methacrylate; hEC, human endothelial cell; hiPSC, human induced pluripotent stem cell; hMSC, human mesenchymal stem cell; HUVEC, human umbilical vein endothelial cell; ICR, Institute of Cancer Research; I/R, ischaemic reperfusion; MI, myocardial infarction; NSG, NOD scid gamma; PCL, poly-(ε-caprolactone); PEGDA, polyethylene glycol diacrylate; PGS, poly-(glycerol sebacate).

For cardiac performance, ejection fraction (EF) was the most commonly recorded indicator and reported in five of the six studies [61–64,66]. In only three studies, the bioprinted patch increased the EF% significantly compared to the control group of animals with MI [61,64,66]; the other two studies [62,63] reported a trend towards improved EF but the findings were not significant. Further to this, in two of the studies, the bioengineered cardiac patch significantly increased fractional shortening % (FS%) post-MI when compared to a control group of mice with MI only [61], or when comparing performance to a treatment group with an acellular patch [64]. Cardiac output (CO) was also recorded in two of the studies but reported non-significant results between 4.55 and 36 mL/min [61,63].

Adhesion and engraftment of the cardiac patch to the transplantation site were reported in four of the studies, and confirmed at the end of the study when the animals were euthanised [61,62,65,66]. No difference was found between different engraftment methods in terms of the patch remaining in place; cellular engraftment between the cardiac patch and native myocardium was tested histologically and confirmed in three of the studies [62,65,66].

Changes to the LV morphology were measured using varying methods and different parameters across all studies in Table 8.2, including *in vivo* using echocardiography and in histology studies after hearts had been excised. None of the studies reported adverse cardiac events post-MI, such as teratoma formation, alloimmunisation or inflammation related to a cardiac patch transplant. It should be noted, however, that only one of the studies included the survival rate of animals with 100% survival in the cardiac patch treatment group and 83.3% survival rate in the control group [63].

Histological analyses demonstrated a significant decrease in the fibrotic area in three studies [61,63,64], and non-significant results in two studies [62,66] after a cardiac patch implantation, when compared to control animals with MI only. Immunostaining was used to quantify markers for cardiomyogenesis and angiogenesis in the transplanted area, as a promising sign of cardiac regeneration. Although two studies had statistically non-significant results [61,65], four studies saw a significant increase in a number and density of the vascularity compared to acellular controls [62–64,66]. In addition, cardiomyocyte proliferation was measured in two studies: a significant increase in the number of cardiomyocytes among an acellular patch group, and the cardiac patch group post-MI was reported in one study [61], while the second returned a non-significant result [62].

8.10 CONSIDERATIONS FOR THE DEVELOPMENT OF PERSONALISED CARDIAC PATCHES

Personalised medicine aims at transforming the standardised healthcare approach to treatments tailored to suit the needs of an individual patient. 3D bioprinting is an ideal method of biofabrication for this purpose; as in wider terms, 3D printing is considered perfect for producing bespoke solutions. To 3D bioprint a patient-specific transplant, the cardiac patch must first be designed to match the patient's genetic and anatomical cardiac profile.

Elements of designing and 3D bioprinting a patient-specific cardiac patch have been described in our previously published review [1]. The process is presented in Figure 8.5, where the left side represents the biological components of the design and the right side considerations regarding the anatomical 3D modelling.

As previously discussed, to tailor the biological basis of the cardiac patch to match individual patients, patient stem cells are reprogrammed to provide the cellular content of the biofabricated cardiac tissue. An autologous approach to the biological design is expected to carry a smaller risk of transplant rejection as the cells originate from the patient. If a hydrogel is used in the construction of the cardiac patch, the material has to support cell viability, ensure the maturation of the cells and maintain cell expression.

Cardiac anatomy and function are typically measured by an echocardiogram, cardiac computed tomography (CT) or cardiac magnetic resonance imaging (MRI). Each imaging modality has its benefits and ideal use. For the purpose of 3D modelling and design, CT scans are used to capture the anatomical features of the heart while MRI identifies the location and severity of MI in the LV wall. Data from the cardiac imaging are segmented using specialised software which produces a detailed digital 3D model of the anatomical

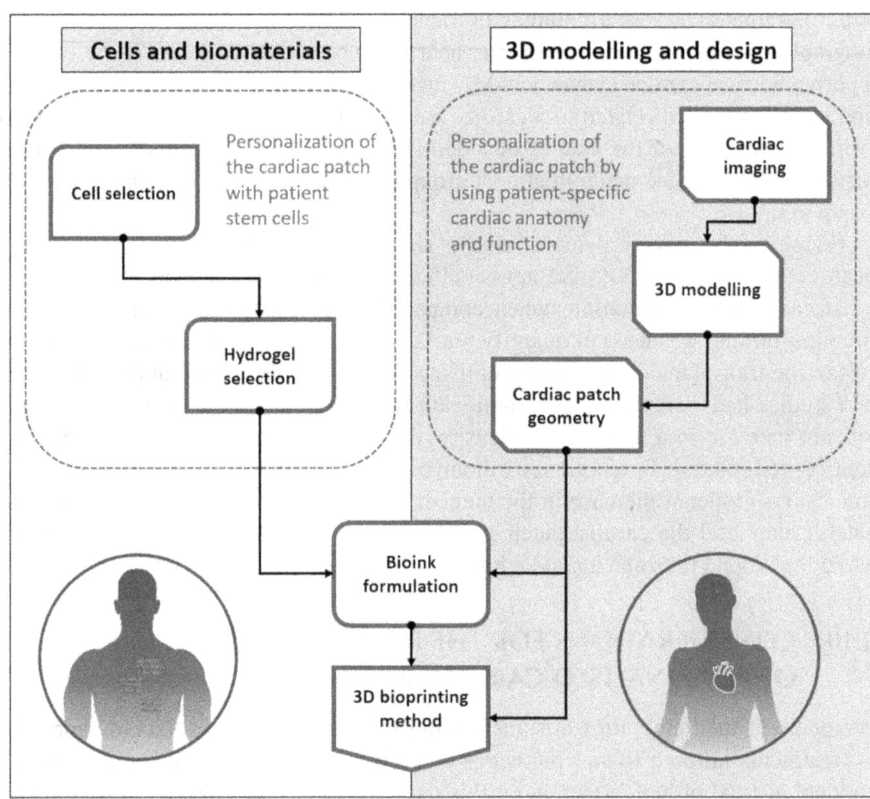

FIGURE 8.5 Biological and design considerations of creating a patient-specific cardiac patch. Selection of the cell line and hydrogel together with the 3D design of the cardiac patch determines optimal bioink formulation and 3D bioprinting method. Source: Matthews et al. [1] used with permission.

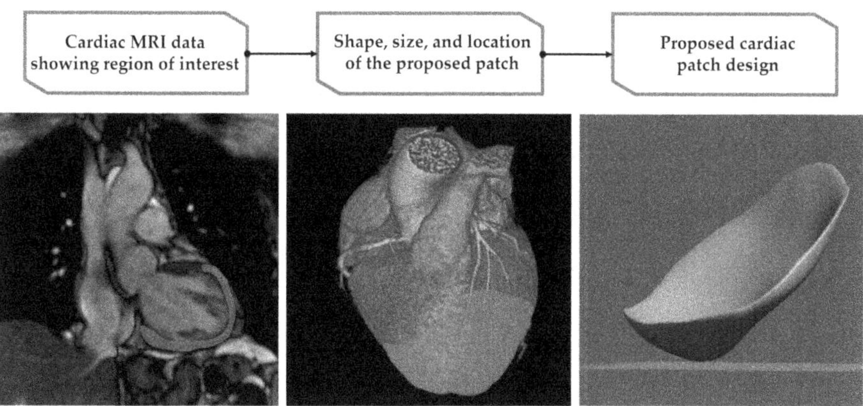

FIGURE 8.6 3D design of personalised cardiac patches using MRI and CT scan data. The infarcted region in the myocardium is identified in a cardiac MRI, and a cardiac CT scan captures the anatomy of the LV wall. Data from the scans are used to create a digital 3D model of a patient-specific cardiac patch. Source: Matthews et al. [1] used with permission.

features. A cardiac patch that conforms to the patient anatomy in the infarcted region is designed using the digital model, typically with a CAD software which produces a file suitable for 3D bioprinting. The concept of the process is presented in Figure 8.6.

Properties of the selected hydrogel and the overall cardiac patch geometry form a basis for the bioink formulation, as it must combine optimal biological and mechanical properties. Biological traits such as biomimicry, cytocompatibility and rate of degradation are required to maintain cell survivability within the patch. Mechanical properties including printability, rheology and swelling behaviour impact the biofabrication of the cardiac patch to a patient-specific 3D geometry. Finally, the bioink composition and the 3D design determine the most favourable 3D bioprinting method. The modality must allow for producing the personalised cardiac patch using the selected biomaterials and be suitable for 3D bioprinting the patch according to its shape and dimensions.

8.11 DISCUSSION

Despite several *in vitro* and *in vivo* preclinical studies, a 3D bioprinted cardiac patch has not been transplanted to a patient's heart. Clinical studies using stem cells for the treatment of MI have so far either utilised cell sheet technology, or stem cells were delivered to the myocardium using an injection. In general, studies conducted to date have been early phase studies that do not provide enough evidence for regulatory approval.

Adapting the method of biofabricating and transplanting a cardiac patch from an animal model to a human study present several challenges. While several studies have been conducted to date to the use of stem cell transplants for treatment of MI, research protocols were designed independently using a variety of methods and materials. In general, standardised test protocols should be developed for assessing the efficacy, feasibility and safety of any type of cardiac patch regardless of the biofabrication method, bioink formulation or cellular/acellular composition [4,67]. Without standardised test protocols, results will remain difficult to compare limiting their usefulness in future studies. There is, therefore, a definite need for better direction in the field of 3D bioprinting in terms of finding best practices to ensure fast and safe translation [4,45,67].

Although studies using 3D bioprinted cardiac patches have already been conducted successfully in small animals, there is still more research to be done before translation to a clinical solution can be achieved. For instance, anatomical and physiological differences to humans are evident as shown in Figure 8.4. Due to the poor comparability, results from small animal models are generally not enough to meet regulatory approval required for progressing to clinical studies [51]. Compared to small animal models, studies using large animals such as pigs have higher resource requirements for carrying out experiments and caring for the animals for the duration of the study. Adding to this, although the anatomical features of the heart are similar between pigs and humans, the age of the test animal is another point of consideration. In juvenile pigs, the growth rate of the animal has to be incorporated to long-term plans as this is likely to result in changes to the myocardial wall [48]. An even bigger obstacle, however, is the lack of established protocols for generating stable pluripotent stem cells for using pigs in cardiac patch studies [2].

All *in vivo* studies discussed in this chapter, including the large animal and clinical studies where 3D bioprinting was not used, had very small sample sizes [53–56,61–66]. The exception is the clinical study by Menasché et al. [58] where a cohort of 120 patients was recruited and the study was conducted in 21 university hospitals across 5 countries. Despite the investment in resources and cross-industry collaboration, the cohort was reduced to 97 patients to fit the study criteria, and the small sample size was reported as a limitation impacting statistical significance of the findings [58].

The enormous effort required for conducting clinically and statistically relevant studies leads to a substantial problem when designing future large animal and clinical studies for 3D bioprinted cardiac patch transplantation. For studies using a large animal model with a statistically significant cohort, the appropriate number of test animals and research facilities will be expensive to obtain [50]. Further to this, recruiting patients for a clinical study of a similar magnitude would call for a multi-centre and multi-disciplinary approach [68]. Such considerations are difficult to resolve. They are, however, necessary to overcome if the method of using 3D bioprinted cardiac patches is to progress to phase I and phase II clinical trials.

In recent years, the materials and methods used in 3D bioprinting have developed significantly. The technology and materials for producing 3D bioprinted cardiac patches are available, but studies undertaken to date are yet to utilise these advances to their full extent. We have presented here a concept for the process of personalising the cardiac patch according to patient biology and cardiac anatomy. A distinct advantage of any 3D printing modality is the potential of prototyping a bespoke design which is ideal for personalised medicine where a patient-specific treatment is the main goal. Medical imaging together with modern design software allow creating personalised cardiac patches as 3D bioprinters use file formats commonly produced by CAD software.

As long as cardiovascular disease (CVD) persists as the primary cause of death globally, medical research will look for alternatives for the treatment of CVD and HF. As described in this book chapter, current lack of consistency in 3D bioprinted cardiac patch studies provides an opportunity to establish clinically relevant approaches to facilitate their testing and translation to the clinic.

REFERENCES

1. Matthews N, Pandolfo B, Moses D, Gentile C. Taking it personally: 3D bioprinting a patient-specific cardiac patch for the treatment of heart failure. *Bioengineering.* 2022;9(3):93.
2. Eschenhagen T, Ridders K, Weinberger F. How to repair a broken heart with pluripotent stem cell-derived cardiomyocytes. *J Mol Cell Cardiol.* 2022;163:106–17.
3. Montero P, Flandes-Iparraguirre M, Musquiz S, Pérez Araluce M, Plano D, Sanmartín C, et al. Cells, materials, and fabrication processes for cardiac tissue engineering. *Front Bioeng Biotechnol.* 2020;8:955.
4. Tian S, Zhao H, Lewinski N. Key parameters and applications of extrusion-based bioprinting. *Bioprinting.* 2021;23:e00156.
5. Wang L, Serpooshan V, Zhang J. Engineering human cardiac muscle patch constructs for prevention of post-infarction LV remodeling. *Front Cardiovasc Med.* 2021;8: 621781.
6. Wang Q, Yang H, Bai A, Jiang W, Li X, Wang X, et al. Functional engineered human cardiac patches prepared from nature's platform improve heart function after acute myocardial infarction. *Biomaterials.* 2016;105:52–65.
7. Nakatani S. Left ventricular rotation and twist: why should we learn? *J Cardiovasc Ultrasound.* 2011;19(1):1–6.
8. Guo R, Morimatsu M, Feng T, Lan F, Chang D, Wan F, et al. Stem cell-derived cell sheet transplantation for heart tissue repair in myocardial infarction. *Stem Cell Res Ther.* 2020;11(1):19.
9. Moore KL, Dalley II, AF, Agur AM. *Clinically Oriented Anatomy.* 6th ed. Philadelphia: Lippincott Williams & Wilkins; 2010.
10. Weinhaus AJ, Roberts KP. Anatomy of the human heart. In: Iaizzo PA, editor. *Handbook of Cardiac Anatomy, Physiology, and Devices.* Totowa, NJ: Humana Press; 2009. pp. 61–88.
11. Lakshmi I. Cardiac function review by machine learning approaches. In: Chauhan K, Chauhan RK, editors. *Image Processing for Automated Diagnosis of Cardiac Diseases.* London (UK): Academic Press; 2021. pp. 49–75.
12. Athanasiou LS, Fotiadis DI, Michalis LK. Introduction. In: Athanasiou LS, Fotiadis DI, Michalis LK, editors. *Atherosclerotic Plaque Characterization Methods Based on Coronary Imaging.* Oxford: Academic Press; 2017. pp. 1–21.
13. Howard BT, Iles TL, Coles JA, Sigg DC, Iaizzo PA. Reversible and irreversible damage of the myocardium: ischemia/reperfusion injury and cardioprotection. In: Iaizzo PA, editor. *Handbook of Cardiac Anatomy, Physiology, and Devices.* Cham: Springer; 2015. pp. 279–93.
14. Jenča D, Melenovský V, Stehlik J, Staněk V, Kettner J, Kautzner J, et al. Heart failure after myocardial infarction: incidence and predictors. *ESC Heart Fail.* 2021;8(1):222–37.
15. Garza MA, Wason EA, Zhang JQ. Cardiac remodeling and physical training post myocardial infarction. *World J Cardiol.* 2015;7(2):52–64.
16. Johnson MJ. Management of end stage cardiac failure. *Postgrad Med J.* 2007;83(980):395–401.
17. Singh D, Singh D, Han SS. 3D printing of scaffold for cells delivery: advances in skin tissue engineering. *Polymers.* 2016;8(1):19. Published 2016 Jan 16. doi:10.3390/polym8010019
18. Vurat MT, Ergun C, Elçin AE, Elçin YM. 3D bioprinting of tissue models with customized bioinks. *Adv Exp Med Biol.* 2020;1249:67–84.
19. Zhang B, Gao L, Ma L, Luo Y, Yang H, Cui Z. 3D bioprinting: a novel avenue for manufacturing tissues and organs. *Engineering.* 2019;5(4):777–94.
20. Kato B, Wisser G, Agrawal DK, Wood T, Thankam FG. 3D bioprinting of cardiac tissue: current challenges and perspectives. *J Mater Sci Mater Med.* 2021;32(5):54–.

21. Highley CB. 3D bioprinting technologies. In: Guvendiren M, editor. 3D *Bioprinting in Medicine: Technologies, Bioinks, and Applications.* Cham: Springer International Publishing; 2019. pp. 1–66.
22. Cho D-W, Kim BS, Jang J, Gao G, Han W, Singh NK. 3D bioprinting techniques. In: Cho D-W, Kim BS, Jang J, Gao G, Han W, Singh NK, editors. 3D *Bioprinting: Modeling In Vitro Tissues and Organs Using Tissue-Specific Bioinks.* Cham: Springer International Publishing; 2019. pp. 25–9.
23. Cui X, Boland T, D'Lima DD, Lotz MK. Thermal inkjet printing in tissue engineering and regenerative medicine. *Recent Pat Drug Deliv Formul.* 2012;6(2):149–55.
24. Jentsch S, Nasehi R, Kuckelkorn C, Gundert B, Aveic S, Fischer H. Multiscale 3D bioprinting by nozzle-free acoustic droplet ejection. *Small Methods.* 2021;5(6):2000971.
25. Papaioannou TG, Manolesou D, Dimakakos E, Tsoucalas G, Vavuranakis M, Tousoulis D. 3D bioprinting methods and techniques: applications on artificial blood vessel fabrication. *Acta Cardiol Sin.* 2019;35(3):284–9.
26. Zhu W, Qu X, Zhu J, Ma X, Patel S, Liu J, et al. Direct 3D bioprinting of prevascularized tissue constructs with complex microarchitecture. *Biomaterials.* 2017;124:106–15.
27. Fatimi A, Okoro OV, Podstawczyk D, Siminska-Stanny J, Shavandi A. Natural hydrogel-based bio-inks for 3D bioprinting in tissue engineering: a review. Gels. 2022;8(3):179.
28. Guvendiren M. 3D Bioprinting in Medicine Technologies, *Bioinks, and Applications.* 1st ed. Cham: Springer International Publishing; 2019.
29. Ouyang L. Pushing the rheological and mechanical boundaries of extrusion-based 3D bioprinting. *Trends Biotechnol.* 2022;40(7):891–902.
30. Camci-Unal G, Annabi N, Dokmeci MR, Liao R, Khademhosseini A. Hydrogels for cardiac tissue engineering. *NPG Asia Mater.* 2014;6(5):e99.
31. Vettori L, Sharma P, Rnjak-Kovacina J, Gentile C. 3D bioprinting of cardiovascular tissues for in vivo and in vitro applications using hybrid hydrogels containing silk fibroin: state of the art and challenges. *Curr Tissue Microenviron Rep.* 2020;1(4):261–76.
32. Lee A, Hudson AR, Shiwarski DJ, Tashman JW, Hinton TJ, Yerneni S, et al. 3D bioprinting of collagen to rebuild components of the human heart. *Science.* 2019;365(6452):482–7.
33. Li H, Liu S, Lin L. Rheological study on 3D printability of alginate hydrogel and effect of graphene oxide. *Int J Bioprint.* 2016;2:54–66.
34. Naghieh S, Sarker MD, Abelseth E, Chen X. Indirect 3D bioprinting and characterization of alginate scaffolds for potential nerve tissue engineering applications. *J Mech Behav Biomed Mater.* 2019;93:183–93.
35. Ouyang L, Highley CB, Sun W, Burdick JA. A generalizable strategy for the 3D bioprinting of hydrogels from nonviscous photo-crosslinkable inks. *Adv Mater.* 2017;29(8):1604983.
36. Cho D-W, Kim BS, Jang J, Gao G, Han W, Singh NK. Conventional bioinks. In: Cho D-W, Kim BS, Jang J, Gao G, Han W, Singh NK, editors. *3D Bioprinting: Modeling In Vitro Tissues and Organs Using Tissue-Specific Bioinks.* Cham: Springer International Publishing; 2019. pp. 31–40.
37. Sionkowska A, Skrzyński S, Śmiechowski K, Kołodziejczak A. The review of versatile application of collagen. Polym Adv *Technol.* 2017;28(1):4–9.
38. Wang X, Ao Q, Tian X, Fan J, Tong H, Hou W, et al. Gelatin-based hydrogels for organ 3D bioprinting. *Polymers.* 2017;9(9):401.
39. Yue K, Trujillo-de Santiago G, Alvarez MM, Tamayol A, Annabi N, Khademhosseini A. Synthesis, properties, and biomedical applications of gelatin methacryloyl (GelMA) hydrogels. *Biomaterials.* 2015;73:254–71.
40. Sharma P, Wang X, Ming CLC, Vettori L, Figtree G, Boyle A, et al. Advanced cardiac models: considerations for the bioengineering of advanced cardiac in vitro models of myocardial infarction. *Small.* 2021;17(15):2170067.

41. Das S, Nam H, Jang J. 3D bioprinting of stem cell-laden cardiac patch: a promising alternative for myocardial repair. *APL Bioeng.* 2021;5(3):031508.
42. Laschke MW, Menger MD. Life is 3D: boosting spheroid function for tissue engineering. *Trends Biotechnol.* 2017;35(2):133–44.
43. Kinney MA, Hookway TA, Wang Y, McDevitt TC. Engineering three-dimensional stem cell morphogenesis for the development of tissue models and scalable regenerative therapeutics. *Ann Biomed Eng.* 2013;42(2):352–67.
44. Fleming P, Argraves WS, Gentile C, Neagu A, Forgacs G, Drake C. Fusion of uniluminal vascular spheroids: a model for assembly of blood vessels. *Dev Dyn.* 2010;239:spcone.
45. Sharma P, Wang X, Ming CLC, Vettori L, Figtree G, Boyle A, et al. Considerations for the bioengineering of advanced cardiac in vitro models of myocardial infarction. *Small.* 2021;17(15):2003765.
46. Polonchuk L, Surija L, Lee M, Sharma P, Liu Chung Ming C, Richter F, et al. Towards engineering heart tissues from bioprinted cardiac spheroids. *Biofabrication.* 2021;13(4):10.1088/1758-5090/ac14ca. Published 2021 Aug 13. doi:10.1088/1758-5090/ac14ca.
47. Chimenti I, Rizzitelli G, Gaetani R, Angelini F, Ionta V, Forte E, et al. Human cardiosphere-seeded gelatin and collagen scaffolds as cardiogenic engineered bioconstructs. *Biomaterials.* 2011;32(35):9271–81.
48. Bianco RW, Gallegos RP, Rivard AL, Voight J, Dalmasso AP. Animal models for cardiac research. In: Iaizzo PA, editor. *Handbook of Cardiac Anatomy, Physiology, and Devices.* Totowa, NJ: Humana Press; 2009. pp. 393–410.
49. Buetow BS, Laflamme MA. Cardiovascular. In: Treuting PM, Dintzis S, Montine KS, editors. *Comparative Anatomy and Histology: A Mouse, Rat, and Human Atlas.* Saint Louis, MO: Elsevier Science & Technology; 2018;570.
50. Silva KAS, Emter CA. Large animal models of heart failure: a translational bridge to clinical success. *JACC Basic Transl Sci.* 2020;5(8):840–56.
51. Hill AJ, Iaizzo PA. Comparative cardiac anatomy. In: Iaizzo PA, editor. *Handbook of Cardiac Anatomy, Physiology, and Devices.* Totowa, NJ: Humana Press; 2009. pp. 87–108.
52. Crick SJ, Sheppard MN, Ho SY, Gebstein L, Anderson RH. Anatomy of the pig heart: comparisons with normal human cardiac structure. *J Anat.* 1998;193(1):105–19.
53. Menasché P, Vanneaux V, Hagège A, Bel A, Cholley B, Parouchev A, et al. Transplantation of human embryonic stem cell-derived cardiovascular progenitors for severe ischemic left ventricular dysfunction. *J Am Coll Cardiol.* 2018;71(4):429–38.
54. Sawa Y, Miyagawa S, Sakaguchi T, Fujita T, Matsuyama A, Saito A, et al. Tissue engineered myoblast sheets improved cardiac function sufficiently to discontinue LVAS in a patient with DCM: report of a case. *Surg Today.* 2012;42(2):181–4.
55. Sawa Y, Yoshikawa Y, Toda K, Fukushima S, Yamazaki K, Ono M, et al. Safety and efficacy of autologous skeletal myoblast sheets (TCD-51073) for the treatment of severe chronic heart failure due to ischemic heart disease. *Circ J.* 2015;79(5):991–9.
56. Yoshikawa Y, Miyagawa S, Toda K, Saito A, Sakata Y, Sawa Y. Myocardial regenerative therapy using a scaffold-free skeletal-muscle-derived cell sheet in patients with dilated cardiomyopathy even under a left ventricular assist device: a safety and feasibility study. *Surg Today.* 2018;48(2):200–10.
57. Herreros J, Prósper F, Perez A, Gavira JJ, Garcia-Velloso MJ, Barba J, et al. Autologous intramyocardial injection of cultured skeletal muscle-derived stem cells in patients with non-acute myocardial infarction. *Eur Heart J.* 2003;24(22):2012–20.
58. Menasché P, Alfieri O, Janssens S, McKenna W, Reichenspurner H, Trinquart L, et al. The Myoblast Autologous Grafting in Ischemic Cardiomyopathy (MAGIC) trial: first randomized placebo-controlled study of myoblast transplantation. *Circulation.* 2008;117(9):1189–200.

59. Pagani FD, DerSimonian H, Zawadzka A, Wetzel K, Edge ASB, Jacoby DB, et al. Autologous skeletal myoblasts transplanted to ischemia-damaged myocardium in humans: histological analysis of cell survival and differentiation. *J Am Coll Cardiol.* 2003;41(5):879–88.
60. Siminiak T, Kalawski R, Fiszer D, Jerzykowska O, Rzeźniczak J, Rozwadowska N, et al. Autologous skeletal myoblast transplantation for the treatment of postinfarction myocardial injury: phase I clinical study with 12 months of follow-up. *Am Heart J.* 2004;148(3):531–7.
61. Jiang X, Feng T, An B, Ren S, Meng J, Li K, et al. A bi-layer hydrogel cardiac patch made of recombinant functional proteins. *Adv Mater.* 2022;34(19):e2201411. doi:10.1002/adma.202201411
62. Cui H, Liu C, Esworthy T, Huang Y, Yu ZX, Zhou X, et al. 4D physiologically adaptable cardiac patch: a 4-month in vivo study for the treatment of myocardial infarction. *Sci Adv.* 2020;6(26).
63. Yeung E, Fukunishi T, Bai Y, Bedja D, Pitaktong I, Mattson G, et al. Cardiac regeneration using human-induced pluripotent stem cell-derived biomaterial-free 3D-bioprinted cardiac patch in vivo. *J Tissue Eng Regen Med.* 2019;13(11):2031–9.
64. Yang Y, Lei D, Huang S, Yang Q, Song B, Guo Y, et al. Elastic 3D-printed hybrid polymeric scaffold improves cardiac remodeling after myocardial infarction. *Adv Healthc Mater.* 2019;8(10):e1900065.
65. Ong CS, Fukunishi T, Zhang H, Huang CY, Nashed A, Blazeski A, et al. Biomaterial-free three-dimensional bioprinting of cardiac tissue using human induced pluripotent stem cell derived cardiomyocytes. *Sci Rep.* 2017;7(1).
66. Gaebel R, Ma N, Liu J, Guan J, Koch L, Klopsch C, et al. Patterning human stem cells and endothelial cells with laser printing for cardiac regeneration. *Biomaterials.* 2011;32(35):9218–30.
67. Ng WL, Chua CK, Shen Y-F. Print me an organ! Why we are not there yet. *Prog Polym Sci.* 2019;97:101145.
68. Menasché P. Cell therapy trials for heart regeneration—lessons learned and future directions. *Nat Rev Cardiol.* 2018;15(11):659–71.

9 3D Bioprinting for Central Nervous System Applications

Denis Scaini
International School for Advanced Studies (SISSA/ISAS)
Basque Foundation for Science
University of Basque Country

CONTENTS

DOI: 10.1201/9781003274568-9

9.1 INTRODUCTION

The study of the human central nervous system (CNS) and the comprehension of the mechanisms regulating the establishment and evolution of its neuropathies have been considerably limited by the difficulty of accessing the human brain tissues (especially nonpathological) and by the absence of reliable *in vitro* models able to summarize CNS characteristics.

Recent technological developments in genetic engineering, such as the development of the CRISPR-Cas9 genome editing technique, and the availability of patient-derived pluripotent cells [1] have changed this scenario. Nowadays, a virtually unlimited number of phenotypically defined cells are available to researchers, offering high representativeness of real physiological or (pre)pathological conditions. Similarly, *in vitro* 3D cellular models have recently received increasing attention, and modern neuroscience is increasingly relying on 3D models to study neuronal circuits, regeneration, and degenerative diseases [2,3]. If, on the one hand, the advent of 3D biofabrication techniques has made a real revolution in tissue modeling; on the other hand, the uncontrolled development of techniques capable of inducing – in a more or less effective way – three-dimensional cellular organizations provided results that are challenging to compare and, consequently, poorly representative. The standardization of procedures or careful morphological and functional characterizations of the model become necessary to extrapolate reliable results from 3D *in vitro* models of the CNS [4].

Currently, *in vitro*, 3D models can be classified into cellular models (*e.g.*, spheroids and organoids) and engineered models (*e.g.*, microfluidic or scaffold-based).

Spheroids are three-dimensional spherical cellular units generally cultured as free-floating aggregates and are characterized by a low complexity in replicating the target tissue organization. They do not require scaffolding to assemble 3D cultures by simply sticking to each other. Organoids are complex clusters of organ-specific cells, such as those from the stomach, liver, or bladder. They originate from stem or progenitor cells and self-assemble when an extracellular scaffolding environment is provided (*e.g.*, Matrigel® or collagen). In this condition, they may grow in 3D to form structural units that partially resemble the target tissue or organ in their structure and function. Both models do not offer direct control over the position of the cells that make up the system, their phenotype, or the level of interconnection. The entire process is endogenously regulated, and the final cellular organization and geometry of the cellular system are mainly stochastically driven. Consequently, only a small fraction of the total number of organoids generated in an experimental run will possess sufficient representativeness of the target tissue or organ.

In contrast, engineering-based models employ artificial guides to control cell culture growth in three dimensions. In microfluidic systems, a liquid flow is used to direct and control the growth environment. In the case of scaffolds, macroporous three-dimensional matrices of predefined size and shape are used to support the development of the artificial tissue model. Cellular models generally offer a better level of cellular complexity and phenotypic likelihood than engineered models, especially when imitating early developmental stages. On the other hand, the engineered models offer greater control of the macroorganization of artificial cellular tissue, which leads to constructs morphologically and dimensionally closer to the tissues they we intend to mimic. However, both models fail to provide control of the spatial position of specific cell phenotypes within the three-dimensional cellular construct. Even the system's topological evolution over time is not controllable.

3D bioprinting is an automated (bio)manufacturing approach that offers high versatility in spatial positioning and phenotypic control of cells within artificial cell constructs (see Figure 9.1) [5].

Several 3D bioprinting methods have been developed; these include inkjet-based, extrusion-based, and laser-assisted devices, each with its characteristics and limitations (a more detailed description is available in Section 9.4). All these techniques have been profitably used to develop artificial three-dimensional models of CNS tissues to perform developmental, pharmacological, or functional studies [6]. A common characteristic of all of them is to offer some level of phenotopological control during the manufacture of a cellular construct, increasing the representativeness and reproducibility of *in vitro* CNS models.

Therefore, starting from the great potential of 3D bioprinting in obtaining *in vitro* 3D neuronal models, this chapter will provide a clear view of the foundations and principles underlying this biofabrication technique when aiming to model in 3D a

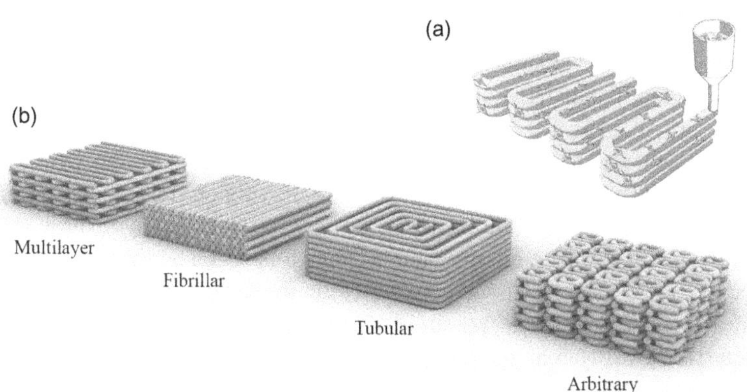

FIGURE 9.1 Examples of the versatility of 3D bioprinting. (a) A schematic of extrusion-based additive biofabrication of neuronal constructs. The bioink loaded with CNS-related cells is organized in a 3D construct through a layer-by-layer process. (b) By exploiting two printheads loaded with two different bioink compositions, it is possible to mimic complex tissue organizations such as laminar, fibrillar, or tubular ones.

portion of the CNS. It also provides insights into the peculiarities associated with the 3D bioprinting of neuronal tissue and some examples of functional 3D models of neuronal tissue obtained using neuronal bioinks and 3D printing.

9.2 THE CENTRAL NERVOUS SYSTEM AS A (BIO)PRINTABLE UNIT

We can define a tissue as an organized three-dimensional assembly of phenotypically distinct cells supported by an extracellular matrix (ECM) and able to perform a specific physiological function. Numerous biological, biochemical, and biophysical phenomena determine the physiological functioning of the tissue by defining cell-cell and cell-microenvironment interactions. The presence of the third dimension is essential to ensure the highest level of functionality. Interestingly, the reduction of the system to 2D models often causes the appearance of aberrant cellular phenotypes and, consequently, the model's failure [7].

Although it is not (yet) possible to duplicate an entire organ in the laboratory, the possibility of generating *in vitro* 3D tissue models that summarize some essential aspects of an organ exists. We will call this structure a *functional unit* of the organ [8]. A functional unit must be able to reproduce on a smaller scale a biofunctional aspect typical of the native tissue. However, even though 3D biofabrication technologies allow for assembling three-dimensional bioconstructs, the tissue biofunctionality can be replicated only if the model incorporates part of the native tissue cellular and ECM composition complexity [9]. The different cells, the mechanical properties of the surrounding environment, and the physicochemical interactions between the cells and the environment represent a complex living system in continuous evolution.

Some CNS tissue features will be described here as a future guideline for designing artificial neuronal tissues.

9.2.1 The Cells Constituting the CNS

Mammalian CNS is a complex 3D structure composed of neuronal and nonneuronal cells embedded in a matrix known as the extracellular matrix (ECM).

The brain ECM is often considered the only aspect to consider when designing a bioink. However, recapitulating the cellular constituents of the CNS tissue is a fundamental step toward printing a successful 3D model. Indeed, it is paramount to gain an overall picture of the complexities and characteristics of the CNS cellular constituents that will become the "active" constituent of a bioink.

The CNS is a complex tissue constituted by the brain and the spinal cord. These two structures developed to pursue distinct functionalities and, consequently, are characterized by different cellular organizations, patterns of connectivity, and ECM compositions. Despite that, both can be recapitulated as a cellular assembly of three cell types: neuronal, glial, and endothelial. Interestingly, recent investigations revealed that, on average, the CNS is composed of roughly the same number of these three cellular constituents. Neurons and glia thus represent more than 2/3 of the cells of the CNS.

In the following, we will focus on the first two classes of cells (neurons and glia) as from them CNS functionality mainly depends. However, it is essential to clarify why so many endothelial cells are present. The CNS is extremely demanding from an energetic point of view. The energy supply is possible through a dense network of arteries, veins, and capillaries – mainly constituted by endothelial cells – embedded within the tissue/organ.

The human CNS comprises approximately 100 billion neurons and slightly more glial cells [10]. Specifically, the brain consists of about 100 billion neuronal cells, and its glial–neuron ratio is slightly less than unity. On the other hand, in the human spinal cord, the presence of 200 million neurons and 2 billion glial cells have been estimated, giving rise to a glia–neuron ratio of about 6 [11,12]. Neurons are electroactive cells capable of collecting, processing, and transmitting electrical signals in the form of changes in their membrane potential (*e.g.*, action potentials). The glia, initially believed to have only a supportive function, subsequently demonstrated to play a crucial role in maintaining CNS homeostasis, assisting neutral signaling, developing the CNS, and many other key aspects. Both cell types are, therefore, essential to ensure the correct CNS functionality.

9.2.1.1 Neuronal Cells

The neuronal composition of the CNS is variegated and compartmentalized.

Neuronal cells composing the spinal cord can be functionally classified into three types: sensory neurons, motor neurons, and interneurons. *Sensory neurons* are nerve cells activated by sensory receptors generally collecting environmental stimuli. They fire and send the information they receive to the rest of the CNS. Most sensory neurons are pseudounipolar, meaning they only have one axon split into two branches. *Motor neurons* of the spinal cord are connected to muscles, glands, and organs. These neurons transmit impulses from the spinal cord to skeletal and smooth muscles and directly drive muscle activation. Motor neurons are multipolar, each with one axon and several dendrites. *Interneurons*, as the name suggests, are the ones in between, connecting motor and sensory neurons. As well as transferring signals between sensory and motor neurons, interneurons can also communicate with each other, forming circuits of various complexities. They are multipolar, just like motor neurons.

The distinction between different types of neuronal cells in the brain is much more complex. For example, there are brain neurons involved in sensory processing – like those in visual or auditory cortexes – and others involved in motor processing – like those in the cerebellum or motor cortex – that can be classified based on their function. However, within these regions, there are tens or even hundreds of different types of neurons. Indeed, part of what gives the brain its complexity (and capability!) is the vast number of specialized neuronal types. Further distinctions possible are, for example, based on morphology, neurotransmitters involved (*e.g.*, γ-aminobutyric acid, glutamate, or acetylcholine), type of synaptic connections originated (*e.g.*, excitatory *vs.* inhibitory), and so on. But the boundaries of such classifications are often confused. Some GABA (γ-aminobutyric acid) neurons send their axon mainly to the cell bodies of other neurons, while others prefer to target dendrites. Furthermore, these neurons could have different electrical properties, shapes, genes expressed, and input/output connection patterns. In other words, a neuronal type (and its function) can be defined only by a particular combination of features.

9.2.1.2 Glial Cells

Glial cells are generally classified into astrocytes, microglia, oligodendrocytes, and ependymal cells [8]. *Astrocytes* have a regulatory role in brain functions implicated in neurogenesis and synaptogenesis, controlling blood–brain barrier (BBB) permeability, and maintaining extracellular homeostasis. *Microglia* represent a specialized population of macrophage-like cells in the CNS acting as immune sentinels capable of orchestrating potent inflammatory responses. Microglia contributes to brain protection and repair, providing synaptic organization cues, neurotrophic support during development, myelin turnover, control of neuronal excitability, and phagocytic debris removal. *Oligodendrocytes* are the myelinating cells of the CNS possessing signal-optimization and metabolic functions. *Ependymal* cells are ciliated-epithelial glial cells that develop from radial glia along the brain's ventricles and spinal canal surfaces. They play a critical role in cerebrospinal fluid (CSF) homeostasis, brain metabolism, and the clearance of waste from the brain.

Therefore, it is clear that to create a representative model of a portion of the CNS, it is necessary to consider a great cellular diversity, each with its characteristic topological organization and cell-to-cell interaction.

9.2.1.3 Sources of CNS Cells

Common cell sources for *in vitro* CNS modeling are primary neuronal cells, immortalized cell lines, and stem cells.

Primary cells are obtained by direct dissociation of living neuronal tissues [7]. Evident ethical concerns limit the availability of human neuronal tissues as a source of primary cells for *in vitro* cultures. Furthermore, most human primary cells have limited regenerative abilities and are difficult to expand *in vitro*. As 3D cultures require very high seeding densities, the problem has been circumvented by using primary cells from other mammals (*i.e.*, rats and mice) [7]. Although cells grown from rodents' CNS have high neurophysiological representativeness and are widely used in 3D neuronal models, they are very fragile and can lose functionality. Therefore, they are not suitable for long-term *in vitro* culturing too [7].

Immortalized cell lines (e.g., those obtained from brain tumors) do not present this problem and are therefore widely used in long-term studies. Unfortunately, these types of cells often cannot recapitulate the neurobiological and physiological characteristics of the nervous tissue.

Recently, the use of neuronal and glial cells derived from human embryonic stem cells, neuronal progenitors, or induced pluripotent stem cells (iPSCs) [13,14] has proven to be an effective alternative to the use of primary and immortalized cells. It has been shown that these cell types can be effectively differentiated into neurons, astrocytes, and oligodendrocytes [7]. They have excellent functional representativeness of the human nervous tissue and can be cultured to obtain high cell densities for a long time.

9.2.2 The CNS Extracellular Matrix

The ECM is a macro- and microfibrous support environment for neurons and glia that contributes to the correct development and functionality of the CNS [15].

The brain tissue ECM can be divided into three main components. The first component, the *basement membrane*, lines the CNS vascular system and, together with endothelial cells, pericytes and astrocytes, forms the blood–brain barrier (BBB) [16]. This layer counts four major proteins, including collagen IV, laminin, entactin, and perlecan. Neurons are integrated within the second component, the *perineuronal network*, a low-fibrously matrix that offers greater mobility to cells and provides the ideal environment for forming neurites and synapses. The perineuronal network comprises proteoglycans, tenascin-R, and other linking proteins [17]. The third component of the brain ECM is the *interstitial component* that connects neurons and the vascular system [18].

From a more general point of view, the CNS matrix is often recapitulated using tenascin, hyaluronic acid, and different proteoglycans [19]. Differently from other tissues, laminin, fibronectin, and collagen are minimally expressed in CNS ECM, while many soluble factors are present (*e.g.*, growth factors, chemokines, and cytokines) [8].

In addition to its (bio)chemical composition, the ECM regulates cellular behavior also through its mechanical properties. The neuronal ECM is characterized by a lower elastic modulus and a greater porosity than other body tissues. The elastic modulus (Young's modulus) of the CNS varies from hundreds of Pa of the most cellularized regions (gray matter) to tens of kPa of regions characterized by the presence of nerve fibers bundles (white matter). It has been demonstrated that environmental stiffness substantially impacts cell behavior and morphology. Similarly, it influences cell development and differentiation as well. For example, neuronal stem cells are prone to differentiate into glial cells when interfaced with rigid matrices (>5 kPa) and into neuronal cells when embedded in soft matrices (<0.5 kPa). Similarly, the porosity of the ECM can significantly influence cellular behavior and metabolism [20]. To develop correctly, a functional neuronal network requires a fine orchestration of all of the aforementioned elements.

Numerous hydrogels (composite or not) have been successfully developed and implemented to create three-dimensional models of CNS via 3D bioprinting. A common feature of these artificial constructs is the presence within them of neuronal cells capable of creating a network (at different levels of complexity). Furthermore, they are functional, meaning the cells they are composed of can generate, process, and transmit electrophysiological signals. The reader may refer to Section 9.3 for a discussion about neuronal bioinks and Section 9.5.3 for more details on the functional aspects connected to bioink-derived cellular assemblies.

A bioink is a construct characterized by a specific viscosity made by a matrix aiming at mimicking the ECM of the target tissue within which native (or representative) cells may be dispersed. From a practical point of view, the most important characteristics a bioink must possess are its ease of printing (printability) and shape stability after printing. In the case of extrusion printing, for example, printability can be associated with the ease with which the material can be extruded through a printing nozzle and deposited on a surface (see Figure 9.1a). This aspect is strongly linked to the degree of viscosity of the material and its thixotropic properties. On the other hand, after printing, material stability expresses its ability to maintain the geometry and mechanical properties set over time when immersed in a liquid environment. Unfortunately, printability and stability are often material properties in conflict. For example, a low viscosity generally improves printability but depresses the final stability of the system. A common approach to overcome this problem is to print the bioink in a non-cross-linked condition and induce cross-linking only once it has been deposited on the surface. In addition to this practical aspect, a good bioink must be suitable and optimized to sustain the development of neuronal tissue (neuronal bioink). The following sections will highlight some of the most critical characteristics biomaterials must have to be used in artificial CNS constructs successfully. Specifically, a range of bioinks that can be used alone or in combination in the 3D bioprinting process will be analyzed.

9.3 BIOMATERIAL FOR A 3D NEURONAL TISSUE MODEL

An important feature a bioink needs to possess to be suitable for 3D *in vitro* cellular reconstructions is that its stiffness can be adjusted to better approach that of the target tissue. In the case of CNS tissues, the final rigidity of the bioink matrix must fall between 0.1 and 10kPa [21,22]. The control of the bioink stiffness can be carried out by inducing a postprinting molecular cross-linking. Among the commonly used natural hydrogels, those based on type I collagen, hyaluronic acid, and chitosan contain endogenous cellular cross-linking sites, such as arginine–glycine–aspartic acid (RGD) moieties or other amino acid sequences [23,24]. On the other hand, synthetic hydrogels are often specifically modified with chemical functional groups that allow cross-linking or covalent anchoring of the proteins that make up natural hydrogels [24].

Several studies have reported the creation of three-dimensional neuronal cultures using hydrogels functionalized with laminin and fibronectin [25,26]. From the functional point of view, many hydrogels sustain a diffusion rate of proteins similar to that of real brain tissue. For example, type I collagen constructs have been shown to have a protein diffusion rate (*e.g.*, for the BSA) of 10^{-4} to 10^{-3} mm^2/s (for collagen concentrations on the order of 1%–5%) [27].

For a long time, type I collagen has been considered the gold standard for creating brain tissue models *in vitro* [28,29]. This was due to the higher neuronal survival and neuritogenesis associated with type I collagen compared to other matrices [30]. As already mentioned, type I collagen has many endogenous RGD sequences in its amino acid sequence that facilitate neuronal cells' focal adhesion (FA) adhesion [31]. Furthermore, when used in conjunction with undifferentiated cells, 3D collagen cultures have been shown to facilitate the differentiation of neuronal stem cells into astrocytes, oligodendrocytes, and neurons. In addition to a correct cellular phenotype, the latter presented neuronal polarity, the expression of neurotransmitters, ion channels, receptors, and, importantly, neuronal membrane excitability [32]. Type I collagen has also been used for 3D bioprinting of hybrid cell systems in which nervous and endothelial cells have been used to recreate 3D models of the brain's blood–brain barrier (BBB) and other vascular compartments [33]. However, collagen is not the main component of CNS ECM. Furthermore, the substantial difficulty of printing this biomaterial makes it unsuitable for creating particularly complex structures requiring higher printing resolution [34]. This difficulty concretizes in the low morphological, physicochemical, and functional reproducibility characterizing different collagen-based bioprinted models.

Another biomaterial widely used to create three-dimensional models of brain tissue is hyaluronic acid (HA) [35]. HA is a particularly interesting biomaterial for 3D bioprinting due to its constitutive abundance in the ECM of the CNS [7]. HA has been used to create 3D models of glioblastoma, and by controlling hydrogel stiffness, it can guide the differentiation of neuronal progenitors toward neuronal or glial phenotypes [36]. Still, in the research field of cell differentiation, 3D bioconstructs of HA embedding fetal and adult progenitors showed the tendency to differentiate into glial cells and neurons, respectively [37]. HA has been demonstrated effective in supporting the development and differentiation of cellular cultures for long periods but has also shown a depressing effect on the growth of neuronal processes (axons and dendrites) and synaptogenesis [38]. These drawbacks make it much more challenging to obtain functional neuronal networks from HA than from other hydrogels. However, on the whole, HA is an attractive biomaterial for 3D bioprinting, especially on its excellent printability and when coupled with other biomaterials. In fact, as a composite constituent, it proves to be a good choice for fabricating morphologically complex models of neuronal tissues.

Agarose and PEG are two non-natural, bioinert synthetic hydrogels that can be easily modified to obtain different stiffnesses. Natural peptides or growth factors derived from the ECM of the target tissue can be used to functionalize the base hydrogels by improving their biological relevance. 3D bioprinted models from these two materials have been exploited to evaluate different aspects of CNS's morphological and functional development [36,39,40]. Unfortunately, these two polymers cannot be modified or degraded by cells unless they are engineered with degradable peptide fractions or cross-linked with chemical groups prone to hydrolysis [41].

9.3.1 Printable Biomaterial

As seen above, a wide range of biomaterials can be successfully used in 3D bioprinting. The most commonly used materials in bioprinting are alginate, poly(ethylene glycol) diacrylate (PEGDA), HA, chitosan, fibrin, silk fibrin, gelatin, agarose, methylcellulose, and collagen. A bioink is usually composed of a combination of these materials to provide the hydrogel with good printability, cytocompatibility, and the ability to mimic the physicochemical characteristics of the target tissue ECM (*e.g.*, stiffness). The good printability and postprinting stability of a bioink are directly associated with the jellification characteristic of the hydrogel. Some gelling mechanisms used in 3D bioprinting are described below. Some are specific to extrusion bioprinting, undoubtedly the most widespread biofabrication technique, while others are related to more techniques. There are three main types of gelling: physical, chemical, and enzymatic. The choice of the best gelling process for 3D bioprinting allows for high-quality prints preserving the shape of the printed structure. The time stability is connected to the gelling mechanism: physical gelling (*e.g.*, changes in temperature, mechanical shear stresses, or ionic strength) induces reversible reticulation, while chemical and enzymatic processes involve the formation of stable covalent chemical bonds (*e.g.*, in the case of photoreticulation).

9.3.1.1 Physical Cross-linking

Physical cross-linking is induced by intertwining high-molecule polymer chains, hydrophilic/hydrophobic interactions, or the formation of hydrogen bonds [42]. Some more common physically cross-linkable hydrogels are agarose, alginate, chitosan, collagen, gelatin, Matrigel®, and pluronic acid (F-127). Physical cross-linking has received significant attention from the 3D (bio)engineering community due to its simplicity and the absence of the need for synthetic/exogenous cross-linking agents. The latter aspect also partly explains the lower cytotoxicity found in cells supported by physically cross-linked bioinks. It should also be noted that these materials, in addition to providing a more favorable environment for incorporated cells and for the diffusion of micro/macro molecules, present reversible gelling, thus allowing post-printing alteration/modulation of the matrix characteristics [43].

9.3.1.2 Chemical Cross-linking

The chemical cross-linking process of a bioink involves the formation of stable covalent bonds between the chains that make up the hydrogel. Chemically cross-linkable hydrogels offer better dimensional/geometric stability and mechanical characteristics than physically cross-linkable hydrogels. However, an external chemical agent must be added to the compound to trigger the gelation reaction. This obviously increases the cost and complexity of the technique and can induce cytotoxicity [43]. One of the most widely used chemical cross-linking mechanisms of a bioink is photocross-linking [44]. Methacrylate gelatin (GelMA) and poly(ethyleneglycol) diacrylate (PEGDA) are two types of light-curing polymers commonly used in CNS 3D bioprinting.

9.3.1.3 Enzymatic Cross-linking

In enzymatic cross-linking reactions, the formation of bonds between the polymer chains of the bioink could be started or accomplished by the action of specific enzymes present within the hydrogel or in the printing medium [45]. This bio-manufacturing approach is undoubtedly the closest to what happens in natural tissue. It is, therefore, particularly appropriate for the manufacture of biocompatible hydrogels, especially for applications in the field of biomedical 3D bioprinting. For this purpose, transglutaminase, tyrosinase, SrtA, phosphopantetheinyl transferase, lysyl oxidase, PAO, phosphatases, thermolysin, β-lactamase, phosphatase/kinase, peroxidases, and α-chymotrypsin have been studied [46]. For example, the high cellular adhesiveness and excellent biocompatibility have made fibrin one of the most widely used enzymatically activated bioinks [47]. In a compound consisting of fibrinogen and thrombin, the former is converted to fibrin by the enzymatic action of the thrombin protease. The fibrin monomers then polymerize spontaneously and non-covalently to form a fibrin gel. The process could be speeded up by the presence of Ca^{2+} in the solution [47].

9.4 APPROACHES TO THE 3D BIOPRINTING OF NERVOUS TISSUES

To date, different bioprinting techniques have been developed and are currently used for the assisted assembly of many artificial three-dimensional tissues for biomedical or research applications. In the field of neuroengineering, in the attempt to fabricate artificial 3D CNS models, the primary technologies used are extrusion-based, inkjet-based, lithography-based, and laser-assisted. Figure 9.2 depicts a schematic recapitulating the working principle of each of these four 3D bioprinting methodologies.

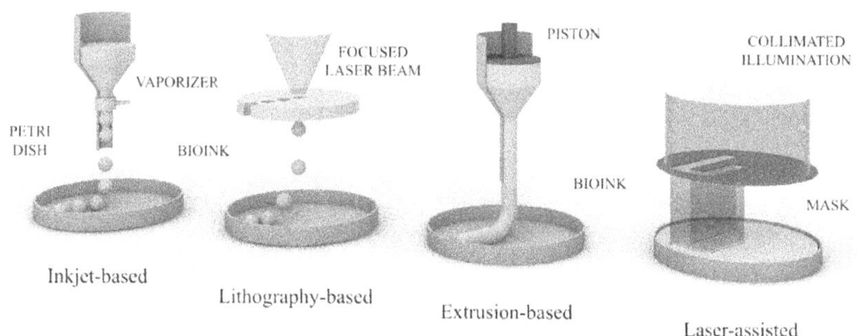

FIGURE 9.2 3D bioprinting technologies for neuronal tissue bioprinting.

Each process is characterized by specific strengths and limitations, making the choice of the most suitable bioprinting methodology a critical aspect when developing 3D cellular models. Generally, 3D bioprinting devices can be endowed with hardware to perform more than a sole technique. For example, a multiple printheads system can be constituted by two (or more) extrusion-based modules to print cells embedded in high-viscosity hydrogels and an inkjet-based module to print cells directly from their culture medium. Importantly, every printhead could be loaded with a different cell phenotype, dramatically increasing the versatility and possibilities during the design and fabrication phases.

9.4.1 Extrusion-Based Bioprinting

Extrusion-based 3D bioprinting is undoubtedly the most widespread biofabrication technique, especially in biomedicine and tissue regeneration laboratories. It is the technique of choice for printing medium-to-high-viscosity materials, such as hydrogels loaded with cells. The printing principle is straightforward: a 3-axis translation system moves a cartridge with a needle dispenser of variable diameter, depositing the printing material in specific areas of a working surface. Usually, the foreground is the surface of a laboratory glass slide, a petri dish, or the well of a multiwell plate. A three-dimensional assembly is obtained in a layer-by-layer fashion by iterating the process with successive overlapping working planes (see Figure 9.1b for some examples of possible geometries). The accurate control of the material supply at the end of the printing nozzle (usually a blunt needle) is made possible by using a mechanical screw plunger (piston) or pneumatically through a digital control unit. The material is generally printed in the form of continuous cylindrical segments whose diameter is a function of the rheological properties of the printed material and the size of the extrusion needle/nozzle [48].

One of the advantages of extrusion bioprinting is its ability to print materials with high viscosity and/or high cell density (from 10 to 10^{-7} mPa·s) [49]. It also offers greater ease of use and versatility than other techniques [50,51] and makes it possible to use chemically, thermally, or optically cross-linkable hydrogels (in this regard, refer to Section 9.3.1). The main drawback of extrusion bioprinting is the low cell viability that can be achieved since the encapsulated cells are exposed to very high mechanical shear stresses during extrusion, especially when using small nozzles (<250 μm) and high printing speeds.

9.4.2 Inkjet-Based Bioprinting

Inkjet 3D bioprinters are very similar to 2D inkjet printers found in many homes and offices. What differentiates them is the ability to use much denser mediums (bioinks) and, above all, the ability to print several times over the same place, accumulating the material in these areas to achieve three-dimensionality [52]. Generally, the printing medium is a liquid solution or low-viscosity hydrogel loaded with cells and stored under controlled conditions inside printing cartridges. The cartridge is connected to a printhead which, through thermal (abrupt temperature changes) or piezoelectric (abrupt changes in pressure) processes, locally vaporizes the bioink giving rise to droplets of different sizes that are projected onto the printing surface [48]. A 3D structure is then produced by stacking the droplets on top of each other following a specific pattern. Also, in this case, the 3D assembly is obtained with a layer-by-layer assembly approach.

The advantages of the 3D inkjet bioprinting method are the high cell viability (80%–90%), which guarantees low operating costs and high printing speeds [53]. Cell viability is greater than extrusion bioprinting because less mechanical stress is exerted on the cells. It should be noted that this printing technique can also be equipped with multiple printheads, thus allowing it to work with various cells simultaneously. As already mentioned, an intrinsic disadvantage of the technique is the inability to print medium- to high-viscosity materials or high cell densities (>10^6 cells/mL). A high cell density is associated with a high bioink viscosity and/or sedimentation of the cells, with consequent printhead nozzle clogging [16].

9.4.3 Lithography-Based Bioprinting

3D biolithography is a technique deriving from the optical lithography techniques commonly used in consumer electronics and microfabrication [54]. It consists in distributing on a surface a thin and uniform layer of a hydrogel loaded with cells which will then be photo-reticulated according to a specific pattern/design using semitransparent masks (raster exposition) or directing a light beam only in specific areas (scanning exposition) [55]. Similarly to the two previously described techniques, the entire operation can be repeated above the previous covering, making it possible to obtain a three-dimensional structure through a layer-by-layer process. The portions of bioink film not photopolymerized can be removed before proceeding with the next layer or at the end of the entire procedure. In the latter case, the uncured portions will act as "sacrificial supports" to obtain suspended structures (bridging).

The main advantage of 3D biolithography is the ability to print very large three-dimensional components (tens of centimeters in side size) at high resolution (<10 μm) in a relatively short time (especially in the case of the raster exposition) [48]. Cell viability depends on printing time (the longer the procedure, the lower the survival rate) and the wavelength of the cross-linked light used (longer wavelengths are usually associated with higher viability but also lower cross-linking efficiency and printing resolution) [56]. The main disadvantage of the technique is the inability to accurately control the position of the cells within a layer (the cell arrangement is stochastic) and the difficulty in extending the fabrication to several different materials (or cellular phenotypes).

9.4.4 Laser-Assisted Bioprinting

Laser-assisted 3D bioprinters originate from microtissue laser dissection and collection systems commonly used in genetics and cell biology laboratories (*e.g.*, the Zeiss PALM MicroBeam). Indeed, a high-power laser beam is used to cut and isolate a specific portion of a starting material, subsequently deposited on a target surface [57]. The donor material is usually made up of a synthetic supporting tape which presents right underneath a bioink layer containing cells (see Figure 9.2). During the printing procedure, the ribbon is slid in front of a focused infrared (IR) laser beam, which is absorbed by the synthetic ribbon and, through a photothermal effect, generates a high-pressure bubble at the interface between the ribbon and the bioink. This pressure pulse detaches a small portion of bioink from the tape, subsequently deposited on a target substrate. The operation is repeated point by point by moving the substrate under the illuminated tape until the desired geometry or pattern is obtained. As in the case of the previous techniques, the iteration of the process on different planes allows for fabricating a three-dimensional structure with a spatial resolution that essentially depends on the size of the excitation laser spot.

One of the main advantages of laser-assisted 3D bioprinting is the high cell viability it guarantees. The reason is related to the absence of physical contact between the projection system and the bioink, significantly reducing the mechanical stress the cells suffered [48]. Another significant advantage is the possibility of using materials with high viscosity or solids. In the latter case, the spatial resolution of the technique significantly improves (about 10 μm). The coupling of the system with cell fluorescence techniques also allows the cells to be manipulated individually and thus arranged in the various layers of the 3D construct according to precise patterns. However, these systems are much more complex and expensive than ones based on nozzles. In addition, the use of high-power lasers can sometimes cause damage to cells or thermal degradation of bioink components [48].

9.4.5 Thermoplastic Materials (Bio)Printing

The possibility of printing thermoplastic materials does not properly fall within the 3D bioprinting techniques. However, given the importance of these materials in supporting the "classical" approaches described above, it has been included at the end of the section. A thermoplastic printing system is nothing more than an extrusion system in which the reservoir containing the printed polymer can be heated up to its glass transition temperature or the melting temperature (usually up to 250°C–300°C). The possibility of printing high-performance biocompatible polymers (*e.g.*, PCL, PVA, or PMMA) offers unique opportunities to extend 3D bioprinting possibilities. For example, among others, (i) printing "hybrid" models in which the cellular phase is supported and/or confined by an internal polymeric framework, (ii) fabricating microfluidic systems that can be easily integrated with 3D CNS models (*e.g.*, 3D laminar models of the neurovascular unit), or (iii) shaping the printing surface to mimic anatomically representative portions of the target tissue (*e.g.*, bioprinting a 3D model of the cornea on a convex surface made with extrusion of thermoplastic polymers instead that a flat one).

9.5 THE NEED FOR FUNCTIONAL AND PHYSIOLOGICAL ASSESSMENT

Like all artificially assembled tissue constructs, even 3D brain models must be accurately evaluated in terms of their representativeness of the target tissue before use. This could be done through the use of appropriate characterization techniques. Model assessment must not be limited only to the evaluation of the viability of the printed cells but also of the correct cellular organization of the construct (both topological and phenotypic) and the actual capacity of the model to recapitulate the functionality of the tissue that pretends to mime. Tissue engineering laboratories often overlook the latter aspect, but it is an essential and critical point in the case of 3D bioprinted CNS models.

If, on the one hand, there are established and reliable techniques for evaluating the vitality, morphology, and functionality of neuronal networks, these have been developed initially to deal with two-dimensional systems and can be translated to the third dimension only with some technical or methodological contrivance. This difficulty makes the characterization of cellular models obtained through 3D bioprinting more demanding than the 2D counterpart. 3D bioprinted CNS models collocate in the space between two-dimensional *in vitro* models and three-dimensional organotypic (or acute) slice models, consequently necessitating the exploitation of "hybrid" technological and methodological approaches for their characterization and study.

The thickness of artificial tissues makes immunofluorescence protocols trickier, hinders our observations by standard optical approaches, or increases the difficulty of measuring the action potential of neuronal cells through external probes. It should be noted that to measure the action potential using electrodes, these must have access to the intracellular side of the cell membrane (or, at least, be in contact with it).

Generally, from the point of view of morphofunctional characterization, all the techniques commonly used to characterize organotypic/acute slices of nervous tissues could be effectively translated to investigate systems obtained by 3D bioprinting. In this regard, it is worth noting that 3D bioprinted models have some advantages over "real" tissues, such as (i) a smaller number of cellular phenotypes generally constitutes the tissue, and cells are potentially located in precise and defined spatial positions; (ii) 3D bioprinted models possess greater transparency to visible light and improved control of the physicochemical properties of the cellular matrix (hydrogel); (iii) the porosity of the extracellular support framework could be modulated, allowing the antibodies used in immunofluorescence to access their target molecules deeply inside the hydrogel easily; and (iv) the three-dimensional neuronal tissue could be fabricated directly above electrodes or sensors, improving the quality of the measurements.

Some of the most critical aspects inherent to the characterization of CNS models obtained using a 3D bioprinter are described below.

9.5.1 Cytotoxicity, Proliferation, and Cell Survival

One of the critical points related to the manufacture and use of artificial three-dimensional models of (nervous) tissue is that nutrients and oxygen may not easily access the innermost regions of the cellular construct, invariably leading to necrosis. Furthermore, to make the (bio)printing procedure possible, the bioinks used to support and convey the cells usually possess properties that are not strictly physiological. For example, cross-linking photocatalysts (often activated by cytotoxic low-wavelength light) or extremely reactive chemical groups could be added to bio-inks, impacting cell survival. Therefore, cell viability in bioprinted 3D models must always be evaluated and, possibly, improved.

Cell viability assays based on prestoBlue or alamarBlue are commonly used to assess living cells within cellular constructs or networks. When added to the culture medium, those chemicals are rapidly reduced by the living cells, giving rise to red fluorescent moieties (Resorufins) and subsequently released into the extracellular space. Both substances are easy to use and allow the evaluation of the entire 3D construct without cell specificity (they could not highlight dead cells). Therefore, they can only be used to evaluate the relative toxicity or proliferation impairment among different 3D hydrogels or additives.

On the other hand, calcein AM and ethidium homodimers can be simultaneously used to evaluate both live and dead cells. Essentially, nonfluorescent calcein AM easily enters living cells, where intracellular esterases hydrolyze the molecule to the intensely green fluorescent calcein. Ethidium homodimers can enter only cells with a damaged plasma membrane and elicit strong red fluorescence upon binding nuclear DNA. Combining these two chemicals allows living and dead cells to be evaluated simultaneously using 3D fluorescence microscopy techniques (see Section 9.5.2 below) and cell counting tools from 3D reconstructions. More relevant to 3D CNS constructs, neuronal progenitor cells and neuron-specific live cell imaging reagents are now commercially available as, for example, the NeuroFluor™ CDr3 and NeuO probes, respectively.

9.5.2 Morphological Characterization

A unique ability of 3D bioprinting is to position specific cellular phenotypes in predetermined three-dimensional spatial coordinates within a 3D construct. This capability enables precise control of the mutual position and density of different cellular phenotypes (*e.g.*, neurons *vs.* glial cells). This theoretical capability is, in practice, limited by various factors such as the difficulty of obtaining single-cell resolution (strictly linked to the printing technique used), the stability of the bioink at the time of printing (in the case of printing by extrusion), and the proliferation and/or migration of cells within the artificial cell construct after printing. For all these reasons, it is essential to evaluate the final construct's dimensional, morphological, and topological characteristics and compare them to the digital theoretical model representing the input of bioprinting processes (refer to Section 9.4). Fluorescence microscopy techniques usually accomplish the characterization of 3D cellular components obtained by 3D bioprinting. Indeed, fluorescence microscopy has become the reference technique in the field because it combines (i) the possibility of acquiring three-dimensional reconstructions of the sample; (ii) a sufficiently large field of view; and (iii) a high spatial resolution (single-molecule) in all the three dimensions.

Confocal microscopy (scanning and spinning disc), multiphoton microscopy (2pi), light sheet microscopy (LSM), and, more recently, light field microscopy (LFM) are among the most commonly used techniques to characterize three-dimensional CNS models. Each technique offers advantages and disadvantages in describing a cellular system, for example, in terms of achievable maximum resolution, speed, or field of view. Although confocal microscopy is the commonly used technique in basic research, its limited ability to penetrate thick cellular constructs restricts its 3D characterization capability. Indeed, for a full description of a 3D biosystem, it is crucial to carefully select the best microscopy technique to use. To this end, refer to the excellent reviews on the subject available in the literature [58,59].

Below is a description of the salient aspects of sample preparation and marking techniques common to all fluorescence microscopy techniques.

9.5.2.1 Sample Transparency

The term "tissue clearing" refers to all those strategies that can be implemented to make a three-dimensional biological sample as transparent as possible to visible light. The sample can be an acute or organotypic tissue section, a cellular organoid, an entire organ, or a whole organism, as a rat fetus, with thickness ranging from hundreds of μm to several tens of millimeters. Typically, samples of this size are not transparent and, therefore, may be challenging to analyze using the visible light of a fluorescence microscope. Three-dimensional fluorescence microscopy techniques, such as confocal, multiphoton, or light sheet microscopy, allow penetrating for 100–800 μm inside a pristine sample, although the image quality rapidly deteriorates at increasing depths. This is mainly due to the multitude of different refractive indices characterizing a heterogeneous material where light interacts differently with all its small components leading to a lack of transparency [60]. To overcome this problem, tissue-clearing methods have been developed to increase three-dimensional samples' transparency by homogenizing their refractive indices. This goal is usually achieved through the removal, replacement, and/or modification of some of the tissue's components (usually the lipids of cell membranes).

Although tissue clearing is a critical aspect for the three-dimensional characterization by fluorescence microscopy of thick samples, the lack-of-transparency problem is less marked in 3D bioprinted *in vitro* models than, for example, in *ex vivo* models (*e.g.*, organotypic or acute tissue slices). The reason for that stays in the smaller number of components that make up a 3D bioprinted system, in the greater control of the physicochemical and optical properties achievable, and on the relatively low density of cells present (in fact, all nonstrictly functional cell phenotypes can be excluded from the model). All these aspects are recapitulated by the general high transparency of the bioink containing the cells.

9.5.2.2 Sample Fluorescent Tagging

The use of fluorescent biomarkers able to specifically target and highlight the different cells that compose the central nervous system is a powerful tool for validating bioprinted CNS models in terms of cellular composition and organization. The knowledge of the exact cell phenotype in every spatial location of an artificial cellular assembly substantiates its topological representativeness. Specific markers can also be used to track the different stages of development, the degree of maturation of the resulting neuronal network (*e.g.*, by visualizing neuronal processes), or the functional constituents of the cells (*e.g.*, by marking excitatory glutamatergic or inhibitory GABAergic synapses). Optical microscopy offers several possible approaches to making cells fluorescent and viewable. For example, it is possible to induce the expression of fluorescent proteins (*e.g.*, GFP or mCherry) through viral or nonviral approaches, by using cells derived from genetically modified organisms able to express fluorescent proteins in CNS cells, or by employing immunofluorescence protocols. The latter technique is undoubtedly the most widespread by ensuring simplicity, versatility, and high quality. The most used markers in immunofluorescence exploit a two-step process in which a primary antibody targeting the protein of interest is subsequently decorated with fluorescent secondary antibodies producing signal amplification. They are generally classified into antibodies for neuronal phenotypes and antibodies that target glial phenotypes. Below, we discuss the most common types of biomarkers used in the fluorescence characterization of artificial CNS 3D models.

9.5.2.3 Immunofluorescence in CNS 3D Models

Targeting biomarkers of CNS cells (*i.e.*, neuronal and glial cells) is a crucial tool to determine the condition and development stage of a 3D CNS model. Moreover, when evaluating the 3D topological organization of a 3D cellular construct, it is essential to tag every cell with its specific phenotype (*e.g.*, motor neuron *vs.* oligodendrocyte), spatial coordinates (x, y, x), and neurites protrusions (*i.e.*, the axon and dendrites). Fluorescence tools can help in highlighting the morphology and connectivity pattern of the neuronal constructs, together with the mutual relationship between neuronal and glial cells. This makes it possible to validate the model system's accuracy from the morphological point of view; compared to the portion of CNS, it pretends to mimic. Below is a (nonexhaustive) list of some of the most common biomarkers used in 3D CNS artificial models.

Neuronal-specific targets:

1. Nestin: An intermediate filament protein present in the cytoskeleton of neuronal stem and progenitor cells. It is expressed in the undifferentiated CNS during development as well as normal and adult CNS and in CNS tumor cells. It requires some attention when a vascularized brain model is made (e.g., by introducing HUVEC cells in the construct) because nestin is also expressed in proliferating endothelial progenitor cells (but not in mature endothelial cells) [61].

2. Beta-tubulin III: It is a neuron-specific constituent of cell microtubules and is used as a general neuronal biomarker to recognize differentiated (but premature) neuronal cells [62]. A more mature neuron biomarker is the microtubule-associated protein 2 (MAP-2), a cytoskeletal protein mainly found in the neuronal soma [63].
3. vGLUT1 and vGLUT2: These are enzymes (glutaminases) producing glutamate in excitatory glutamatergic neurons and contribute to its accumulation in the presynaptic vesicles at the nerve ending [64]. Alternative targets are the NMDAR1 and NMDA2B glutamate-gated ion channels, which produce intracellular calcium transient upon glutamate binding.
4. GABA (gamma-aminobutyric acid): It is a neurotransmitter released by GABAergic (usually inhibitory) neurons [65], and it is considered a mature neuronal marker. Alternative targets for mature GABAergic neurons are GAD65 and GAD67, two enzymes involved in the production of GABA.
5. TH (tyrosine hydroxylase): It is an enzyme that produces dopamine and norepinephrine and is generally used as a target to mark mature dopaminergic neurons. ChAT (cCholine acetyltransferase) is an enzyme involved in the production of the neurotransmitter acetylcholine and used as a target to highlight mature differentiated cholinergic neurons [66].

Glial-specific targets:

1. GFAP (glial fibrillary acidic protein): It is a cytoskeletal component found only in astrocytes and is generally considered a good target for this cell phenotype [67].
2. OLIG1 and OLIG2 (oligodendrocyte transcription factors 1 and 2): They are specific helix–loop–helix factors for oligodendrocytogenesis and are possible targets to mark mature oligodendrocytes [68]. Myelin oligodendrocyte glycoprotein (MOG) is also a potential target to highlight mature oligodendrocytes.
3. CD11b and CD45: They are cell surface antigens targeted to highlight microglia cells, the immunocompetent cells in the brain [69]. Notably, microglia could be "activated" by external stimuli in the pro-inflammatory phenotype M1 (expressing CD86) or in the neuroprotective M2 microglia (expressing, instead, CD206).

9.5.3 Functional Characterization

The functional validation of an artificial three-dimensional construct of cells is one of the most important (and often overlooked) aspects that must be addressed once a model has been (bio)fabricated. Fortunately, in the case of artificial tissues that contain neuronal cells and in the hypothesis that the objective of the construct is to give rise to a mature neuronal network, a basic functional validation is easily achievable by evaluating the establishment and characteristics of spontaneous electrical activity within the three-dimensional network. Neuronal cells can alter their membrane potential in a structured way by generating electrical events (action potentials) that can be detected and analyzed in terms of intensity, frequency, shape, and characteristic pattern of activity. The establishment of electrophysiological phenomena in an artificial 3D construct similar to those that characterize the tissue we propose to replicate could be considered an excellent functional validation of the model.

Among the different approaches available to measure the electrical activity of neuronal networks, those easily translatable to three-dimensional *in vitro* systems include optical techniques, microelectrodes, multielectrode arrays, and the exploitation of *in vivo* probes.

9.5.3.1 Calcium Imaging

Calcium imaging is a technique widely used in many fields of cell biology and physiology allowing the visualization of tiny variations in the local calcium concentration (Ca^{2+}) through fluorescence microscopy techniques [70]. In neuroscience, calcium imaging is commonly used to indirectly measure the electrical activity of the cells that make up a neuronal network (single-cell resolution) or the dynamics of calcium within presynaptic terminals (subcellular resolution) [71,72]. This is made possible because the establishment of action potentials in a neuronal cell is accompanied by changes in the intracellular calcium concentration. Therefore, fluorescent probes with a high affinity for calcium, which can modify their excitation/emission spectrum due to this interaction, are used. Fluorescence microscopy allows the observation and recording of these variations in fluorescence intensity, emerging as "flashes" within the cells. Each light blink can thus be associated with the variation in intracellular calcium induced by a burst of action potentials in the cell. The frequency, shape, and intensity (in the case of ratiometric calcium probes) of these calcium transients can be used to obtain information on spontaneous or induced electrical activity in neurons, on the type of cell (*e.g.*, neuronal *vs.* glial cells), or precisely quantify calcium concentrations in subcellular compartments.

Two main classes of calcium probes are available: chemical indicators and genetically encoded calcium indicators (GECI) [73]. The former are small molecules introduced into the culture medium and are able to penetrate inside the cell. This category includes Indo-1, Fura-2, Oregon Green, Fluo-3, and Fluo-4 calcium indicators. The latter are fluorescent proteins derived from fluorescent proteins (GFP or variants) that may be genetically expressed in target cells through, for example, transfection [74]. It is also possible to make transgenic animals that express the dye in all or only part of the cells that constitute the CNS [75].

The sensitivity and temporal resolution of the calcium signals will depend on the type and characteristics of the calcium probe and the fluorescence microscopy technique used. It will be advisable to select the microscopy technique that best suits the experimental needs of the experiment in progress in terms of, for example, maximum acquisition speed, effective field of vision, quality of the three-dimensional reconstruction, and ability to penetrate within the 3D bioprinted system (refer to Section 9.5.2.1 for more details on that aspect).

9.5.3.2 Microelectrodes

Artificial 3D neuronal constructs should be validated in the electrophysiological response of their embedded neuronal networks. When in some region of a neuronal cell, the membrane potential exceeds the threshold value, and it generates an abrupt, stereotyped, rise in the potential named action potential (AP). An AP causes neurotransmitters to be released from the presynaptic side into the synaptic cleft and, ultimately, the generation of excitatory or inhibitory subthreshold events (STP) on the postsynaptic side. STPs propagate in the neuronal tree undergoing summation and/or integration until they eventually overcome the threshold generating a new AP. APs and STPs are unit events of variable intensity and very short duration (1–5 ms) that could be detected using electrodes. Patch clamping is the most meaningful electrode-based detection system of electrophysiological signals [76]. It allows the detection and fine characterization of APs and STPs with ultimate temporal resolution (>100 kHz). It requires special equipment, such as an optical microscope, a micromanipulator, a microelectrode (glass micropipette), and a dedicated electrical detection system. The technique provides unmatched knowledge of membrane electrodynamics phenomena but requires experienced users to take advantage of all its capabilities. Moreover, to be effective, it is necessary that the end of the glass electrode physically touches the plasma membrane of the target cell, making a tight junction with it (gigaseal). No obstructions have to interpose between the pipette and the cell. Therefore, it could be exploited to characterize the 3D bioprinted model only by evaluating its electrical activity from the more marginal neurons, the only ones freely accessible by the probe. Thus, unfortunately, a patch clamp system is not suitable for accurately characterizing the inner parts of an artificial 3D model since it cannot easily reach deeply embedded neurons.

9.5.3.3 Multielectrodes Arrays

Multielectrode arrays (MEAs) are also used to detect the electrical activity of multiple neurons in organotypic or acute brain slices [77]. In the planar configuration, they consist of microscopic planar circular electrodes (a few μm in diameter) distributed on an insulating surface (usually transparent glass), each of which is connected to an amplification system that allows the detection of tiny variations (μV) of the proximal electric potential. As in the case of patch clamping, this system does not make possible the detection of the electrical activity from neurons located deeply inside a 3D CNS model. However, the electrodes of an MEA can detect the local field potentials (LFPs) which are generated by the action potentials of groups of neurons close to (or in contact with) the electrode surface. An MEA system generally can only measure events associated with changes in suprathreshold neuronal membrane potentials. MEAs can be classified into two groups: passive electrode MEAs, where a few tens (usually 64) electrodes are distributed on a surface at a distance of a few hundred microns, and active MEA systems, based on CMOS devices (complementary metal-oxide semiconductor), much smaller and with electrodes interdistances of a few tens of microns. The formers are cheaper but have a lower spatial resolution (they often detect the neuronal activity of multiple cells with a single electrode). Instead, CMOS-based MEAs are much more expensive.

Still, they offer higher spatial resolution and the ability to flexibly select the electrodes from which to record signals based on the expected neuronal activity. Both systems allow simultaneously stimulate and record the electrical activity of the network. They are suitable for the long-term analysis of neuronal networks (*i.e.*, for network development and maturation studies). Recently, 3D-MEA systems have been developed in which the electrodes protrude from the surface into the third dimension so that the active region of the electrode, located at the end of the protrusion, can slip into the three-dimensional tissues reaching the innermost cell layers (approximately 40–100 μm) [78].

9.5.3.4 *In Vivo* Probes

The methods used for *in vivo* brain analysis can also be applied to studying artificial brain tissue obtained by 3D bioprinting. This strategy is particularly appealing when it is necessary to functionally characterize three-dimensional models of considerable size. For example, the Utah array, developed by Normann et al. in 1992 [79], is a standard worldwide when there is the need to record local field potentials from live animals. It is composed of an array of 10 × 10 microscopic silicon needles of variable length (usually a few mm) distributed over an area of approximately $4 \times 4\,mm^2$. Each needle presents a conductive conical metal tip at its very end, connected independently to an electrical amplification system. It is placed chronically onto the cerebral cortex and the needles, sticking into the underlying neuronal regions, detect multiunit electrical activity. This type of device is particularly invasive since all the tissue crossed by the needles is damaged. Still, it is a key tool in basic research to electrophysiologically characterize three-dimensional models of large CNS.

9.6 EXAMPLES

Bioprinting of neurons and glial cells is challenging. Neurons are vulnerable cells *in vitro*, and the intrinsic environmental conditions of the printing process (*i.e.*, mechanical or thermal stress) can impact the viability of nerve cells or affect their differentiation, development, and physiological functionality. In this section, the reader can find some examples of 3D bioprinting in which a careful optimization of the bioprinting process and an accurate design of the bioink composition have made it possible to generate three-dimensional artificial tissues of various portions of the CNS. The examples proposed do not claim to be exhaustive of the real possibilities of the technique, especially since, in all three cases, the biofabrication was conducted through extrusion-based 3D bioprinting. However, these are representative examples of the different origins that the cells used in a bioprinting process may have (*i.e.*, primary cells from animals, stem cells from cell lines, or human-derived pluripotent cells). Furthermore, in all cases, the bioprinting process was followed by a morphological and functional validation of the cellular construct thus obtained. As we have seen previously, the physiological validation of a tissue (or portion of an organ) obtained through 3D bioprinting is an essential aspect aiming at its exploitation in biomedical or biotechnological research.

In (D), the variation in compressive modulus (mean ± SD) was measured at 10% strain corresponding to 3.5%, 5.0%, and 7.5% w/v polymer concentrations post-equilibrium swelling. In (E) page images of a 3D cell-free crosshatch structures made with GelNB-PEGdiSH bioink at 3.5% (w/v) printed at 15 °C with a constant pressure of 150 kPa and a printing speed of 2.5 mm s^{-1}. In (F) confocal live/dead assay of primary cortical neurons hosted within a GelNB-PEGdiSH bioink at 3.5% w/v. Live cells were stained after 7 days post-printing in green with calcein, while dead cells were stained in red with propidium iodide (from Yao et al. 2022).

In (G), an electron microscopy image of a lyophilized HBC/HA/MA-based bioink. In (H), the same bioink endowed with NSCs has been bioprinted and cultured *in vitro*. Live/Dead staining of the 3D bioprinted NSC-laden HBC/HA/MA scaffold has been done after 7 days post-printing (calcein, in green). In (I), the survival and differentiation of NSCs bioprinted within an SCI lesioned area three months post-implantation. Double immunostaining with GFP (green) and Tuj1 (red) to illustrate the survival and neuronal differentiation (top), and GFP (green) and NF (red) to highlight the survival and mature neuron formation (bottom) within the construct (from Liu et al. 2021).

9.6.1 Cortical Constructs from Human-Derived iPSC

Bioprinted 3D neuronal construct could be fabricated from cortical neurons and glial cells derived from human-induced pluripotent stem cells (hiPSCs). The resulting cortical constructs develop in three-dimensional networks characterized by molecular, morphological, and functional properties resembling real neuronal tissues. The possibility to derive pluripotent stem cells from human patients opens unprecedented possibilities in modeling and studying the onset and evolution of neurodegenerative diseases.

In 2019, A. Rosa and coworkers [80] described a method to obtain long-term 3D cortical constructs in which human cortical neurons hold their cellular characteristics and functional properties (see Figure 9.3a). Compared to other approaches, bioprinting specific cell types obtained by predifferentiating pluripotent stem cells generated by reprogrammed somatic cells (hiPSC) is more advantageous, allowing better control of the resulting bioprinted construct in terms of cell phenotype spatial localization, cell survival, and, importantly, cell functionality.

A bioink made of Matrigel® and alginate has been used to recreate a cortical portion of CNS. The selection of the most suitable bioink for cell viability within a 3D construct remains a critical aspect of the bioprinting process. Matrigel®, a matrix preparation extracted from the Engelbreth-Holm-Swarm mouse sarcoma, has demonstrated effectiveness as a bioink component for the generation of hiPSC-derived cardiac and spinal cord bioprinted constructs [81,82]. However, the exact composition of this xenogeneic component is somewhat unknown. This represents a significant limitation for basic and translational applications of bioprinted models, including those of the CNS. Future studies must identify more physiological, standardized, and defined alternatives to Matrigel®. In this direction, the exploitation of xeno-free compounds or decellularized extracellular matrices could represent an exciting option for the bioprinting of neuronal constructs.

The bioprinting procedure exploited here assured the survival of 70%–80% of printed human cells for up to 70 days postprinting. This is one of the most extended maintenance times reported for hiPSC-derived neurons in 3D bioprinted constructs. The obtained cortical 3D model displayed morphological (see Figure 9.3b) and

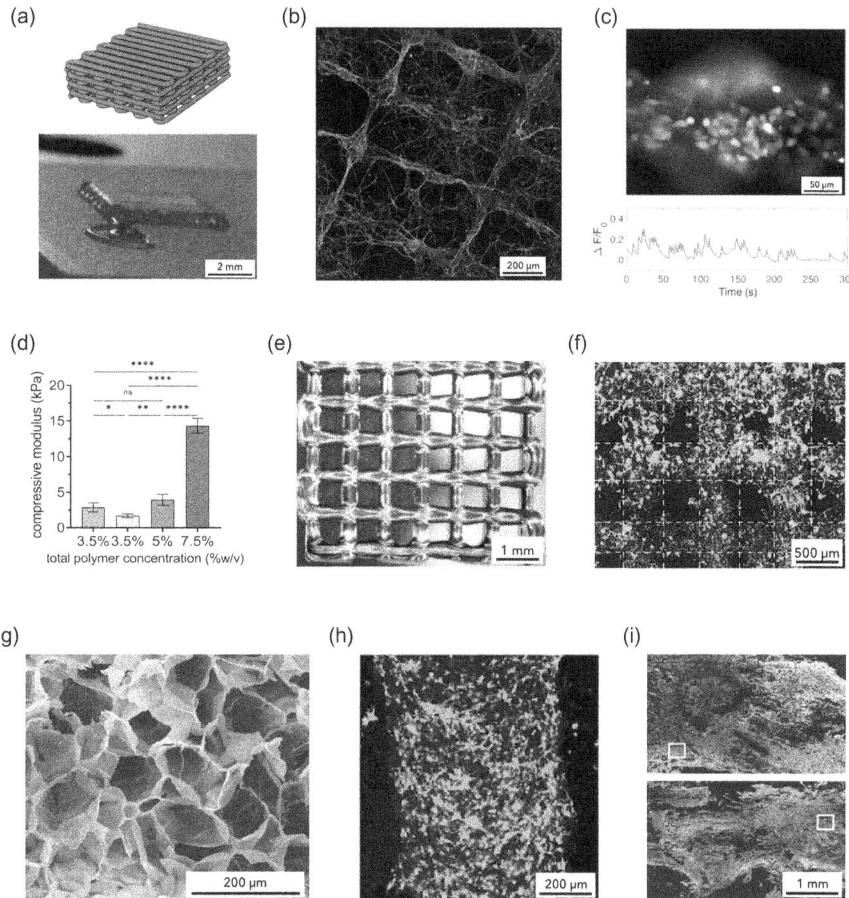

FIGURE 9.3 3D bioprinting approaches for neuronal tissue modeling. In (a), digital representation of a 3D biomodel (top) and an image of the final bioprinted 3D construct (bottom). In (b), a confocal reconstruction of bioprinted neuronal cells at 7 days postprinting, stained with a neuronal marker (MAP2 antibody) and DAPI (highlighting cell's nuclei). (c) Calcium image (top) and trace (bottom) of cortical neurons isolated within the 3D network at 7 days postprinting. Source: Salaris et al. [80] used with permission.

functional properties typical of immature neuronal networks. Indeed, calcium imaging experiments showed sustained calcium spontaneous activity after 7 days from the printing procedure, thus suggesting that the printing process does not prevent the development of a functional network (see Figure 9.3c). However, passive and active neuronal properties, analyzed at the single-cell level through patch-clamping experiments, were typical of immature neuronal cells.

An essential aspect of this example is that it demonstrated the possibility of generating artificial 3D human neuronal constructs. Indeed, the ability to mimic a native tissue could be improved, for instance, by printing mixed populations with precise ratios of neuronal and glial cells or by printing iPSCs carrying pathogenic mutations associated with neurological diseases. Different neuronal subtypes can be obtained from iPSC and used as the cellular components of 3D constructs for disease models and drug screening. In the case of diseases characterized by a complex pathological cell-to-cell interaction, CNS and non-CNS cells could be printed together, increasing artificial tissue representativeness. In the long term, further development of this technology could provide bioprinted cortical neuronal constructs that can be exploited as customized, standardized, and scalable preclinical models for drug development and evaluation.

9.6.2 Mechanoadaptive 3D Models from Primary CNS Cells

Many *in vitro* models exploited in neuronal biology and physiology studies utilize neuronal networks established on rigid two-dimensional substrates. Despite the simplicity of these models, the two-dimensional confinement and the substrate stiffness may influence cell morphology, network formation, and neuronal communication. With this perspective, 3D bioprinting of gel-enfolded primary cells could be a powerful approach to overcome the abovementioned limitations and recapitulate relevant aspects of *in vivo* features. Yet, such an approach has sometimes been limited in terms of the level of resolution and feature size achievable, lacking the possibility of modeling some critical topological aspects of brain architecture, especially when attempting to simultaneously recapitulate microenvironment mechanical cues too. The main reason for this difficulty relates to the mismatch between the optimal mechanical properties a bioink has to possess to provide good printability and the physiological mechanical properties characterizing the target CNS tissue (refer to Section 9.3 for more details about this aspect).

The availability of bioinks swearing high-resolution bioprinting of soft neuronal tissue structures remains scarce due to the challenges associated with filament formation and shape retention using biomaterials with low mechanical properties. In 2022, Forsythe J. S. and coworkers reported three-dimensional constructs obtained by 3D bioprinting of rat primary cortical neuronal cells using a hydrogel medium composed of gelatin norbornene (GelNB) and poly(ethylene glycol)dithiol (PEGdiSH) [83]. This bioink benefits from rapid photo-click chemistry, yielding stable crosshatch three-dimensional neuronal scaffolds with a filament width of about 300 μm. Under printing conditions, the cell viability of bioprinted primary neurons was comparable to the 2D control group (about 80%). In the case of GelNB–PEGdiSH precursors, the printing temperature was found to profoundly influence the intrinsic rheological properties of the bioink, which concomitantly impacted printability and shape fidelity. These findings underscore the importance of precise temperature control. A bioink composed of 3.5% w/v GelNB–PEGdiSH loaded with cells has been successfully used to fabricate 3D neuronal models characterized by compliance similar to the native brain tissue (see Figure 9.3d). This bioink was amenable to fabricating free-standing scaffolds without internal collapse or the need for exploiting supporting sacrificial materials (see Figure 9.3e). Indeed, one of the advantages of thiolene-based chemistry lies in its synergy with light-assisted photocuring. The combination of the temperature sensitivity of the gelatin and the hydrogel stability imparted by covalent photo-cross-linking allows the generation of multilayered neuronal constructs for long-term culture (see Figure 9.3f).

The correct amount of illumination during the printing, the specificity of the cross-linking reaction, and the speed of the thiolene reaction play a critical role in the print times achievable. This is relevant for 3D bioprinting, as rapid cross-linking kinetics not only imparts shape retention after the printing process but also minimizes the exposure time of cells to the cytotoxic UV irradiation required for efficient photo-cross-linking. By modulating the degree of photocuring, the rheological and mechanical properties of the final GelNB–PEGdiSH scaffold can fit the physiological values of the target tissue or, alternatively, mimic (pro)pathological mechanical conditions.

9.6.3 Spinal Cord Constructs Made through NSC Bioprinting

Spinal cord biomodeling may play a relevant role in studying neuronal and axonal regeneration processes throughout the damaged portion of a spinal cord injury (SCI). In this regard, the bioprinting technique offers a versatile and powerful platform for precisely building complex neuronal tissue constructs by printing bioinks consisting of suitable biomaterials and functional cells. The distinct advantage of the 3D bioprinting technology is that a cellularized scaffold could be fabricated with cells (*e.g.*, neuronal stem cells – NSC) spatially arranged to mimic the spinal cord cytoarchitecture, providing morphological cues that favor local cell differentiation and axonal (re) connection. Moreover, in the field of SCI treatment, a 3D bioconstruct with precisely the shape and dimensions of the damaged portion it proposes to replace could be fabricated. However, to achieve this goal, it is essential to develop bioinks that can assure the long-term viability of embedded NSCs.

In 2021, Z. Zhang and coworkers developed an innovative 3D bioprinting strategy to create a living neuronal scaffold via 3D bioprinting [84]. Their bioprinted scaffolds, mimicking the native spinal cord from a micro-to-macro scale, not only provided an ideal microenvironment for the growth and neuronal differentiation of NSCs but also simulated the parallel linear structure of white matter of the spinal cord for optimal neuronal processes regeneration (see Figure 9.3g).

The ideal bioinks for NSC bioprinting should possess specific properties, such as excellent printability, good mechanical properties, and negligible cytotoxicity. A novel biocompatible bioink fulfilling all the requirements mentioned above consists of a mixture of hydroxypropyl chitosan (HBC), thiolated hyaluronic acid (HA-SH), vinyl sulfonated hyaluronic acid (HA-VS), and Matrigel® (MA). The HBC/HA/MA bioink could be coprinted with NSCs to create a stable scaffold by a single-step bioprinting method. The viability of the NSCs within 3D bioprinted scaffolds remained extremely high (about 95%), indicating the little adverse effect of the 3D printing procedure on cell survival. Besides good printability and stable mechanical support, the scaffold provided a favorable physiological milieu for NSC growth and differentiation. Another remarkable aspect of the proposed approach is the possibility of controlling the porosity and stiffness of the printed scaffolds by varying the concentrations of bioink components. Indeed, it has been demonstrated that 3D-bioprinted HBC/HA/MA scaffolds with appropriate porosity and mechanical strength can promote the proliferation and differentiation of NSCs in both neuronal and glial directions (see Figure 9.3h). But the most remarkable result obtained by this 3D construct was the demonstration that, when implanted in an SCI animal model, besides neuronal differentiation, the exogenous NSCs also secreted multiple neurotrophic molecules able to increase the survival and neurogenesis of endogenous NSCs. Therefore, NSCs grafted within the 3D bioprinted scaffold significantly promoted axon regeneration through the collective effect of exogenous and endogenous neuritogenesis (see Figure 9.3i).

Overall, this study demonstrated the feasibility of 3D bioprinted models to promote the morphological structure of the spinal cord and the use of NSC-laden scaffolds for SCI repair *in vivo*. In the future, 3D bioprinting may move toward clinical applications in neuronal tissue engineering, dealing not only with SCI but also other CNS neurodegenerative conditions.

9.7 OUTLOOKS AND FUTURE CHALLENGES

The 3D bioprinting technique possesses all the potential to revolutionize the study of the CNS not only in the basic research field but also in more applicative and translational terms too.

Thanks to its simplicity of use and the possibility to define a predefined cellular and/or ECM composition for each of its volumetric units, this technique allows the creation of physiologically relevant brain constructs for applications ranging from the study of CNS development to drug screening. An area in which the potential of 3D bioprinting could play a crucial role is in the field of *in vitro* artificial tissues obtained from stem cells, the so-called organoids. Indeed, this additive (bio)assembly technique may provide the necessary structural, geometrical, and mechanical cues to drive the correct development of organoids. However, to achieve these results, it is necessary to have access to bioinks specifically optimized for neuronal tissues. Many popular bioinks used in 3D bioprinting for tissue engineering applications do not show sufficient optimization to be used with neuronal cells. Although collagen-based hydrogels, Matrigel®, HA, and laminin show good neuronal biocompatibility, they do not offer good printability when used in pure form. High-resolution 3D bioprinting of neuronal tissues can be obtained by mixing the aforementioned hydrogels with high printability ones.

The three-dimensional revolution promised by the 3D bioprinting technique for CNS applications will concretize only from progress in developing new neuronal-oriented bioinks. When research on bioinks will be able to provide recipes for neuronal bioinks capable of ensuring optimal neuronal survival and/or driving coupled with high printability, the possibilities of 3D bioprinting to reproduce (functional) portions of the CNS will be limited only by the needs of researchers or clinicians.

Future materials science efforts will likely be directed toward developing and synthesizing new highly bioprintable neurocompatible hydrogels.

REFERENCES

1. Yu J, Vodyanik MA, Smuga-Otto K, Antosiewicz-Bourget J, Frane JL, Tian S, et al. Induced pluripotent stem cell lines derived from human somatic cells. *Science.* 2007;318(5858):1917–20.
2. Thomas M, Willerth SM. 3-D bioprinting of neural tissue for applications in cell therapy and drug screening. *Front Bioeng Biotechnol.* 2017;5:69.

3. Hsieh FY, Hsu S. 3D bioprinting: A new insight into the therapeutic strategy of neural tissue regeneration. *Organogenesis*. 2015;11(4):153–8.
4. Lin H, Li Q, Lei Y. Three-dimensional tissues using human pluripotent stem cell spheroids as biofabrication building blocks. *Biofabrication*. 2017;9(2):025007.
5. Dai X, Ma C, Lan Q, Xu T. 3D bioprinted glioma stem cells for brain tumor model and applications of drug susceptibility. *Biofabrication*. 2016;8(4):045005.
6. Gu Q, Tomaskovic-Crook E, Lozano R, Chen Y, Kapsa RM, Zhou Q, et al. Functional 3D neural mini-tissues from printed gel-based bioink and human neural stem cells. *Adv Healthc Mater.* 2016;5(12):1429–38.
7. Hopkins AM, DeSimone E, Chwalek K, Kaplan DL. 3D in vitro modeling of the central nervous system. *Prog Neurobiol*. 2015;125:1–25.
8. Zhuang P, Sun AX, An J, Chua CK, Chew SY. 3D neural tissue models: From spheroids to bioprinting. *Biomaterials*. 2018;154:113–33.
9. Tam RY, Fuehrmann T, Mitrousis N, Shoichet MS. Regenerative therapies for central nervous system diseases: A biomaterials approach. *Neuropsychopharmacology*. 2014;39(1):169–88.
10. Benam KH, Dauth S, Hassell B, Herland A, Jain A, Jang KJ, et al. Engineered in vitro disease models. *Annu Rev Pathol Mech Dis*. 2015;10(1):195–262.
11. von Bartheld CS, Bahney J, Herculano-Houzel S. The search for true numbers of neurons and glial cells in the human brain: A review of 150 years of cell counting: Quantifying neurons and glia in human brain. *J Comp Neurol*. 2016;524(18):3865–95.
12. Bahney J, von Bartheld CS. The cellular composition and glia-neuron ratio in the spinal cord of a human and a nonhuman primate: Comparison with other species and brain regions: Number of cells in spinal cord. *Anat Rec*. 2018;301(4):697–710.
13. Dubois-Dauphin ML, Toni N, Julien SD, Charvet I, Sundstrom LE, Stoppini L. The long-term survival of in vitro engineered nervous tissue derived from the specific neural differentiation of mouse embryonic stem cells. *Biomaterials*. 2010;31(27):7032–42.
14. Gage FH. Mammalian neural stem cells. *Science*. 2000;287(5457):1433–8.
15. Lam D, Enright HA, Cadena J, Peters SKG, Sales AP, Osburn JJ, et al. Tissue-specific extracellular matrix accelerates the formation of neural networks and communities in a neuron-glia co-culture on a multi-electrode array. *Sci Rep*. 2019;9(1):4159.
16. Xu L, Nirwane A, Yao Y. Basement membrane and blood–brain barrier. *Stroke Vasc Neurol*. 2019;4(2):78–82.
17. Lau LW, Cua R, Keough MB, Haylock-Jacobs S, Yong VW. Pathophysiology of the brain extracellular matrix: A new target for remyelination. *Nat Rev Neurosci*. 2013;14(10):722–9.
18. Kim Y, Meade SM, Chen K, Feng H, Rayyan J, Hess-Dunning A, et al. Nano-architectural approaches for improved intracortical interface technologies. *Front Neurosci*. 2018;12:456.
19. Barros CS, Franco SJ, Muller U. Extracellular matrix: Functions in the nervous system. *Cold Spring Harb Perspect Biol*. 2011;3(1):a005108.
20. Her GJ, Wu HC, Chen MH, Chen MY, Chang SC, Wang TW. Control of three-dimensional substrate stiffness to manipulate mesenchymal stem cell fate toward neuronal or glial lineages. *Acta Biomater.* 2013;9(2):5170–80.
21. Ahearne M, Yang Y, El Haj AJ, Then KY, Liu KK. Characterizing the viscoelastic properties of thin hydrogel-based constructs for tissue engineering applications. *J R Soc Interface*. 2005;2(5):455–63.
22. Man AJ, Davis HE, Itoh A, Leach JK, Bannerman P. Neurite outgrowth in fibrin gels is regulated by substrate stiffness. *Tissue Eng Part A*. 2011;17(23–24):2931–42.
23. Kardestuncer T, McCarthy MB, Karageorgiou V, Kaplan D, Gronowicz G. RGD-tethered silk substrate stimulates the differentiation of human tendon cells. *Clin Orthop*. 2006;448:234–9.

24. Rice JJ, Martino MM, De Laporte L, Tortelli F, Briquez PS, Hubbell JA. Engineering the regenerative microenvironment with biomaterials. *Adv Healthc Mater.* 2013;2(1):57–71.
25. Hou S, Tian W, Xu Q, Cui F, Zhang J, Lu Q, et al. The enhancement of cell adherence and inducement of neurite outgrowth of dorsal root ganglia co-cultured with hyaluronic acid hydrogels modified with Nogo-66 receptor antagonist in vitro. *Neuroscience.* 2006;137(2):519–29.
26. Stabenfeldt SE, LaPlaca MC. Variations in rigidity and ligand density influence neuronal response in methylcellulose–laminin hydrogels. *Acta Biomater.* 2011;7(12):4102–8.
27. Ramanujan S, Pluen A, McKee TD, Brown EB, Boucher Y, Jain RK. Diffusion and convection in collagen gels: Implications for transport in the tumor interstitium. *Biophys J.* 2002;83(3):1650–60.
28. Tang-Schomer MD, White JD, Tien LW, Schmitt LI, Valentin TM, Graziano DJ, et al. Bioengineered functional brain-like cortical tissue. *Proc Natl Acad Sci.* 2014;111(38):13811–6.
29. Bercu MM, Arien-Zakay H, Stoler D, Lecht S, Lelkes PI, Samuel S, et al. Enhanced survival and neurite network formation of human umbilical cord blood neuronal progenitors in three-dimensional collagen constructs. *J Mol Neurosci.* 2013;51(2):249–61.
30. Zhou W, Blewitt M, Hobgood A, Willits RK. Comparison of neurite growth in three dimensional natural and synthetic hydrogels. *J Biomater Sci Polym Ed.* 2013;24(3):301–14.
31. Mobasseri R, Tian L, Soleimani M, Ramakrishna S, Naderi-Manesh H. Bio-active molecules modified surfaces enhanced mesenchymal stem cell adhesion and proliferation. *Biochem Biophys Res Commun.* 2017;483(1):312–7.
32. Ma W, Fitzgerald W, Liu QY, O'Shaughnessy TJ, Maric D, Lin HJ, et al. CNS stem and progenitor cell differentiation into functional neuronal circuits in three-dimensional collagen gels. *Exp Neurol.* 2004;190(2):276–88.
33. Chrobak KM, Potter DR, Tien J. Formation of perfused, functional microvascular tubes in vitro. *Microvasc Res.* 2006;71(3):185–96.
34. Antoine EE, Vlachos PP, Rylander MN. Review of collagen I hydrogels for bioengineered tissue microenvironments: Characterization of mechanics, structure, and transport. *Tissue Eng Part B Rev.* 2014;20(6):683–96.
35. Pedron S, Becka E, Harley BAC. Regulation of glioma cell phenotype in 3D matrices by hyaluronic acid. *Biomaterials.* 2013;34(30):7408–17.
36. Seidlits SK, Khaing ZZ, Petersen RR, Nickels JD, Vanscoy JE, Shear JB, et al. The effects of hyaluronic acid hydrogels with tunable mechanical properties on neural progenitor cell differentiation. *Biomaterials.* 2010;31(14):3930–40.
37. Aurand ER, Wagner JL, Shandas R, Bjugstad KB. Hydrogel formulation determines cell fate of fetal and adult neural progenitor cells. *Stem Cell Res.* 2014;12(1):11–23.
38. Bignami A, Hosley M, Dahl D. Hyaluronic acid and hyaluronic acid-binding proteins in brain extracellular matrix. *Anat Embryol* (Berl). 1993;188(5). Available from: http://link.springer.com/10.1007/BF00190136.
39. Wang C, Tong X, Yang F. Bioengineered 3D brain tumor model to elucidate the effects of matrix stiffness on glioblastoma cell behavior using PEG-based hydrogels. *Mol Pharm.* 2014;11(7):2115–25.
40. Bellamkonda R, Ranieri JP, Bouche N, Aebischer P. Hydrogel-based three-dimensional matrix for neural cells. *J Biomed Mater Res.* 1995;29(5):663–71.
41. Chwalek K, Levental KR, Tsurkan MV, Zieris A, Freudenberg U, Werner C. Two-tier hydrogel degradation to boost endothelial cell morphogenesis. *Biomaterials.* 2011;32(36):9649–57.
42. Malda J, Visser J, Melchels FP, Jüngst T, Hennink WE, Dhert WJA, et al. 25th anniversary article: Engineering hydrogels for biofabrication. *Adv Mater.* 2013;25(36):5011–28.

43. Hennink WE, van Nostrum CF. Novel crosslinking methods to design hydrogels. *Adv Drug Deliv Rev.* 2002;54(1):13–36.
44. Wang Z, Abdulla R, Parker B, Samanipour R, Ghosh S, Kim K. A simple and high-resolution stereolithography-based 3D bioprinting system using visible light crosslinkable bioinks. *Biofabrication.* 2015;7(4):045009.
45. Heck T, Faccio G, Richter M, Thöny-Meyer L. Enzyme-catalyzed protein crosslinking. *Appl Microbiol Biotechnol.* 2013;97(2):461–75.
46. Sood A, Ji SM, Kumar A, Han SS. Enzyme-triggered crosslinked hybrid hydrogels for bone tissue engineering. *Materials.* 2022;15(18):6383.
47. Ehsan SM, Welch-Reardon KM, Waterman ML, Hughes CCW, George SC. A three-dimensional in vitro model of tumor cell intravasation. *Integr Biol.* 2014;6(6):603.
48. Mandrycky C, Wang Z, Kim K, Kim DH. 3D bioprinting for engineering complex tissues. *Biotechnol Adv.* 2016;34(4):422–34.
49. Jiang T, Munguia-Lopez JG, Flores-Torres S, Kort-Mascort J, Kinsella JM. Extrusion bioprinting of soft materials: An emerging technique for biological model fabrication. *Appl Phys Rev.* 2019;6(1):011310.
50. Murphy SV, Atala A. 3D bioprinting of tissues and organs. *Nat Biotechnol.* 2014;32(8):773–85.
51. Lee JS, Hong JM, Jung JW, Shim JH, Oh JH, Cho DW. 3D printing of composite tissue with complex shape applied to ear regeneration. *Biofabrication.* 2014;6(2):024103.
52. Tuan RS, Boland G, Tuli R. Adult mesenchymal stem cells and cell-based tissue engineering. *Arthritis Res Ther.* 2003;5(1):32.
53. Cui X, Gao G, Qiu Y. Accelerated myotube formation using bioprinting technology for biosensor applications. *Biotechnol Lett.* 2013;35(3):315–21.
54. Pimpin A, Srituravanich W. Review on micro- and nanolithography techniques and their applications. *Eng J.* 2012;16(1):37–56.
55. Chen Y. Nanofabrication by electron beam lithography and its applications: A review. *Microelectron Eng.* 2015;135:57–72.
56. Gauvin R, Chen YC, Lee JW, Soman P, Zorlutuna P, Nichol JW, et al. Microfabrication of complex porous tissue engineering scaffolds using 3D projection stereolithography. *Biomaterials.* 2012;33(15):3824–34.
57. Guillotin B, Souquet A, Catros S, Duocastella M, Pippenger B, Bellance S, et al. Laser assisted bioprinting of engineered tissue with high cell density and microscale organization. *Biomaterials.* 2010;31(28):7250–6.
58. Brenna C, Simioni C, Varano G, Conti I, Costanzi E, Melloni M, et al. Optical tissue clearing associated with 3D imaging: Application in preclinical and clinical studies. *Histochem Cell Biol.* 2022;157(5):497–511.
59. Yoon S, Cheon SY, Park S, Lee D, Lee Y, Han S, et al. Recent advances in optical imaging through deep tissue: Imaging probes and techniques. *Biomater Res.* 2022;26(1):57.
60. Richardson DS, Lichtman JW. Clarifying tissue clearing. *Cell.* 2015;162(2):246–57.
61. Suzuki S, Namiki J, Shibata S, Mastuzaki Y, Okano H. The neural stem/progenitor cell marker nestin is expressed in proliferative endothelial cells, but not in mature vasculature. *J Histochem Cytochem.* 2010;58(8):721–30.
62. Lee MK, Rebhun LI, Frankfurter A. Posttranslational modification of class III beta-tubulin. *Proc Natl Acad Sci.* 1990;87(18):7195–9.
63. Vallee R. Structure and phosphorylation of microtubule-associated protein 2 (MAP 2). *Proc Natl Acad Sci.* 1980;77(6):3206–10.
64. Glasgow SM, Henke RM, MacDonald RJ, Wright CVE, Johnson JE. Ptf1a determines GABAergic over glutamatergic neuronal cell fate in the spinal cord dorsal horn. *Development.* 2005;132(24):5461–9.
65. Li Y, Lei Z, Xu ZC. Enhancement of inhibitory synaptic transmission in large aspiny neurons after transient cerebral ischemia. *Neuroscience.* 2009;159(2):670–81.

66. Nishimura K, Kitamura Y, Inoue T, Umesono Y, Yoshimoto K, Takeuchi K, et al. Identification and distribution of tryptophan hydroxylase (TPH)-positive neurons in the planarian Dugesia japonica. *Neurosci Res.* 2007;59(1):101–6.
67. Hol EM, Pekny M. Glial fibrillary acidic protein (GFAP) and the astrocyte intermediate filament system in diseases of the central nervous system. *Curr Opin Cell Biol.* 2015;32:121–30.
68. Marques S, Zeisel A, Codeluppi S, van Bruggen D, Mendanha Falcão A, Xiao L, et al. Oligodendrocyte heterogeneity in the mouse juvenile and adult central nervous system. *Science.* 2016;352(6291):1326–9.
69. Havla J, Kümpfel T, Schinner R, Spadaro M, Schuh E, Meinl E, et al. Myelin-oligodendrocyte-glycoprotein (MOG) autoantibodies as potential markers of severe optic neuritis and subclinical retinal axonal degeneration. *J Neurol.* 2017;264(1):139–51.
70. Barreto-Chang OL, Dolmetsch RE. Calcium imaging of cortical neurons using Fura-2 AM. *J Vis Exp.* 2009;(23):1067.
71. Rusakov DA. Heterogeneity and specificity of presynaptic Ca^{2+} current modulation by mGluRs at individual hippocampal synapses. *Cereb Cortex.* 2004;14(7):748–58.
72. Smith SJ, Buchanan J, Osses LR, Charlton MP, Augustine GJ. The spatial distribution of calcium signals in squid presynaptic terminals. *J Physiol.* 1993;472(1):573–93.
73. Stosiek C, Garaschuk O, Holthoff K, Konnerth A. *In vivo* two-photon calcium imaging of neuronal networks. *Proc Natl Acad Sci.* 2003;100(12):7319–24.
74. Grienberger C, Konnerth A. Imaging calcium in neurons. *Neuron.* 2012;73(5):862–85.
75. Kovalchuk Y, Homma R, Liang Y, Maslyukov A, Hermes M, Thestrup T, et al. In vivo odourant response properties of migrating adult-born neurons in the mouse olfactory bulb. *Nat Commun.* 2015;6(1):6349.
76. Kornreich BG. The patch clamp technique: Principles and technical considerations. *J Vet Cardiol.* 2007;9(1):25–37.
77. Simeone TA, Simeone KA, Samson KK, Kim DY, Rho JM. Loss of the Kv1.1 potassium channel promotes pathologic sharp waves and high frequency oscillations in in vitro hippocampal slices. *Neurobiol Dis.* 2013;54:68–81.
78. Spira ME, Huang SH, Shmoel N, Erez H. Multisite intracellular recordings by MEA. In: Chiappalone M, Pasquale V, Frega M, editors. *In Vitro Neuronal Networks.* Cham: Springer International Publishing; 2019. pp. 125–53. (Advances in Neurobiology; vol. 22). Available from: http://link.springer.com/10.1007/978-3-030-11135-9_5.
79. Jones KE, Campbell PK, Normann RA. A glass/silicon composite intracortical electrode array. *Ann Biomed Eng.* 1992 Jul;20(4):423–37.
80. Salaris F, Colosi C, Brighi C, Soloperto A, Turris V, Benedetti MC,, et al. 3D bioprinted human cortical neural constructs derived from induced pluripotent stem cells. *J Clin Med.* 2019;8(10):1595. doi: 10.3390/jcm8101595. PMID: 31581732; PMCID: PMC6832547.
81. Koch L, Deiwick A, Franke A, Schwanke K, Haverich A, Zweigerdt R, et al. Laser bioprinting of human induced pluripotent stem cells—The effect of printing and biomaterials on cell survival, pluripotency, and differentiation. *Biofabrication.* 2018;10(3):035005.
82. Joung D, Truong V, Neitzke CC, Guo SZ, Walsh PJ, Monat JR, et al. 3D printed stem-cell derived neural progenitors generate spinal cord scaffolds. *Adv Funct Mater.* 2018;28(39):1801850.
83. Yao Y, Molotnikov A, Parkington HC, Meagher L, Forsythe JS. Extrusion 3D bioprinting of functional self-supporting neural constructs using a photoclickable gelatin bioink. *Biofabrication.* 2022;14(3):035014.
84. Liu X, Hao M, Chen Z, Zhang T, Huang J, Dai J, et al. 3D bioprinted neural tissue constructs for spinal cord injury repair. *Biomaterials.* 2021;272:120771.

10 3D Bioprinting for Ocular Applications

Idoia Gallego, Markel Lafuente-Merchan, Myriam Sainz-Ramos, Iván Maldonado, Jon Zarate Sesma, Laura Saenz del Burgo Martínez, Gustavo Puras Ochoa, and Jose Luis Pedraz Muñoz
University of the Basque Country UPV/EHU
Institute of Health Carlos III
Bioaraba

Hodei Gómez-Fernández
University of the Basque Country UPV/EHU
AJL Ophthalmic S.A.

CONTENTS

10.1 INTRODUCTION

Ocular diseases and vision impairment (VI) are an increasing reality in worldwide society. Among them, congenital disorders, age-related diseases, retinopathies, corneal damage, trachoma and other visual abnormalities are the main causes of VI and blindness. In particular, according to the 2010 Global Survey by the World

DOI: 10.1201/9781003274568-10

Health Organization (WHO), around 39 million people suffer from blindness [1], while the updated estimation of this population increased by 4.3 million more in the past decade, as reported by the 2019 Global Burden of Disease [2]. The affected population is even higher when talking about VI, where it is estimated that 1.1 billion people presented this medical problem in 2020, with worryingly increasing rates in the near future [2]. All of these ocular diseases and VI result in high healthcare costs [3], but beyond the economic costs derived from treatments and ocular surgeries, patients' life quality is critically compromised, especially in the case of some vision/ocular diseases that can lead to VI and even blindness. In these scenarios, patients frequently develop depressive disorders associated with ocular disabilities [4], jeopardising their life quality and well-being. In addition, as shown by the high prevalence and incidence rates, the currently available treatments do not manage to diminish the rates of affected patients worldwide, and advanced therapies, such as gene therapy and cell therapy, are still in the early stages to reach clinical practice in the ophthalmologic field, or are not affordable. A clear example of this issue is the retinal gene therapy drug LUXTURNA®, used to treat Leber's congenital amaurosis type 2, at a cost of $850,000 per one-time treatment.

Three-dimensional (3D) technology arises as a promising tool in ophthalmology, not only for eye tissue engineering by the use of bioinks aimed at mimicking the target tissue with its specific extracellular matrix (ECM) and cell types by 3D bioprinting [5] but also for the development of prostheses, diagnostic tools, drug release systems, surgical simulators and medical education by 3D printing [6]. Of note, this technology presents several advantages such as self-tailored therapies, low-cost production and relatively easy design and development [7]. In addition, the eye has several physiological barriers, such as tear film, corneal epithelium, conjunctival tissue and blood–ocular barriers, i.e. the blood–aqueous barrier, which protects the anterior segment of the eye, and the blood–retinal barrier, which protects the posterior one. These particular features make the eye an immune-privileged organ, representing an attractive target for 3D printing and bioprinting, since the probability of rejection and immunologic side effects after transplanted grafts is reduced. In addition, the implementation of this strategy could potentially diminish the existing imbalance between organ donors and the demand of transplantation [7].

10.1.1 Target Eye Structures for 3D Bioprinting

It is noteworthy that each of the structures that form the eye presents its own particular biological and architectural features. The eye is a complex organ composed of an intricate network of cell types and layers, which are represented in Figure 10.1. It can be anatomically divided into two major parts: the anterior segment composed of the conjunctiva, cornea, pupil, iris, ciliary body and lens, and the posterior segment composed of the choroid, retina, macula and optic nerve. For its part, the sclera surrounds the eye in both segments. The integrity and proper functioning of each structure enable vision. In case of disease, generally one of the mentioned eye layers is affected [8], which would turn into the target tissue to substitute using 3D bioprinting or 3D printing, depending on whether the structure to resemble has cells or not,

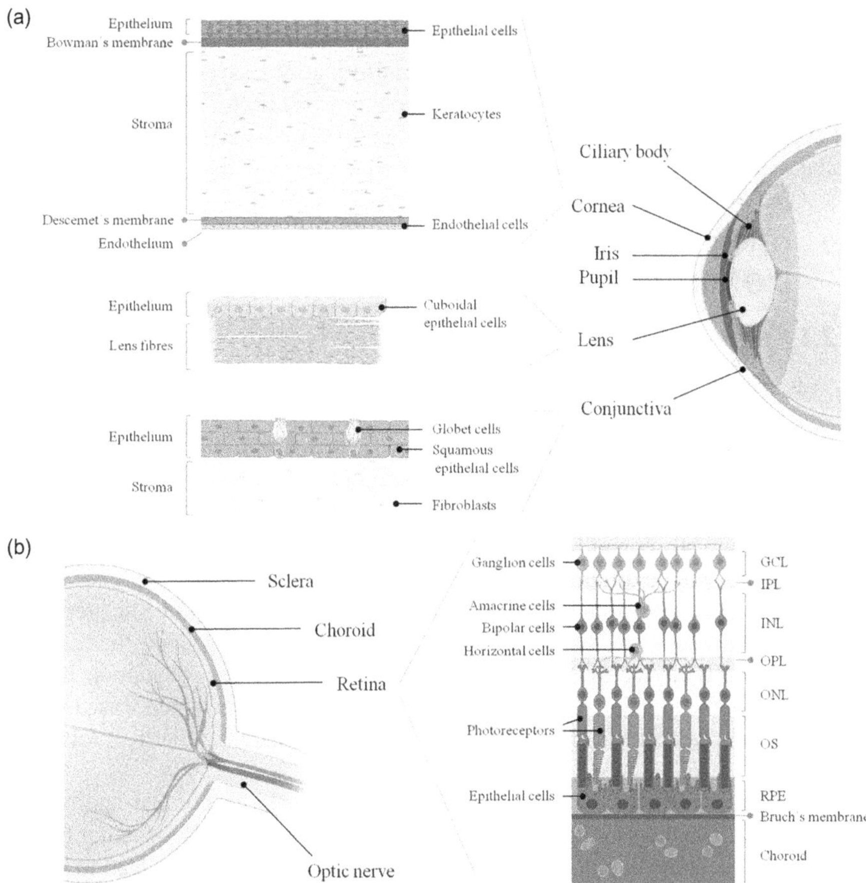

FIGURE 10.1 Overview of the ocular anatomy showing the potential target layers that can be manufactured using 3D bioprinting and their specific cell types. (a) Anterior segment. (b) Posterior segment. GCL, ganglion cell layer; IPL, inner plexiform layer; INL, inner nuclear layer; ONL, outer nuclear layer; OPL, outer plexiform layer; OS, outer segment; RPE, retinal pigment epithelium.

respectively. The only acellular structure in the eye is the sclera, which is a fibrous membrane. Hence, in the case of tissue engineering approaches, the technology of choice would be 3D bioprinting in almost all cases, by including in the bioink the specific cell type(s) of the target eye layer.

Concerning the different layers and cell types that form the eye, they range from the simplest structure with only a single cell type to the most complex one (Figure 10.1). In this sense, the eye's lens (or crystalline lens) is surrounded by a only layer of cuboidal epithelial cells, while the retina is composed of more than 100 cell types [9], making this last structure the most complex tissue in terms of cell composition, interconnections and biological function, which is comprehensively taking into account that it is part of the central nervous system and responsible for the phototransduction process.

Besides the biologically functional eye structures, "inert" or acellular eye parts can also be custom tailored using 3D printing. This is the case of prostheses such as sclera or eyeballs for patients with inherited malformations, severe ocular injury and those that require enucleation due to several circumstances [6,7]. In addition, as we will explain in greater depth afterwards, this additive manufacturing technique can also be used to evaluate and improve drug-based therapies in the eye.

10.2 GENERAL REMARKS RELATED TO 3D BIOPRINTING EYE STRUCTURES

10.2.1 Materials and Biomaterials

It is reasonable that the type of materials and biomaterials used in the 3D bioprinting process is critical and will determine the biomechanical and physical properties of the specific 3D printed or bioprinted eye structure. Hence, their selection and proportion in the ink's mixture will define the stiffness, printability and biocompatibility, among other properties, depending on the required features of the target structure to mimic, as much as possible, the native one (Table 10.1). It has also been taken into consideration that these materials will be different in the case of 3D printing or 3D bioprinting, since the last one's ink must have a suitable microenvironment for cell survival while preserving biological properties. In this sense, alginate [10–15], gelatine and gelatine methacrylate (GelMA) [15–21] are the most widely employed biomaterials for ophthalmic 3D bioprinting, while the function of other materials and biomaterials is more focused to give the specific mechanical and physical properties of each ocular tissue, such as follows:

- *Transparency*: this feature is of particular relevance for corneal and conjunctival 3D bioprinting to allow proper vision. An excess of particular biomaterials in the bioink, as occurs with collagen and elastin, can lead to loss of transparency, which is usually analysed using light transmittance. Also, the accuracy of collagen fibre arrangement in the 3D scaffold, which can be modulated by the proteoglycan (PG) content, is a key parameter that affects transparency [22] and optical quality, also known as visual sharpness, which is analysed in the 3D bioprinted scaffolds using the polychromatic modulation transfer function (PMTF). In this regard, the smoothness of the biomaterial and the 3D bioprinting technique used are critical factors to achieve good optical quality.
- *Stiffness*: the top biomaterial to add this property to the 3D bio-scaffold is collagen type I, but its use is normally limited to low concentrations of <2% w/v [23], while the native cornea presents >14% [24]. This limitation of its use is referred to avoid excessive viscosity, turbidity and the cytotoxicity produced by its low pH value. Besides, stiffness must not be too high to permit the deformation of the scaffold to the target tissue morphology. A significant aspect that merges with the scaffold stiffness is suturability. In the cases where the bioprinted graft has to be implanted in the target ocular tissue, materials that allow suturing while avoiding tearing are of great importance. This is the case of GelMA [25], which can be considered a hybrid material that results from the combination of natural and synthetic

TABLE 10.1
Biomaterials Employed to Manufacture Ocular Tissues Using 3D Bioprinting

Materials	Origin	Target Tissue	Properties						Observations	Ref.
			T	S	E	Bc	Bd	CA		
Agarose	Natural	Cornea	+	++	+	++	++	–	Temperature sensitivity; simple gelation	[31]
Alginate	Natural	Cornea Retina	+++	++	++	+++	++	+	Depending on the concentration; control of cross-linking; high viscosity	[17]
Carboxymethyl chitosan (CMC)	Natural	Cornea	+++	–	–	++	+++	++	Soluble in a wide range of pH	[36,37]
Elastin	Natural	Conjunctiva	–	+	+++	+++	++	++	ECM component	[18]
GelMA	Hybrid	Conjunctiva	+++	++	++	+++	++	+++	Modifiable ink/hydrogel stiffness and elasticity	[21,25]
HA	Natural	Cornea Retina	+++	+	+++	+++	+++	+++	ECM component; modifiable ink/hydrogel stiffness	[32,33]
Polyethylene glycol diacrylate (PEGDA)	Synthetic	Cornea	++	+++	+	++	+	–	Photopolymerisation; Its molecular weight (MW) influences in properties; biocompatibility decreasing when concentration >25%	[33,34]
Poly(vinyl alcohol) (PVA)	Synthetic	Cornea	+++	++	–	++	+	+		[35]
Type I collagen	Natural	Cornea	–	+++	+++	+	++	++	Mimics native ECM; bioink acidification could affect biocompatibility; high viscosity and turbidity	[30]

T, transparency; S, stiffness; E: elasticity; Bc, biocompatibility; Bd, biodegradability; CA, cellular adhesion.
– Poor, + medium, ++ high, +++ very high.

polymers. Stiffness and suturability are especially desirable for corneal and conjunctival 3D bioprinted tissues. Hence, the fine-tuning of materials and proportions should be balanced to achieve the proper stiffness while enabling the suturability of the 3D bioprinted scaffold in these target tissues.

- *Elasticity*: it is of special interest for conjunctival 3D bioprinting. The use of materials such as elastin, a naturally derived polymer, can confer elastic behaviour to the 3D scaffold in order to mimic the target tissue.
- *Biodegradability*: this feature will depend on the final goal of the bioprinted scaffold. In the cases where it is intended to substitute a target tissue, as permanently as possible, biodegradability is not desired to avoid repeated interventions for the patient. For such purposes, resins and synthetic materials could be employed in the bioink using 3D printing. On the contrary, for regenerative medicine purposes, the aim is to achieve progressive biodegradation of the scaffold while regenerating the target ocular tissue. In this sense, biomaterials such as alginate, GelMA and hyaluronic acid (HA) are the most adequate ones in 3D bioprinting approaches.

In addition to the aforementioned features, there are some common properties necessary for all the ocular bioprinted scaffolds, which are biocompatibility, sterility and cellular adhesion. It is desirable that the used materials are biocompatible and sterile to avoid potential side effects after the implant of the 3D bio-scaffold, as well as cytotoxicity of the cells in the bioink. In this sense, as commented before, the natural polymer alginate and the hybrid material GelMA are the most widely used biomaterials, but the addition of HA to bioinks for ocular applications [18,26,27] helps to regulate cellular signalling and performance. In particular, this native ECM derivative promotes cell viability, proliferation and migration [28], features collectively referred to as cellular adhesion, which is also facilitated by porous and rough scaffolds that allow nutrients and oxygen interchange.

Finally, there can be other tissue-specific features as occurs with the cornea, where it is demanded that the 3D bioprinted scaffold has a particular curvature, which goes hand in hand with the scaffold stiffness, to maintain this precise shape and fit with the patient corneal arch to enable correct light refraction [29].

10.2.2 Cell Types

In terms of cell complexity, eye structures range from a single cell type, as in the case of the eye's lens, to an intricate system of more than 100 cell types arranged in different layers, orientations and interconnections, as is the case of retina [9]. Hence, depending on the eye tissue to resemble, specific cell layers, cell types and even cell orientation must be considered in 3D bioprinting, as shown in Figure 10.1. Although cell orientation is the most difficult feature to reproduce when developing a 3D scaffold, current 3D bioprinting technology enables certain control over this parameter by fine-tuning the layer thickness and printing orientation with proper computer-aided design (CAD) programming. Anyway, it is expected that arising technologies can improve the precision to guide cell disposition in complex 3D bioprinted tissues.

In 3D bioprinting for ocular applications, the main target tissues to resemble are the cornea, conjunctiva, retina and eye's lens. Each structure and even each layer of the structure have specific cell types that need to be included in the bioink. Table 10.2 shows the cell types employed to 3D bioprint different layers of the aforementioned eye tissues. In general terms, these cell types consist of epithelial cells, stem cells, keratocytes (for cornea), photoreceptor (PR) cells (for retina) and ganglion cells (for retina).

TABLE 10.2
Cell Types Employed to Manufacture Ocular Tissues Using 3D Bioprinting

Cell Type	Origin	Target Tissue	*In Vitro*	*In Vivo*	Ref.
Encapsulated differentiated keratocytes from human turbinate-derived mesenchymal stem cells (hTMSCs)	Human	Corneal stroma	Cell viability	No	[22]
Human conjunctival stem cells (hCjSCs)	Human	Conjunctiva	Cell viability Quantitative polymerase chain reaction (qPCR): analyse proliferation, stemness, ocular lineage and mesenchymal lineage	No	[21]
Human limbal epithelial progenitor cells (hLEPCs)	Human	Conjunctiva	Cell viability Cell attachment Proliferation assays	Epithelialisation, inflammation, scar tissue formation and presence of granulation tissue	[18]
Human retinoblastoma cell line (Y79)	Human	Retina	Cell viability (PrestoBlue assay) Cell staining	No	[38]
Photoreceptor cells (PRCs) isolated from pig ocular globes	Pig	Retina	Actin cytoskeleton staining Immunohistochemical analysis	No	[20]
PRCs differentiated from human foetal retinal progenitor cells (fRPCs)	Human	Retina	Immunostaining of PR-specific marker to evaluate the differentiation PR-specific protein expression quantification (Western blot) qPCR to analyse PR maturation	No	[27]

(Continued)

TABLE 10.2 (*Continued*)
Cell Types Employed to Manufacture Ocular Tissues Using 3D Bioprinting

Cell Type	Origin	Target Tissue	*In Vitro*	*In Vivo*	Ref.
Rabbit adipose-derived mesenchymal stem cells (rASCs)	Rabbit	Corneal stroma	Cell viability (3-(4,5-dimethylthiazol-2-yl)-2,5-diphenyltetrazolium bromide (MTT) and live/dead assay)	Anterior lamellar keratoplasty (ALK) in the rabbit keratectomy model	[34]
Rabbit corneal epithelial cells (rCECs)	Rabbit	Corneal epithelium	Cell viability (MTT and live/dead assay)	ALK in the rabbit keratectomy model	[34]
Retinal ganglion cell (RGC) neurons	Rat	Retina	Cell viability Electrophysiological properties Immunostaining for cell orientation	No	[14]
Retinal glial cells	Rat	Retina	Cell viability after bioprinting Immunocytochemistry	No	[39]
Retinal pigment epithelial cell line (ARPE-19)	Human	Retina (RPE layer)	Cell metabolic activity evaluation Actin cytoskeleton staining Immunohistochemical analysis VEGF release quantification	No	[20]
			Cell viability (PrestoBlue assay) Cell staining (DAPI; haematoxylin/eosin)	No	[38]
PRs differentiated from induced pluripotent stem cells (IPSCs)	Human	Retina	Immunocytochemistry to observe differentiation from IPSCs and cell alignment inside the scaffold	No	[40]
RPE cells	Unknown	Retina (RPE layer)	Cell viability (live/dead assay)	No	[27]

10.3 3D BIOPRINTING OF EYE STRUCTURES

10.3.1 Cornea

The cornea is an external tissue located in the anterior hemisphere of the eye and is the first barrier protecting the intraocular structures from the environment. It is transparent and avascular, and its morphology has a dome-shaped structure, having a relevant role in transmittance and light diffraction [41]. The outermost layer is the epithelium, with an average thickness of 58 μm [42], which provides refractive power to the eye by forming part of the tear film–corneal interface [41]. Next, Bowman's layer is a 10 μm acellular structure mainly composed of a randomly arranged fibre network of collagen, which provides stability to the cornea [43]. The middle and main layer is the stroma, comprising 90% of the corneal thickness [44], with ECM elements, keratocytes and orthogonally aligned collagen fibres, fundamental due to the relation to the shape, mechanical properties [45] and optical properties such as transparency [46]. The next layer is called Dua's layer or pre-Descemet's membrane, an acellular tissue of 10 μm composed mainly of collagen type I oriented transversely, longitudinally and obliquely [47], followed by the Descemet membrane. The deeper layer is the endothelium, of 5 μm thickness, which confers stiffness to the organ and regulates corneal hydration [44] (Figure 10.1a).

Major diseases affecting this tissue include keratoconus, which worsens visual acuity (VA) and causes irregular astigmatism. Keratoconus is the leading indication for corneal transplantation [48], affecting approximately 1 in 2,000 people in the general population. The corneal mechanical stability is threatened in this bilateral pathology, conducting progressive morphological changes [49]. The main change appears in the disposition of the stromal lamellae, due to a decrease in the ECM's glycosaminoglycan (GAG) number, leading to a change in the PG arrangement and, finally, a distortion in the collagen fibre organisation [50]. This results in a progressive thinning of the corneal stroma, central/paracentral posterior ectasia and rupture in the Bowman membrane, in addition to a significant decrease in the collagen fibre elasticity [51].

The corneal transplant is the primary treatment for keratoconus so far, and although a procedure called corneal cross-linking (CLX) has greatly improved the detention of the ectasia process of the cornea [52], it does not achieve regeneration or healing. Hence, current treatments are not sufficient to meet the demand for corneas globally. In this sense, the tissue engineering field is investing to create biomimetic corneas starting from mimicking isolated layers such as stroma [13,16,22,31], epithelium [12,15] and endothelium [17] using principally extrusion 3D bioprinting.

At present, only two works from Sorkio et al. and He et al. have reported a 3D bioprint of two layers (epithelium and stroma) of the cornea. The first one employed human embryonic stem cell-derived limbal epithelial stem cells (hESC-LESCs) and human adipose tissue-derived stem cells (hASCs) in two different bioinks for scaffolding by laser-assisted 3D bioprinting. However, although successful, this study was limited to *in vitro* assays [26]. Recently, a 3D scaffold composed of GelMA and polyethylene glycol diacrylate (PEGDA) has been designed as a bilayer hydrogel with promising results *in vivo* [34]. In this study, the stromal layer contained rabbit adipose-derived mesenchymal stem cells (rASCs), and the epithelial section contained rabbit corneal epithelial cells (rCECs). The chosen printing technology was digital light processing (DLP) or photo-initiated copolymerisation, a light-assisted technology based on the layer-by-layer local photopolymerisation of a photocuring bioink. The main advantages of this printing technology were the high cellular viability, high resolution (1 μm) and high printing velocity (Figure 10.2a). Furthermore, the bioprinted scaffold showed good cell adhesion, proliferation and migration properties.

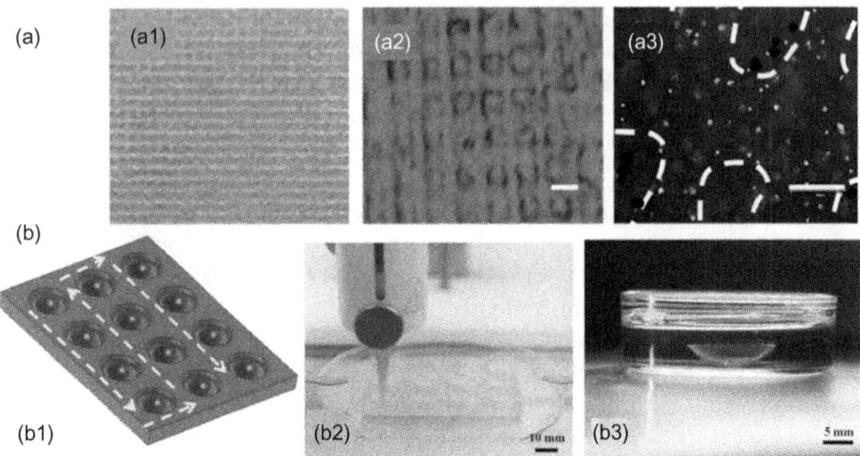

FIGURE 10.2 (a) PEGDA/GelMA hydrogel. (a1) Digital photograph and (a2) micrograph of the printed orthogonally aligned fibrous structure. (a3) Representative image of a live/dead rCEC assay in an orthogonally aligned fibrous object after culturing for 2 days. Reproduced with permission from Ref. [34]. (b) High-throughput corneal bioprinting. (b1) Support scaffold with printing path in yellow arrows. (b2) Process of corneal scaffolds bioprinting using a BIO X printer. (b3) 3D bioprinted cornea after cross-linking. Reproduced with permission from Ref. [53].

It exhibited high light transmittance, appropriate swelling degree, permeability and degradation rate. Also, *in vivo* assays were performed to verify the healing effects of the biomimetic tissue through ophthalmic and histopathological tests, observing effective wound healing in the corneal defects and adequate re-epithelisation and stromal regeneration [34].

Research efforts have also been focused on developing large-scale 3D bioprinted corneas (Figure 10.2b). In this sense, Kutlehria S. et al. designed and printed by stereolithography a polylactic acid (PLA) support scaffold that allowed the printing of 6–12 corneas at a time. Then, by extrusion technique, 3D scaffolds consisting of sodium alginate, gelatine type B from bovine skin, collagen type I and human corneal keratocytes (hCKs) were bioprinted. The bioprinted corneas were transparent, smooth, had adequate curvature and supported cell growth for 2 weeks. This research work offers a new avenue for optimisation and design to obtain printed tissue on a large scale [53].

Advances in the 3D bioprinting field focused on corneal tissue and have evolved to even reach clinical trials. In this regard, a clinical trial developed in 2019 by Kim H. et al. proved high capacity in controlling the orientation of the collagen fibres. In this study, decellularised corneal ECM (Co-dECM) hydrogel at 2% concentration was designed, with an extracted matrix from corneas dissected from bovine eyeballs. The cell types selected for this study were differentiated and encapsulated human keratocytes from human turbinate-derived mesenchymal stem cells (hTMSCs). The mechanical characterisation showed optimal viscoelastic properties for extrusion bioprinting. The printing pressure has to be controlled since, despite improving the collagen alignment, cell viability can be threatened. For this reason, the parameters taken into account are the bioink viscosity, the printer flow rate and the internal diameter of the needle. In conclusion, the corneal biomimetic tissue designed in this article demonstrated efficiency as a corneal native transparent tissue [22].

10.3.2 Conjunctiva

The conjunctiva is the outermost part of the eye and is composed of two cell layers (Figure 10.1a). The stratified epithelium contains goblet cells capable of secreting mucins, which provide lubrication and protection against external agents. The stroma, which has nerves and blood vessels, is in turn composed of two layers, a superficial adenoid layer with lymphocytes and reticular connective tissue and a deeper fibrous layer that covers the entire eyeball composed of collagen and elastin fibres [54]. One of the most critical diseases of the conjunctiva with 10% prevalence is pterygium, which consists of uncontrolled growth of its epithelium, causing chronic inflammation. This affects the innermost layers and can lead to blindness. At present, the exact cause of the disease is not known, since in each individual the factors of the immune response that end up causing the homeostatic imbalance of the conjunctiva are different [55].

A bioprinting model capable of simulating the pathological conditions of conjunctiva with pterygium has recently been developed. The bioprinting technique used was DLP, and the cells employed in the bioink were human conjunctival stem cells (hCjSCs), which can be differentiated into the two main types of the conjunctival epithelium (keratocytes and goblet cells), macrophages and vascular endothelial cells. The structural component of the scaffold was made by GelMA, HA glycidyl methacrylate (HAGM) and lithium phenyl-2,4,6-trimethylbenzoylphosphinate (LAP). Through these scaffolds, it was possible to simulate the evolution of the disease *ex vivo* by analysing the genetic expression of the factors in the immune response that cause the disease. This technique gives us the opportunity to treat future patients with pterygium in a personalised way by performing scaffolds with cells extracted from the patient [21].

However, the conjunctiva can be damaged by external agents, which requires surgery for its repair. Currently, amniotic tissue is the most common structure used for conjunctival grafts, but recently, a study carried out by Dehghani et al. developed a synthetic membrane using 3D bioprinting [18] (Figure 10.3a). The scaffold was made of collagen type IA, gelatine from porcine skin, soluble elastin (MW 60 kDa) and sodium hyaluronate, with human limbal epithelial progenitor cells (hLEPCs) embedded in the bioink. The results showed that this membrane had the capacity for conjunctival regeneration with a greater effect on decreasing inflammation in the first days after surgery (Figure 10.3b).

10.3.3 Crystalline Lens

The crystalline lens is made up mainly of protein (60%) and is covered by a collagen capsule with epithelial cells on its surface (Figure 10.1a). The epithelial cells form in layers, with the deepest layers being the oldest and located in the nucleus of the lens. The lens epithelial cells synthesise crystallins and lens-specific proteins and further degrade into transparent organelles and eventually become fibrous cells [56]. One of

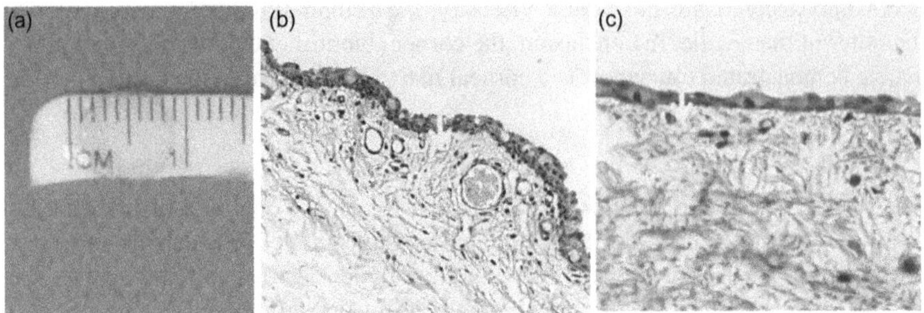

FIGURE 10.3 (a) Gelatine-based 3D scaffold; (b) gelatine-based membrane-treated rabbit eye: three- to five-layer epithelium (between yellow arrows) was repaired with normal cellular morphology and (c) non-treated rabbit eye: the epithelium was not repaired from the conjunctival damage. Reproduced with permission from Ref. [18].

the most common diseases of the crystalline lens is cataracts, which is a clouding of the lens that leads to loss of vision. Cataracts can be congenital or late onset after the age of 55 due to cumulative damage caused by external agents such as ultraviolet rays or internal oxidative processes [57]. The most common treatment is surgery in which the lens is removed and replaced with an intraocular lens. Nowadays, research is being carried out into the development of lenses using 3D printing, where the challenge is to develop lens with a smooth surface, to avoid current post-surgery medication [58].

Such an approach has been followed by Li J. W. et al. in which the crystalline lens has been replaced by a lens manufactured by 3D printing with poly(acrylamide-co-sodium acrylate) hydrogel [59]. It was observed, in New Zealand white rabbit eyes, that this material offered sufficient transparency to allow light rays to pass without causing damage to the surrounding ocular tissue (Figure 10.4). In addition, it showed that the cells in contact with the 3D printed lens suffered cell death, thus preventing the lens from suffering cell invasion, which would cause its loss of transparency.

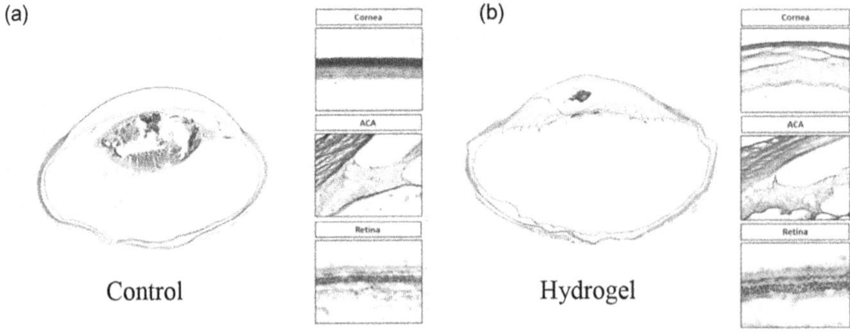

FIGURE 10.4 Histological sections of the cornea, anterior chamber angle and retina of a rabbit eye 3 months after intraocular implantation of the 3D printed lens. The hydrogel (b) improved the connectivity of cells and layered lamination compared with the control (a). Reproduced with permission from Ref. [59].

10.3.4 Retina

The retina is a complex tissue placed at the back of the eye. Its complexity resides in its multi-layered structure where many cell types are arranged in a specific way to be functional [60] (Figure 10.1b). The most important cell types are the PRs, bipolar cells, horizontal cells, retinal ganglion cells and glial cells [61]. The retina is supported by a specialised monolayer known as retinal pigment epithelium (RPE). It provides nutrients and growth factors to PRs and physical support to the retina [62]. The retina's function is related to vision by converting light signals into electrical pulses that are conducted to the brain. Consequently, any disease in this area may lead to blindness. Glaucoma, retinitis pigmentosa and age-related macular degeneration (AMD) are the most common and prevalent diseases. Glaucoma is related to retinal ganglion cell loss [63]. Likewise, retinitis pigmentosa is characterised by cone and rod PR death [64]. On the contrary, AMD is a disorder in the medium part of the retina, causing progressive degeneration along with increased inflammation of the retina [65].

Retinal cell recovery has been considered the ideal solution for retinal diseases; however, their culture *in vitro* is a challenge. For example, PRs undergo apoptosis without specific retinal ECM components or co-culture with another supportive retinal cell [26]. Furthermore, it has been reported cell death and unusual behaviour in implanted cells [66]. Scaffolding through 3D bioprinting has arisen as a solution to these problems. In fact, high cell viability may be obtained using retinal ECM-alike scaffolds. In addition, scaffolds can be bioprinted to simulate the multi-layered structure of the retina. Moreover, the bioprinting technique admits a great range of cell types that could be oriented in the same manner as in the native retina [11].

Several research works have focused on fabricating retinal scaffolds using 3D bioprinting technology. Masaeli E. et al. manufactured a GelMA layer to simulate the acellular retinal Brunch's membrane. Then, two different cell types were deposited on it using piezoelectric inkjet bioprinting. First, retinal pigment epithelial cell line (ARPE-19) cells were seeded to simulate the RPE, and afterwards, PRs isolated from pig ocular globes were deposited. After bioprinting, both cell types were evaluated by immunostaining (Figure 10.5a). ARPE-19 cells showed high cell viability and good distribution throughout the GelMA layer. However, PRs maintained their phenotype after bioprinting. Finally, human vascular endothelial growth factor (hVEGF) release was observed from the scaffold, suggesting that the 3D bioprinted scaffold resembled the native retina [20].

A similar approach was performed by Wang P. et al. They manufactured a scaffold with two layers using a bioink composed of methacrylated HA by glycidyl-hydroxyl reaction and polyethylene glycol-Arg-Gly-Asp-Ser peptide (PEG-RGDS). The bioprinting process was carried out using a laser-assisted 3D bioprinter. The first layer was composed of RPE cells to simulate the RPE layer, while the upper layer was based on foetal retinal progenitor cells (fRPCs) that were differentiated into PRs (Figure 10.5b). As in the native retina, both layers differed in their thickness, with the upper layer thicker than the RPE layer. The results showed that the stiffness of the scaffold was similar to that of the native retina. Moreover, cell viability was high (above 70%) and fRPCs were successfully differentiated into PRs. Consequently,

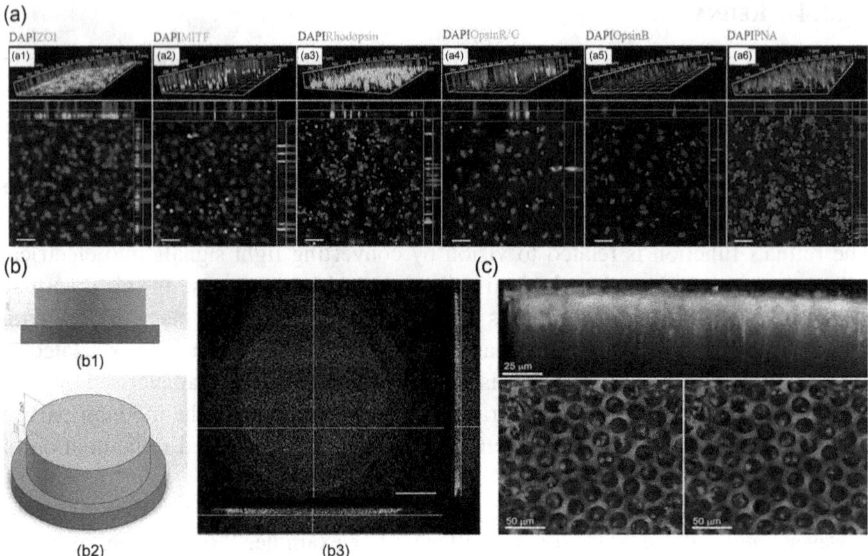

FIGURE 10.5 3D bioprinted retinal structures. (a) Confocal fluorescence microscopy images of bioprinted constructs immunolabelled with (a1) zonula occludens-1 (ZO1), (a2) melanocyte inducing transcription factor (MITF), (a3) rhodopsin, (a4) opsin R/G, (a5) opsin B and (a6) peanut agglutinin (PNA). Nuclei are counterstained with 4',6-diamidino-2-fenilindol (DAPI). The top images show a 3D view and the bottom images show an ortho view of the constructs. Scale bars: 50 µm. Reproduced with permission from Ref. [20]. (b) Bilayer bioprinted scaffold (b1) top view and (b2) side view of structural design from SOLIDWORKS®; (b3) confocal fluorescent images showing bilayer construct. Scale bar: 500 µm. Reproduced with permission from Ref. [27]. (c) Side view and top-down images of retinal progenitor cells (RPCs) differentiated from IPSCs nettled in scaffold pores. Scale bars: 25 µm and 50 µm. Reproduced with permission from Ref. [40].

they achieved a 3D bioprinted scaffold that simulates a niche similar to that of the retina in which PR maturation was promoted [27].

In another research work, Shi P. et al. used an alginate/pluronic bioink to fabricate a retinal structure through inkjet-based bioprinting. The bioprinted structure was composed of two layers: a monolayer based on ARPE-19 cells to simulate RPE and over it and a layer with Y79 cells. The results demonstrated that both cell types were highly viable after bioprinting and that they proliferated over time. Furthermore, scaffolds with different cell densities were achieved to obtain structures with similar characteristics to those of the native retina [38].

Cell orientation is a key factor to obtain a functional retinal structure. In fact, several studies have focused on aligning cells inside printed scaffolds to simulate the native retina. For example, Worthington et al. used a two-photon polymerisation 3D printing technique to manufacture scaffolds using an ink composed of indium tin oxide-coated glass. They optimised the hatching type and distance, as well as slicing distance, to achieve scaffolds with different pore sizes on which retinal progenitor cells differentiated from induced pluripotent stem cells (IPSCs) were seeded. The results showed that scaffolds with larger pore sizes were the best option to seed the cells since neural structures aligned in parallel to pores were observed [40]

(Figure 10.5c). Likewise, Kador et al. combined two promising manufacturing techniques such as electrospinning and thermal inkjet 3D bioprinting to create scaffolds with appropriate cell orientation. For manufacturing electrospinning fibres, PLA and Matrigel™ were used, and for thermal inkjet bioprinting, the bioink was composed of alginate and retinal ganglion cells (RGCs). The authors showed good cell viability after bioprinting by combining both techniques. Moreover, cells exhibited excellent electrophysiological properties after bioprinting. Importantly, they obtained a proper orientation of the cells inside scaffolds since a radial arrangement of the axons was observed [14]. Hence, these studies demonstrated a feasible approach to achieving scaffolds with a cell orientation similar to those of the native retina.

10.4 OCULAR PROSTHESIS BY 3D PRINTING

Aside from mimicking eye tissues with biological performance by 3D bioprinting, 3D additive manufacturing of ocular acellular structures, as prosthetics, is at the fingertips using 3D printing. The beneficiaries of such technology are overall patients presenting severe ocular damage, loss of eyeball or congenital malformations [6,7]. In these cases, enucleation, evisceration and facial disfigurement are associated with emotional and psychological traumas that improve with ocular prosthesis wearing [67], which also confers anatomical orbital support.

Until the emergence of 3D printing, eyeball prosthesis elaboration was a very time-consuming and laborious process. For many decades, it has consisted of an expensive artisanal procedure with few material options for eyeball elaboration (acrylics or PLEXIGLAS®, with potential allergic reactions and unrealistic aspect, respectively), hand painting of the iris and fine silk fibres gluing to emulate veins. Besides, previous to eye prosthesis, patients' eye socket had to be moulded by an invasive approach, such as alginate-based impression moulding. Fortunately, nowadays this has been substituted by non-invasive imaging techniques to 3D scan the eye socket with light scanners, computed tomography scanners or optical coherence tomography [68–71]. Afterwards, this digital computerised information is converted to a 3D design of the scanned eye anatomy and 3D printed in full colour [72]. Figure 10.6 shows a diagram summarising the steps to manufacture an ocular prosthesis, with an iris and sclera, by 3D printing.

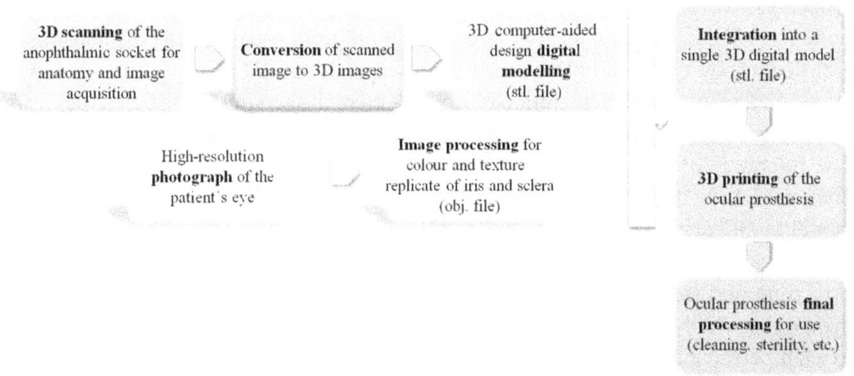

FIGURE 10.6 General workflow to design and 3D print an ocular prosthesis.

Among the materials used for ocular prosthetics, vulcanites and celluloids employed two centuries ago gave way to mixes of sand and iron oxide for glass eye fabrication. Since the middle of the twentieth century, the use of acrylic resins began to stand out to develop ocular prosthesis due to their attractive features such as adaptability, high resistance to fracture, translucence, lightweight and enabling colouring [73]. The types of resins more reported at the moment are the biocompatible polymethyl methacrylate [70,74] and Bio-Compatible PolyJet™ materials (Bio-Compatible MED610) [69,72]. In fact, this last material was used to 3D print the first ocular prosthesis in a case report by Ruiters et al. [69]. However, their implementation in clinical practice will require further research to enhance material lifespan and biocompatibility, since this type of resin allows one month of skin contact and short term (24 hours) of mucous membrane contact. In addition, along with biocompatible resins, photopolymers are employed to 3D print in different colours (mainly to resemble the iris) while maintaining strength, stiffness and translucency in the ocular prosthetics, as in the work developed by Groot A. L. W. et al. [72]. Nevertheless, also here research efforts must be made to enhance colour stability over time in the ocular prosthesis.

Thus, the rapid evolution of 3D technology to print ocular prosthesis might reach, in the near future, a more biocompatible and realistic appearance of the prosthesis along with time–cost reduction in the manufacturing process, which will increasingly provide many improvements to the ophthalmic area.

10.5 3D PRINTING AND BIOPRINTING FOR DRUG AND NEW THERAPY TESTING

Nowadays, the development of non-invasive medical devices to ensure people's health is gaining prominence. These advances, in the field of vision, are mainly based on the development of contact lenses (CLs) that can be used to treat diseases such as glaucoma, bacterial or allergic conjunctivitis, corneal infections or keratitis, and for the diagnosis or monitoring of various health conditions such as dry eye, intraocular pressure, diabetes and glucose levels, in which the development of smart contact lenses (SCLs) is involved [75–78].

Generally, CLs are obtained by spin casting, moulding and lathe machining processes, which present several problems when producing personalised and functionalised SCLs. For this reason, to control with great precision the dimensions and architecture by CAD and obtain reproducible products, 3D printing has been implemented. The most used techniques are selective laser sintering, fused deposition modelling, photocuring stereoscopic printing, stereolithography and DLP [79,80]. The tolerance of the eye to these lenses is important to the patient. In this regard, Phan et al. have developed an eye model provided with tear film simulation and blink model by 3D printing, to test them [81,82].

CLs can also be used for drug delivery in a non-invasive route, enhancing exposure time and treatment compliance. These lenses are usually 3D-printed gelatine hydrogels, which must fulfil appropriate characteristics such as optimal mechanics, oxygen permeability and transparency. To maintain transparency, in some cases the drug will only be integrated on the outside, leaving a hollow centre [58]. In fact, it was found that the inclusion of PEG diacrylate in CLs prolonged the release of dexamethasone to reduce inflammation and irritation from eye infections or after surgery [83]. Apart from CLs, a 3D-printed drug-loaded rod consisting of a polymeric shell and hydrogel core, loaded with bevacizumab and dexamethasone, respectively, has been developed by coaxial printing. This strategy enables to release both drugs with controlled kinetics inside the vitreous to face retinal vascular diseases. The versatility of this 3D printing technique allows for modulating the rod dimensions, drug loading and release profile of the loaded drugs [84].

3D printing may serve not only to produce the lenses or delivery devices but also to fabricate the moulds used to print those devices. Kojima H. et al. successfully developed a self-sustaining drug delivery device for continuous secretion of brain-derived neurotrophic factor (BDNF) for at least 16 days. This device, aimed at the treatment of retinal degenerative diseases, was made of a semi-porous capsule with two 3D printed photo-curable polymers that protected human ARPE-19 cells, allowing cellular survival, and the sustained release of the therapeutic BDNF from these cells [85].

Regarding SCLs, the incorporation of electronic sensors and their interconnections can be performed by 3D printing [86]. However, the 3D printed moulds can be used to create microchannels in polymeric hydrogels, which will host biosensors, to form these SCLs [87]. In this sense, 3D printed CLs can include sensors that may be able to obtain information from patients to diagnose or monitor diseases in a non-invasive way [58,79,88].

Finally, it must be taken into account that for the design and development of CLs, it is necessary to be clear about the objective to be addressed to select the appropriate materials. After material characterisation (mechanical aspects, biocompatibility, elasticity, transparency and flexibility) and 3D CAD template design, good printability must be demonstrated to proceed to 3D printing, as well as the incorporation of the embedded sensors or drugs. Finally, CL characterisation is needed to demonstrate suitable shape, curvature, flexibility, transparency, adaptation, biocompatibility or roughness. In addition, in the case of drug delivery, drug absorption and release tests are required [77,82].

10.6 FUTURE PROSPECTS, CHALLENGES AND CONCLUSIONS

Progress in additive manufacturing in the medical field has led to a revolution in regenerative medicine in the last decades. In particular, ophthalmology represents a clear beneficiary of such technology to face the current lack of efficient treatments related to the damage and/or loss of specific eye tissues, or even the whole eyeball. To date, the most efficient approach to recover the functionality of eye tissue is transplantation; however, the great imbalance between donors and patients demanding this replacement makes this solution untenable.

3D bioprinting arises as a promising tool with encouraging results in eye tissue replacement and regeneration with special emphasis on the conjunctiva, cornea and retina. In these scenarios, the optimisation of bioinks using different, and increasingly more specialised, materials and biomaterials at suitable proportions has greatly evolved to mimic the special eye tissues' physical and mechanical features. Although considerable efforts have been made by the scientific community, we are still at the beginning to achieve translation to clinical practice. At present, scaffolds with only two layers have been 3D bioprinted, presenting a particular cell orientation in some cases. The great complexity of some eye tissues, such as the retina, makes these advancements insufficient, and further research and investment of funds are needed to overcome this issue.

Future research lines to achieve the goal of bioprinting a full eye tissue will be very likely focused on the design and implementation of new natural, synthetic or hybrid biomaterials to enable easier printability while preserving cell viability in the scaffold. Along with the highly probable development of new 3D bioprinting techniques, it is feasible to achieve in the near future 3D bioprinted eye tissue scaffolds that reach clinical practice. However, this fact will require the regulatory approval of the Food and Drug Administration (FDA) agency, which at the moment has no classification for 3D bioprinted scaffolds nor for 3D additive manufacturing technology. Also, ethical concerns related to the use of these bioprinted eye grafts will need further consideration before their use in clinics can become a reality. Finally, efforts on cost-effectiveness and time efficiency will enable affordable 3D bioprinted and 3D printed products for patients.

Hence, it can be concluded that 3D bioprinting in the ophthalmologic field has the potential to make huge progress in the treatment of VI and in the design of realistic and durable eye prosthetics and drug delivery systems by 3D printing. In fact, it represents a versatile technology that can be further refined and improved to solve eye malignancies with no treatment to date.

ACKNOWLEDGEMENTS

This project was supported by the Basque Country Government (Consolidated Groups, IT1448-22) by the University of Basque Country UPV/EHU (pre-doctoral grant PIF17/79) and by the Spanish Ministry of Science and Innovation (Grant PID2019-106199RB-C21). This research was also supported by CIBER – Consorcio Centro de Investigación Biomédica en Red-CB06/01/1028, Instituto de Salud Carlos III, Ministerio de Ciencia e Innovación. The authors wish to thank the intellectual and technical assistance from the ICTS (Infraestructuras Científico-Tecnológicas Singulares, Spain) "NANBIOSIS," more specifically the Drug Formulation Unit (U10) of the CIBER in Bioengineering, Biomaterials and Nanomedicine (CIBER-BBN) at the University of the Basque Country (UPV/EHU).

REFERENCES

1. Pascolini D, Mariotti SP. Global estimates of visual impairment: 2010. *Br J Ophthalmol* 2012;96(5):614–618.
2. GBD 2019 Blindness and Vision Impairment Collaborators, Vision Loss Expert Group of the Global Burden of Disease Study. Trends in prevalence of blindness and distance and near vision impairment over 30 years: An analysis for the Global Burden of Disease Study. *Lancet Glob Health* 2021;9(2):e130–e143.
3. Marques AP, Ramke J, Cairns J, Butt T, Zhang JH, Jones I, et al. The economics of vision impairment and its leading causes: A systematic review. *EClinicalMedicine* 2022;46:101354.

4. Abdolalizadeh P, Ghasemi Falavarjani K. Correlation between global prevalence of vision impairment and depressive disorders. *Eur J Ophthalmol* 2022;32(6): 3227–3236. DOI: 10.1177/11206721221086152. Epub 2022 Mar 11. PMID: 35275499.
5. Ruiz-Alonso S, Villate-Beitia I, Gallego I, Lafuente-Merchan M, Puras G, Saenz-Del-Burgo L, et al. Current insights into 3D bioprinting: An advanced approach for eye tissue regeneration. *Pharmaceutics* 2021;13(3). DOI:10.3390/pharmaceutics13030308.
6. Tsui JKS, Bell S, Cruz LD, Dick AD, Sagoo MS. Applications of three-dimensional printing in ophthalmology. *Surv Ophthalmol* 2022; 67(4):1287–1310. DOI: 10.1016/j.survophthal.2022.01.004. Epub 2022 Jan 24. PMID: 35085588.
7. Sommer AC, Blumenthal EZ. Implementations of 3D printing in ophthalmology. *Graefes Arch Clin Exp Ophthalmol* 2019;257(9):1815–1822.
8. Fenton OS, Paolini M, Andresen JL, Müller FJ, Langer R. Outlooks on three-dimensional printing for ocular biomaterials research. *J Ocul Pharmacol Therapeut* 2020;36(1):7–17.
9. Rizzolo LJ, Nasonkin IO, Adelman RA. Retinal cell transplantation, biomaterials, and in vitro models for developing next-generation therapies of age-related macular degeneration. *Stem Cells Transl Med* 2022;11(3):269–281.
10. Lee KY, Mooney DJ. Alginate: Properties and biomedical applications. *Prog Polym Sci* 2012;37(1):106–126.
11. Shi P, Edgar TYS, Yeong WY, Laude A. Hybrid three-dimensional (3D) bioprinting of retina equivalent for ocular research. *Int J Bioprint* 2017;3(2):008.
12. Zhang B, Xue Q, Hu H, Yu M, Gao L, Luo Y, et al. Integrated 3D bioprinting-based geometry-control strategy for fabricating corneal substitutes. *J Zhejiang University B Sci* 2019;20(12):945–959.
13. Isaacson A, Swioklo S, Connon CJ. 3D bioprinting of a corneal stroma equivalent. *Exp Eye Res* 2018;173:188–193.
14. Kador KE, Grogan SP, Dorthé EW, Venugopalan P, Malek MF, Goldberg JL, et al. Control of retinal ganglion cell positioning and neurite growth: Combining 3D printing with radial electrospun scaffolds. *Tissue Eng Part A* 2016;22(3–4):286–294.
15. Wu Z, Su X, Xu Y, Kong B, Sun W, Mi S. Bioprinting three-dimensional cell-laden tissue constructs with controllable degradation. *Sci Rep* 2016;6(1):24474.
16. Kilic Bektas C, Hasirci V. Cell loaded 3D bioprinted GelMA hydrogels for corneal stroma engineering. *Biomater Sci* 2020;8(1):438–449.
17. Kim KW, Lee SJ, Park SH, Kim JC. Ex vivo functionality of 3D bioprinted corneal endothelium engineered with ribonuclease 5-overexpressing human corneal endothelial cells. *Adv Healthcare Mater* 2018;7(18):1800398.
18. Dehghani S, Rasoulianboroujeni M, Ghasemi H, Keshel SH, Nozarian Z, Hashemian MN, et al. 3D-Printed membrane as an alternative to amniotic membrane for ocular surface/conjunctival defect reconstruction: An in vitro & in vivo study. *Biomaterials* 2018;174:95–112.
19. Rajabi N, Rezaei A, Kharaziha M, Bakhsheshi-Rad HR, Luo H, RamaKrishna S, et al. Recent advances on bioprinted gelatin methacrylate-based hydrogels for tissue repair. *Tissue Eng Part A* 2021;27(11–12):679–702.
20. Masaeli E, Forster V, Picaud S, Karamali F, Nasr-Esfahani MH, Marquette C. Tissue engineering of retina through high resolution 3-dimensional inkjet bioprinting. *Biofabrication* 2020;12(2):025006. DOI: 10.1088/1758-5090/ab4a20. PMID: 31578006.
21. Zhong Z, Wang J, Tian J, Deng X, Balayan A, Sun Y, et al. Rapid 3D bioprinting of a multicellular model recapitulating pterygium microenvironment. *Biomaterials* 202;282:121391.
22. Kim H, Jang J, Park J, Lee K, Lee S, Lee D, et al. Shear-induced alignment of collagen fibrils using 3D cell printing for corneal stroma tissue engineering. *Biofabrication* 2019;11(3):035017.

23. Diamantides N, Wang L, Pruiksma T, Siemiatkoski J, Dugopolski C, Shortkroff S, et al. Correlating rheological properties and printability of collagen bioinks: The effects of riboflavin photocrosslinking and pH. *Biofabrication* 2017 Jul 5;9(3):034102. DOI: 10.1088/1758-5090/aa780f. PMID: 28677597.
24. Leonard DW, Meek KM. Refractive indices of the collagen fibrils and extrafibrillar material of the corneal stroma. *Biophys J* 1997;72(3):1382–1387.
25. Klotz BJ, Gawlitta D, Rosenberg AJWP, Malda J, Melchels FPW. Gelatin-methacryloyl hydrogels: Towards biofabrication-based tissue repair. *Trends Biotechnol* 2016;34(5):394–407.
26. Sorkio A, Koch L, Koivusalo L, Deiwick A, Miettinen S, Chichkov B, et al. Human stem cell based corneal tissue mimicking structures using laser-assisted 3D bioprinting and functional bioinks. *Biomaterials* 2018;171:57–71.
27. Wang P, Li X, Zhu W, Zhong Z, Moran A, Wang W, et al. 3D bioprinting of hydrogels for retina cell culturing. *Bioprinting* 2018;11:e00029. DOI: 10.1016/j.bprint.2018.e00029. Epub 2018 Sep 5. PMID: 31903439; PMCID: PMC6941869.
28. Noh I, Kim N, Tran HN, Lee J, Lee C. 3D printable hyaluronic acid-based hydrogel for its potential application as a bioink in tissue engineering. *Biomater Res* 2019 Feb 6;23:3. DOI: 10.1186/s40824-018-0152-8. PMID: 30774971; PMCID: PMC6364434.
29. Iyamu E, Iyamu J, Obiakor CI. The role of axial length-corneal radius of curvature ratio in refractive state categorization in a Nigerian population. *ISRN Ophthalmology* 2011;2011:138941.
30. Gibney R, Ferraris E. Bioprinting of collagen type I and II via aerosol jet printing for the replication of dense collagenous tissues. *Front Bioeng Biotechnol* 2021;9:786945.
31. Duarte Campos DF, Rohde M, Ross M, Anvari P, Blaeser A, Vogt M, et al. Corneal bioprinting utilizing collagen-based bioinks and primary human keratocytes. *J Biomed Mater Res A* 2019;107(9):1945–1953.
32. Widjaja LK, Bora M, Chan PN, Lipik V, Wong TT, Venkatraman SS. Hyaluronic acid-based nanocomposite hydrogels for ocular drug delivery applications. *J Biomed Mater Res A* 2014;102(9):3056–3065.
33. Bhusal A, Dogan E, Nguyen HA, Labutina O, Nieto D, Khademhosseini A, et al. Multi-material digital light processing bioprinting of hydrogel-based microfluidic chips. *Biofabrication* 2021;14(1). DOI:10.1088/1758-5090/ac2d78.
34. He B, Wang J, Xie M, Xu M, Zhang Y, Hao H, et al. 3D printed biomimetic epithelium/stroma bilayer hydrogel implant for corneal regeneration. *Bioact Mater* 2022;17:234–247.
35. Ulag S, Sahin EA, Yilmaz BK, Kalaskar DM, Ekren N, Kilic O, et al. 3D printed artificial cornea for corneal stromal transplantation. *Eur Polym J* 2020;133:109744.
36. de Abreu F.R., Campana-Filho S.P. Characteristics and properties of carboxymethylchitosan. *Carbohydr Polym* 2009;75(2):214–221.
37. Xu W, Liu K, Li T, Zhang W, Dong Y, Lv J, et al. An in situ hydrogel based on carboxymethyl chitosan and sodium alginate dialdehyde for corneal wound healing after alkali burn. *J Biomed Mater Res A* 2019;107(4):742–754.
38. Shi P, Tan YSE, Yeong WY, Li HY, Laude A. A bilayer photoreceptor-retinal tissue model with gradient cell density design: A study of microvalve-based bioprinting. *J Tissue Eng Regen Med* 2018;12(5):1297–1306.
39. Lorber B, Hsiao W, Martin KR. Three-dimensional printing of the retina. *Curr Opin Ophthalmol* 2016;27(3):262–267.
40. Worthington KS, Wiley LA, Kaalberg EE, Collins MM, Mullins RF, Stone EM, et al. Two-photon polymerization for production of human iPSC-derived retinal cell grafts. *Acta Biomater* 2017;55:385–395.
41. DelMonte DW, Kim T. Anatomy and physiology of the cornea. *J Cataract Refract Surg* 2011;37(3):588–598.

42. Prakash G, Agarwal A, Mazhari AI, Chari M, Kumar DA, Kumar G, et al. Reliability and reproducibility of assessment of corneal epithelial thickness by fourier domain optical coherence tomography. *Invest Ophthalmol Vis Sci* 2012;53(6):2580–2585.
43. Downie LE, Bandlitz S, Bergmanson JPG, Craig JP, Dutta D, Maldonado-Codina C, et al. CLEAR - Anatomy and physiology of the anterior eye. *Cont Lens Anterior Eye* 2021;44(2):132–156.
44. Thomasy SM, Raghunathan VK, Winkler M, Reilly CM, Sadeli AR, Russell P, et al. Elastic modulus and collagen organization of the rabbit cornea: Epithelium to endothelium. *Acta Biomater* 2014;10(2):785–791.
45. Boote C, Dennis S, Huang Y, Quantock AJ, Meek KM. Lamellar orientation in human cornea in relation to mechanical properties. *J Struct Biol* 2005;149(1):1–6.
46. Maurice DM. The transparency of the corneal stroma. *Vision Res* 1970;10(1):107–108.
47. Dua HS, Said DG. Clinical evidence of the pre-Descemets layer (Dua's layer) in corneal pathology. *Eye* (Lond) 2016;30(8):1144–1145.
48. Xeroudaki M, Thangavelu M, Lennikov A, Ratnayake A, Bisevac J, Petrovski G, et al. A porous collagen-based hydrogel and implantation method for corneal stromal regeneration and sustained local drug delivery. *Sci Rep* 2020 Oct 9;10(1):16936. DOI: 10.1038/s41598-020-73730-9. PMID: 33037282; PMCID: PMC7547117.
49. Scarcelli G, Besner S, Pineda R, Yun SH. Biomechanical characterization of keratoconus corneas ex vivo with Brillouin microscopy. *Invest Ophthalmol Vis Sci* 2014;55(7):4490–4495.
50. Meek KM, Tuft SJ, Huang Y, Gill PS, Hayes S, Newton RH, et al. Changes in collagen orientation and distribution in keratoconus corneas. *Invest Ophthalmol Vis Sci* 2005;46(6):1948–1956.
51. Santodomingo-Rubido J, Carracedo G, Suzaki A, Villa-Collar C, Vincent SJ, Wolffsohn JS. Keratoconus: An updated review. *Cont Lens Anterior Eye* 2022;45(3):101559.
52. Imbornoni LM, McGhee CNJ, Belin MW. Evolution of keratoconus: From diagnosis to therapeutics. *Klin Monbl Augenheilkd* 2018;235(6):680–688.
53. Kutlehria S, Dinh TC, Bagde A, Patel N, Gebeyehu A, Singh M. High-throughput 3D bioprinting of corneal stromal equivalents. *J Biomed Mater Res B Appl Biomater* 2020;108(7):2981–2994.
54. Diebold Y, Garcia-Posadas L. Is the conjunctiva a potential target for advanced therapy medicinal products? *Pharmaceutics* 2021;13(8). DOI:10.3390/pharmaceutics13081140.
55. Shahraki T, Arabi A, Feizi S. Pterygium: An update on pathophysiology, clinical features, and management. *Ther Adv Ophthalmol* 2021;13:25158414211020152. DOI: 10.1177/25158414211020152. PMID: 34104871; PMCID: PMC8170279.
56. Hejtmancik JF, Shiels A. Overview of the lens. *Prog Mol Biol Transl Sci* 2015;134:119–127.
57. Shiels A, Hejtmancik JF. Biology of inherited cataracts and opportunities for treatment. *Annu Rev Vis Sci* 2019;5:123–149.
58. Larochelle RD, Mann SE, Ifantides C. 3D printing in eye care. *Ophthalmol Ther* 2021;10(4):733–752.
59. Li JW, Li YJ, Hu XS, Gong Y, Xu BB, Xu HW, et al. Biosafety of a 3D-printed intraocular lens made of a poly(acrylamide-co-sodium acrylate) hydrogel in vitro and in vivo. *Int J Ophthalmol* 2020;13(10):1521–1530.
60. Grossniklaus HE, Geisert EE, Nickerson JM. Chapter twenty-two - Introduction to the retina. In: Hejtmancik JF, Nickerson JM, editors. *Progress in Molecular Biology and Translational Science*. Academic Press; 2015. pp. 383–396.
61. Holmes D. Reconstructing the retina. *Nature* 2018;561(7721):S2–S3.
62. Ao J, Wood JP, Chidlow G, Gillies MC, Casson RJ. Retinal pigment epithelium in the pathogenesis of age-related macular degeneration and photobiomodulation as a potential therapy? *Clin Exp Ophthalmol* 2018;46(6):670–686.

63. Gupta D, Chen PP. Glaucoma. *Am Fam Physician* 2016;93(8):668–674.
64. Tsang SH, Sharma T. Retinitis pigmentosa (non-syndromic). *Adv Exp Med Biol* 2018;1085:125–130.
65. Mitchell P, Liew G, Gopinath B, Wong TY. Age-related macular degeneration. *Lancet* 2018;392(10153):1147–1159.
66. Barber AC, Hippert C, Duran Y, West EL, Bainbridge JWB, Warre-Cornish K, et al. Repair of the degenerate retina by photoreceptor transplantation. *Proc Natl Acad Sci U S A* 2013;110(1):354–359.
67. Chin K, Margolin CB, Finger PT. Early ocular prosthesis insertion improves quality of life after enucleation. *Optometry* 2006;77(2):71–75.
68. Ko J, Kim SH, Baek SW, Chae MK, Yoon JS. Semi-automated fabrication of customized ocular prosthesis with three-dimensional printing and sublimation transfer printing technology. *Sci Rep* 2019 Feb 27;9(1):2968. DOI: 10.1038/s41598-019-38992-y. PMID: 30814585; PMCID: PMC6393501.
69. Ruiters S, Sun Y, de Jong S, Politis C, Mombaerts I. Computer-aided design and three-dimensional printing in the manufacturing of an ocular prosthesis. *Br J Ophthalmol* 2016;100(7):879–881.
70. Alam MS, Sugavaneswaran M, Arumaikkannu G, Mukherjee B. An innovative method of ocular prosthesis fabrication by bio-CAD and rapid 3-D printing technology: A pilot study. *Orbit* 2017;36(4):223–227.
71. Sagoo MS, Bell S, Carpenter D, Bott G, Hara N, Schmidt U, et al. Anterior segment optical coherence tomography for imaging the anophthalmic socket. *Eye* (Lond) 2020;34(8):1479–1481.
72. Groot ALW, Remmers JS, Hartong DT. Three-dimensional computer-aided design of a full-color ocular prosthesis with textured iris and sclera manufactured in one single print job. *3D Print Addit Manuf* 2021;8(6):343–348.
73. Dyer NA. The artificial eye. *Aust J Ophthalmol* 1980;8(4):325–327.
74. Rokaya D, Kritsana J, Amornvit P, Dhakal N, Khurshid Z, Zafar MS, et al. Magnification of iris through clear acrylic resin in ocular prosthesis. *J Funct Biomater* 2022;13(1). DOI:10.3390/jfb13010029.
75. Park J, Kim J, Kim SY, Cheong WH, Jang J, Park YG, et al. Soft, smart contact lenses with integrations of wireless circuits, glucose sensors, and displays. *Sci Adv* 2018;4(1):eaap9841.
76. Wang Y, Zhao Q, Du X. Structurally coloured contact lens sensor for point-of-care ophthalmic health monitoring. *J Mater Chem B* 2020;8(16):3519–3526.
77. Zhu Y, Li S, Li J, Falcone N, Cui Q, Shah S, et al. Lab-on-a-contact lens: Recent advances and future opportunities in diagnostics and therapeutics. *Adv Mater* 2022 Jun;34(24):e2108389. DOI: 10.1002/adma.202108389. Epub 2022 Apr 11. PMID: 35130584; PMCID: PMC9233032.
78. Mirzajani H, Mirlou F, Istif E, Singh R, Beker L. Powering smart contact lenses for continuous health monitoring: Recent advancements and future challenges. *Biosens Bioelectron* 2022;197:113761.
79. Alam F, Elsherif M, AlQattan B, Salih A, Lee SM, Yetisen AK, et al. 3D printed contact lenses. *ACS Biomater Sci Eng* 2021;7(2):794–803.
80. Alam F, Elsherif M, AlQattan B, Ali M, Ahmed IMG, Salih A, et al. Prospects for additive manufacturing in contact lens devices. *Adv Eng Mater* 2021;23:2000941.
81. Phan CM, Walther H, Gao H, Rossy J, Subbaraman LN, Jones L. Development of an in vitro ocular platform to test contact lenses. *J Vis Exp* 2016 Apr 6;(110):e53907. DOI: 10.3791/53907. PMID: 27078088; PMCID: PMC4841367.
82. Phan CM, Shukla M, Walther H, Heynen M, Suh D, Jones L. Development of an in vitro blink model for ophthalmic drug delivery. *Pharmaceutics* 2021;13(3). DOI:10.3390/pharmaceutics13030300.

83. Zidan G, Greene CA, Etxabide A, Rupenthal ID, Seyfoddin A. Gelatine-based drug-eluting bandage contact lenses: Effect of PEGDA concentration and manufacturing technique. *Int J Pharm* 2021;599:120452.
84. Won JY, Kim J, Gao G, Kim J, Jang J, Park YH, et al. 3D printing of drug-loaded multi-shell rods for local delivery of bevacizumab and dexamethasone: A synergetic therapy for retinal vascular diseases. *Acta Biomater* 2020;116:174–185.
85. Kojima H, Raut B, Chen LJ, Nagai N, Abe T, Kaji H. A 3D printed self-sustainable cell-encapsulation drug delivery device for periocular transplant-based treatment of retinal degenerative diseases. *Micromachines* (Basel) 2020;11(4). DOI:10.3390/mi11040436.
86. Kim H, Kim J, Kang J, Song YW. Three-dimensionally printed interconnects for smart contact lenses. *ACS Appl Mater Interfaces* 2018;10(33):28086–28092.
87. Chen Y, Zhang S, Cui Q, Ni J, Wang X, Cheng X, et al. Microengineered poly(HEMA) hydrogels for wearable contact lens biosensing. *Lab Chip* 2020;20(22):4205–4214.
88. Yuan M, Das R, Ghannam, R, Wang Y, Reboud J, Fromme R, et al. Electronic contact lens: A platform for wireless health monitoring applications. *Adv Intell Syst* 2020;2:1900190.

11 Bioreactors for Tendon Constructs

Janne Spierings and J. Foolen
Eindhoven University of Technology

CONTENTS

DOI: 10.1201/9781003274568-11

11.1 INTRODUCTION: TENDON ANATOMY, PATHOLOGY, AND CLINICAL IMPORTANCE OF DEVELOPING TENDON CONSTRUCTS

Worldwide, over four million incidences of tendon injuries are reported annually, accounting for almost 30% of all musculoskeletal injuries [1]. These injuries can result in joint instability, pain, reduced function and disability, early onset of osteoarthritis, and eventually, joint replacement [2]. With the current aging society and the engagement of an increasing amount of people, also elderly, in (extreme) sports, tendon disorders occur more often and are considered a major societal, clinical, and financial burden [1,3].

Tendons (Figure 11.1) are fibrous connective tissues that link muscles to bones [4]. They transmit forces, store energy, and help to maintain posture and enable joint movement [4]. The most abundant cell type in tendons is the tenocyte, a spindle-shaped specialized fibroblast interspersed between the collagen fibrils and primarily aligned along the long axis of the tendon [4]. They produce the extracellular matrix (ECM) components and regulate homeostasis of tendon tissue [4]. The most abundant protein, collagen type I, has a remarkable hierarchy at multiple length scales (Figure 11.1) and is responsible for the tensile strength of tendons. Collagen type III contributes to the elasticity of tendons by forming thin and loosely organized fibrils [5]. Together with elastin and proteoglycans, collagen gives tendons their characteristic mechanical behavior [4]. This mechanical behavior is often reflected by a stress–strain relation consisting of four regions: a toe region, a linear region, microdamage, and macrodamage. The toe region represents the uncrimping of the collagen fibers. In the linear region, the fibers lose their crimp pattern and align with the direction of the load. Subsequently, beyond the linear region, the first microtears can occur, resulting in microdamage of the tendon tissue. When the strain further increases, more and more fibers will break, leading to macroscopic failure of the tendon [6].

In pathological tendons, the cells are more stellate-shaped, and the collagen matrix is disorganized and contains higher levels of collagen type III [7]. Since the healing

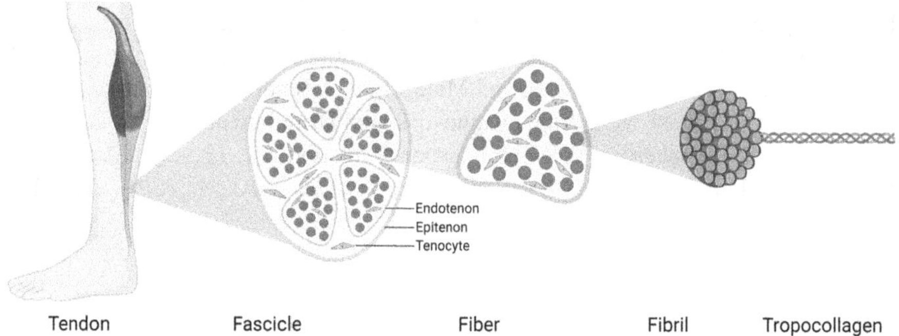

FIGURE 11.1 Schematic overview of the hierarchical organization of tendons. Tendons consist of bundles that contain fascicles, which in turn consist of fibers, containing fibrils, and finally collagen molecules. The cells, tenocytes, are interspersed between the fibrils. Created with BioRender.com.

capacity of tendons is both poor and slow, ruptured tendons are often replaced with an autograft, an allograft, or a xenograft [1,8]. Unfortunately, there is a high chance of graft rupture. Additionally, autografts result in donor site morbidity, and allografts and xenografts are often low in availability and are at risk for immune rejection and disease transmission [1]. These drawbacks led to an increased popularity in the development of tissue-engineered tendon grafts [1].

In short, tissue engineering can be described as the development of materials to create scaffolds that, in combination with cells and bioactive molecules, can restore or replace damaged biological tissues [4]. To properly restore or replace tendons, tissue-engineered grafts should have properties similar to native tissue. With the emerging field of tissue engineering, bioreactors became useful tools. Bioreactors are devices in which biological and/or biochemical processes can be recreated in a highly controlled *in vitro* culture environment [9,10]. They can be used to study both physiology and pathophysiology and create understanding of mechanical and biological factors that regulate tendon formation, homeostasis, or degeneration [8,11]. Over the past decades, they evolved from a tool to study these mechanisms fundamentally, to a device that can be used to create novel tissue-engineered constructs for clinical applications or as an *in vitro* model to predict *in vivo* outcomes of engineered constructs [8,10,11].

A large variety of (tendon) bioreactors have been developed for different purposes. In this chapter, we will focus on and discuss those that provide the possibility for applying mechanical loading to tendon constructs. In doing so, we will define ways in which tendon bioreactors are used and can be used. Often, a more detailed description of scientific output from published work is included. These more in-depth descriptions are meant to provide the reader with an understanding of the possibilities, limitations, and future challenges in tendon research, when exploiting bioreactor systems. They are based on a random selection of articles, and by no means have we attempted to give a complete overview of the existing literature (Table 11.1).

11.2 THE PREREQUISITE OF APPLYING MECHANICAL LOAD TO TENDONS AND TENDON CONSTRUCTS

11.2.1 Dynamic versus Static Mechanical Culturing of Tendons and Tendon Constructs

Tendons experience dynamic mechanical load *in vivo*, which is essential to maintain their native tissue structure and composition, and to prevent excessive tissue degradation [8,12,13]. Tenocytes sense and respond to mechanical stimuli by translating them into biological responses. This can result in ECM remodeling to alter the structure, composition, and mechanical properties to adapt to the new loading environment [13]. When static loading conditions are applied to tendon constructs, by fixing both tissue ends in space and time, an inhomogeneous cell distribution has been observed to develop, with the majority of cells being present and growing at the periphery of the tendon construct [14–18]. Nutrient transport toward the center of the construct is also compromised, resulting in ECM deposition mostly at the periphery of the construct [14,15,19]. Moreover, static

TABLE 11.1
Overview of the Studies Using Tendon Bioreactors That Are Highlighted in This Chapter

Reference	Scaffold Material	Cell Type	Type of Bioreactor	Loading Regime	Biological Effects
[21]	Rabbit Achilles tendon	Rabbit tenocytes	'3D' custom-made bioreactor	Uniaxial cyclic strain of 3%, 6%, or 9% at 0.25 Hz for 8 hours a day for 6 days	Tendons subjected to 6% strain were able to maintain their native structural integrity and cellular function
[22]	Murine tendon fascicle	Murine tenocytes	'3D' custom-made bioreactor	Uniaxial cyclic strain of 1% at 1 Hz for 8 hours a day for 6 days	Tendon fascicles were able to maintain their native cell phenotype and morphology, and elastic modulus
[39]	Collagen type I-coated silicone membrane	Human MSCs	STREX loading device	Uniaxial cyclic strain of 4%, 8%, or 12% at 1 Hz for 6, 24, 48, or 72 hours	Cells subjected to 8% strain for 72 hours differentiated toward spindle-shaped cells with TNC, SCX, and TNMD gene expression levels similar to native tenocytes
[34]	Collagen type I	Human ASCs	'3D' custom-made bioreactor	Uniaxial cyclic strain of 2%, 4%, or 6% at 0.1 or 1 Hz for 2 hours a day for 7 days	Cells subjected to 2% strain at 0.1 Hz showed an elongated morphology and increased COL I, COL III, DCN, ACAN, TNC, SCX, and TNMD gene expression
[30,37]	Decellularized equine tendon	Equine BMSCs and ASCs	'3D' custom-made bioreactor	Uniaxial cyclic strain of 3% at 0.33 Hz for 1 hour a day for 10 days	Both cell types showed an elongated and tenocytic morphology, expressed tendon marker genes, and showed an increased elastic modulus
[44]	PEG-fibrinogen	Murine fibroblasts	'3D' custom-made bioreactor	Uniaxial cyclic strain of 10% at 0.5 Hz for 8 hours a day for 15 days	Cells deposited collagen fibers along the stretching direction and the elastic modulus of the scaffold increased
[45]	PCL fibers	Human MSCs	'3D' custom-made bioreactor	Uniaxial cyclic strain of 3% for 4 hours a day for 21 days	Cyclic strain resulted in more collagen and ECM production and an increased elastic modulus

(*Continued*)

TABLE 11.1 (*Continued*)
Overview of the Studies Using Tendon Bioreactors That Are Highlighted in This Chapter

Reference	Scaffold Material	Cell Type	Type of Bioreactor	Loading Regime	Biological Effects
[42]	Decellularized porcine tendon	N/A	'3D' custom-made bioreactor	Cyclic strain of 10% with 90° torsion at 1 Hz for 12 hours a day for 7 days	Tendons subjected to load improved ultimate tensile strength beyond that of native tendons
[26]	Fibronectin-coated silicone membrane	Rabbit tenocytes, fibroblasts, BMSCs, and ASCs	Flexcell® Uniflex®	Uniaxial cyclic strain of 4% or 8% at 0.1 or 1 Hz for 8 hours a day for 7 days	Cells subjected to 4% strain at 0.1 Hz showed increased cell proliferation and collagen type I production
[67]	Gelatin-coated silicone membrane	Rat BMSCs	'2D' custom-made bioreactor	Uniaxial cyclic strain of 10% at 1 Hz for 12 or 24 hours	After 24 hours, cells were elongated with upregulated COL I, COL III, and TNC gene expression
[73,75]	Silicone membrane with microgrooves	Rabbit TSCs	'2.5D' custom-made bioreactor	Uniaxial cyclic strain of 4% or 8% at 0.5 Hz for 12 hours	Cells subjected to 4% strain elongated, proliferated, and aligned along the microgrooves in the axis of stretching. Cells subjected to 8% strain differentiated into non-tenogenic lineages
[76]	Collagen type I	Avian tendon cells	Flexcell® TissueTrain®	Uniaxial cyclic strain of 1% at 1 Hz for 1 hour a day for 2 weeks	The elastic modulus improved but was still far from native tendon tissue
[40]	Collagen type I	Human BMSCs	Flexcell® TissueTrain®	Uniaxial cyclic strain of 1% at 1 Hz for 30 minutes a day for 7 days	Cells subjected to 1% strain maintained their SCX expression over time
[78,79]	Canine flexor tendon	Canine tenocytes	'3D' custom-made bioreactor	Uniaxial cyclic strain of ~1.5% at 0.017 Hz for 12 hours a day for 4 weeks	Tendons subjected to mechanical loading were able to maintain their native structure and mechanical properties

(*Continued*)

TABLE 11.1 (*Continued*)
Overview of the Studies Using Tendon Bioreactors That Are Highlighted in This Chapter

Reference	Scaffold Material	Cell Type	Type of Bioreactor	Loading Regime	Biological Effects
[77]	Collagen type I	Human tenocytes	Flexcell® TissueTrain®	Uniaxial cyclic strain of 5% at 1 Hz for 2 days with or without TGFβ addition	Cells stimulated with either strain or TGFβ showed similar gene expression profiles. TGFβ-inhibition abrogated the strain-induced changes
[120]	Rat flexor tendon	Rat tenocytes	'3D' custom-made bioreactor	Overloading using 8% strain for 72 hours with or without VEGF receptor inhibitor	Overloading resulted in nuclear rounding and collagen degradation. When VEGF receptor 3 was inhibited, nuclear morphology and collagen degradation were similar to native tendons
[106]	Rabbit Achilles tendon	Rabbit TSCs	'3D' custom-made bioreactor	Underloading using 3% strain at 0.25 Hz for 8 hours a day for 20 days	Multiple ossification sites were found, and the maximum load and stiffness decreased
[123]	Hyaluronate fibers	Human BMSCs	'3D' custom-made bioreactor	Uniaxial cyclic strain of 10% at 1 Hz for 3 days with or without hGDF-5 addition	Cells subjected to both strain and hGDF-5 showed increased tenogenic gene expression (COL1A1, COL1A3, DCN, SCX, and TNC)
[124]	PCL fibers	Human BMSCs	'3D' custom-made bioreactor	Uniaxial cyclic strain of 10% at 1 Hz for 4 hours a day for 7 days with or without BMP-12 addition	Cells subjected to 10% strain showed increased TNMD, DCN, and TNC gene expression. Cyclic mechanical loading and BMP-12 treatment synergistically increased cell viability, proliferation, and alignment
[85]	PLLA fibers	Human BMSCs	ElectroForce 5200 BioDynamic	Uniaxial cyclic strain of 10% at 1 Hz for 2 hours a day for 10 days in osteogenic differentiation medium	Cells subjected to mechanical loading showed upregulation of tendon-specific genes rather than bone-specific markers
[32]	Decellularized human umbilical vein	Rat BMSCs	'3D' custom-made bioreactor	Uniaxial cyclic strain of 2% at 0.017, 0.033, or 0.083 Hz for 0.5, 1, or 2 hours a day for 7 days	Cells subjected to slower frequencies and load durations showed more cellular proliferation and tenogenesis

(*Continued*)

TABLE 11.1 (*Continued*)
Overview of the Studies Using Tendon Bioreactors That Are Highlighted in This Chapter

Reference	Scaffold Material	Cell Type	Type of Bioreactor	Loading Regime	Biological Effects
[35]	Collagen type I	Murine MSCs	Flexcell® TissueTrain®	Uniaxial cyclic strain of 2.5%, 5%, 7.5%, or 10% at 0.1 Hz for 2 hours a day for 2 weeks	Cells subjected to maximal cyclic strain and duration showed the biggest increase in tenocytic gene expression and an elastic modulus similar to native tendon
[84]	Decellularized rabbit flexor tendon	Rabbit tenocytes	Ligagen L30-4C	Uniaxial cyclic strain of 1.25 N at 0.017 Hz for 2 hours a day for 5 days	Constructs subjected to mechanical loading showed improved mechanical properties and better cellularity of the tendon, which was beneficial for *in vivo* implantation
[96,109]	Collagen type 1	Rabbit BMSCs	'3D' custom-made bioreactor	Uniaxial cyclic strain of 2.4% at 0.2 Hz for 8 hours a day for 2 weeks	Constructs subjected to mechanical loading showed increased mechanical properties both *in vitro* and *in vivo*
[112]	Decellularized equine flexor tendon	Equine ASCs	'3D' custom-made bioreactor	Uniaxial cyclic strain of 2% at 1 Hz for 45 minutes a day for 3 days in an inflammatory environment	Cells dynamically cultured in the inflammatory environment showed increased cell dead and lower cell integration
[33]	PDMS	Rat tendon-derived cells	'2D' custom-made bioreactor	Overloading using 8% strain at 0.5 Hz for 8 hours with or without the addition of EGCG or piracetam	Cells subjected to overloading showed increased gene expression of non-tenocyte lineages. With the addition of EGCG or piracetam, this increase was reduced
[133]	Collagen type I	Human tenocytes	Flexcell® TissueTrain®	Uniaxial cyclic strain of 1% at 1 Hz for 1 hour a day for 7 days with or without nandrolone decanoate addition	Mechanical load and nandrolone decanoate synergistically increased ultimate tensile stress and strain

culture results in matrix disruption [20–22]. Together, they reveal the inability to engineer or maintain tendon constructs with native-like structural, compositional, and mechanical properties [14]. When aiming to develop tendon constructs that mimic native-like properties or maintain tendon constructs at homeostasis, dynamic mechanical loading is vital.

11.2.2 Effects of Dynamic Mechanical Loading on Tendons and Tendon Constructs

The effect of different cyclic tensile strains on tendons or tendon constructs has been examined by multiple researchers, as a delicate balance exists where too much and too little mechanical load can result in an adverse response [18,21,23–35]. In 2013, Wang and coworkers investigated the impact of different mechanical stimulation regimes on rabbit Achilles' tendons [21]. They found that a low-magnitude strain of 3% for 6 days did not prevent matrix deterioration and that a high-magnitude strain of 9% resulted in major matrix rupture, while a cyclic tensile strain of 6% maintained cellular function and structural integrity of the tissue [21]. With these results in mind, they proposed a model describing the effect of mechanical loading on tendon homeostasis. The model (Figure 11.2) proposes that with increasing strain, individual collagen fibers rupture with eventual complete rupture at the failure point. However, with this increasing strain, the tissue also responds by producing matrix to compensate for the increased load. In this model, an optimal strain range is defined that promotes

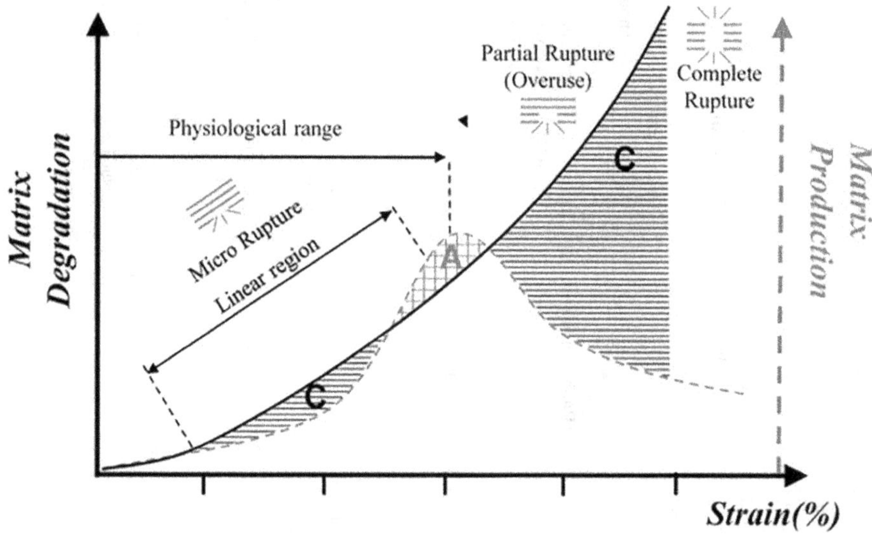

FIGURE 11.2 Proposed model showing matrix degradation (solid line) and matrix production (dashed line) affected by mechanical loading (*x*-axis). A is the anabolic zone in which the biological repair response as a result of strain exceeds the matrix damage caused by the same strain. C is the catabolic zone in which there is either too little load to stimulate matrix production or too much mechanical damage because of excessive tensile loading that cannot be compensated for by additional matrix production. Source: Wang (2017), with permission.

matrix production to result in net tissue repair. In this anabolic zone, the biological repair response as a result of strain exceeds the matrix damage caused by the same strain, and the tendon can maintain its structural integrity. Contrary, in the catabolic zones, there is either too little load to stimulate matrix production or too much mechanical damage because of excessive tensile loading that cannot be compensated for by additional matrix production [21].

Next to that, Wang et al. cultured rabbit Achilles' tendons in an *ex vivo* loading deprivation culture system for 6 days and revealed that tenocytes started to lose their elongated morphology with increased incidences of apoptosis [20]. After 12 days of load deprivation, the collagen fibers became disoriented, the ECM was disrupted, and the collagen fiber architecture lost its strong anisotropy. Load deprivation also resulted in a decreased maximum tensile load and stiffness of the tissue. However, when a 6-day cyclic mechanical loading of 6% strain was applied to the tendons, after being load deprived for 6 days, the initial degenerative changes of the tendons recovered. The spindle-shaped morphology of tenocytes was restored, the apoptotic rate was reduced, and the collagen fiber architecture and mechanical properties were regained [20]. Similarly, Wunderli and colleagues cultured murine tail tendon fascicles *ex vivo* with and without applied mechanical load [22]. They showed that minimal *ex vivo* loading of 1% at 1 Hz for 8 hours a day could maintain native cell phenotype and morphology for up to 6 days, while complete load deprivation resulted in a disarranged actin cytoskeleton and nuclear rounding. Moreover, load deprivation downregulated tendon marker genes, such as tenomodulin (TNMD), and upregulated matrix remodeling markers, such as matrix metalloproteinase (MMP)-3 and MMP-9 [22]. Together, these results show that mechanical loading is essential for tendon homeostasis *ex vivo*, but that a delicate balance exists where the absence of mechanical stimulation results in disadvantageous tissue degradation and excessive loading also has detrimental effects.

Not only do *ex vivo* cultures benefit from the addition of mechanical loading, but also studies aiming to create novel tendon constructs can benefit from applying mechanical load [36]. Mesenchymal stem cells (MSCs), especially bone marrow-derived stem cells (BMSCs) and adipose-derived stem cells (ASCs), are often used to create tissue-engineered tendon grafts [34,37]. These cells have a high proliferative capacity and are able to undergo xenogenesis [34,37], among others when provided with the adequate type of mechanical stimulation [38]. Mechanical loading increases tenogenic differentiation of both human BMSCs [39,40] and human ASCs [34,41]. For example, Nam et al. showed that human BMSCs stimulated with 8% uniaxial cyclic strain at 1 Hz for 72 hours, in a collagen type I-coated silicon chamber, resulted in spindle-shaped cells with tenogenic marker tenascin C (TNC), scleraxis (SCX), and TNMD, gene expression levels close to native tenocyte levels [39]. Similarly, Subramanian et al. found that when they mechanically stimulated human ASCs, embedded in 3D collagen scaffolds, with physiological loading (2% stretch at 0.1 Hz for 2 hours a day for 7 days), the cells elongated and displayed increased gene expression levels of collagen type I (COL I), collagen type III (COL III), decorin (DCN), aggrecan (ACAN), TNC, SCX, and TNMD compared to unloaded constructs [34]. Hereby, there was no upregulation found in osteogenic, chondrogenic, and myogenic gene expression levels [34]. Moreover, the collagen matrix consisted of collagen fibers that ran parallel to the direction of the applied load [34]. In 2016, Young Strom and colleagues investigated tenogenesis of both BMSCs and ASCs. They seeded decellularized tendon constructs with either equine BMSCs or ASCs and mechanically stimulated the constructs (3% strain at 0.33 Hz for 1 hour a day for 10 days). They found that both cell types infiltrated the decellularized tendon construct, showed an elongated and tenocytic morphology, and expressed tendon marker genes [37]. Next to that, for both cell types, mechanical loading was found to increase the failure stress of the constructs, relative to native tendons [37].

In fact, mechanical stimulation is often used to increase the mechanical properties of a tendon construct [36,42,43]. For example, Testa et al. mechanically loaded polyethylene glycol (PEG) fibrinogen scaffolds, seeded with mouse fibroblasts in a bioreactor (for 15 days under 10% strain at 0.5 Hz for 8 hours a day) [44]. They showed an increase in elastic modulus compared to unloaded constructs. The elastic modulus further increased after a combination of mechanical loading and biochemical stimulation with transforming growth factor beta (TGFβ) and ascorbic acid [44]. Banik et al. also found an increased elastic modulus when they mechanically loaded electrospun poly-(ε-caprolactone) (PCL) scaffolds, seeded with human MSCs (3% strain for 4 hours a day for 21 days), compared to statically loaded constructs [45]. When the laboratory of James Chang decellularized rabbit flexor tendons, the ultimate tensile strength and elastic modulus decreased due to the decellularization [46]. Though, when they reseeded the decellularized tendons with either rabbit tenocytes, ASCs, or fibroblasts and mechanically conditioned the constructs (intermittent loading at 1.25 N at 1 Hz; 1-hour load and 1-hour rest, for 5 days), the ultimate tensile strength and elastic modulus increased toward native levels [46,47]. On that note, Youngstrom and coworkers mechanically stimulated equine decellularized tendons, seeded with either equine BMSCs or ASCs (3% strain for 1 hour a day for 10 days), and found that the failure stress and elastic modulus were similar to those of a native tendon [30,37]. Also, Lee et al. improved the ultimate tensile strength of decellularized porcine tendons beyond that of native tendons after a 7-day bioreactor culture (10% strain, with axial rotation; 45° clockwise and 90° counterclockwise for 12 hours each day) [42].

Combining all these results, applying mechanical load to constructs during culture can be considered beneficial in producing a tissue-engineered tendon graft with mechanical properties that mimic native tendon tissue. Therefore, bioreactors are of great importance in the tissue engineering and regenerative medicine field, as they create a dynamic mechanical culture environment.

11.3 TENDON BIOREACTORS

In the 1980s, bioreactors were initially developed and used to produce cell-derived drugs and therapeutics or to obtain large cell populations [38]. Nowadays, they are being used for many more applications; for an overview, we refer to Selden and Fuller [48] and Drapal et al. [49]. In the tendon field, bioreactors are designed to perform at least one of the following functions: (i) control culture conditions, such

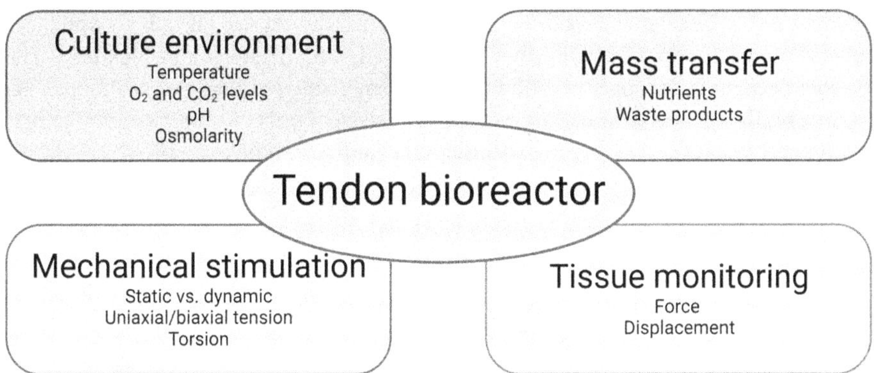

FIGURE 11.3 Schematic overview of tendon bioreactors and their main functions. Created with BioRender.com.

as temperature, pH, osmolarity, oxygen concentration, and nutrient and metabolite levels; (ii) assist in the mass transfer of nutrients and waste products; (iii) provide a physiologically relevant environment, for example, mechanical loading; and/or (iv) provide information about the condition of the tissue [38,50]. A schematic overview can be found in Figure 11.3.

11.3.1 Different Types of Tendon Bioreactors

Bioreactors with the capacity to apply dynamic loading are either based on dynamic flow or mechanical load [14]. Within the dynamic flow-based bioreactors, there are three different types: spinner flask bioreactors; rotating wall vessel bioreactors; and flow perfusion bioreactors [14]. Spinner flask bioreactors are based on the principle of impeller mixing of the culture media, mostly created by a magnetic stirrer. This maintains cells in suspension and facilitates mass transport of nutrients and waste products [14,51]. Rotating wall vessel bioreactors, for example, the one developed by NASA [52], allow cells to grow into three-dimensional (3D) cell aggregates in a constant free fall and low shear environment, created by a rotating culture chamber [14,53]. Lastly, flow perfusion bioreactors percolate culture media through constructs to enable the mass transport of nutrients and waste products using a pump system [14]. However, to better mimic the dynamic mechanical load, experienced by tendons *in vivo* [54], bioreactors that apply mechanical load are more suitable to use for tendon-related purposes and will be the main focus of the remainder of this chapter.

In these bioreactors, a specific mechanical loading protocol is applied to the construct. This loading protocol consists of several characteristics, which are the amplitude of the load, the frequency of the load, the loading duration, the shape of the loading cycle, and the total culture time. The amplitude is the magnitude of the applied load. Most of the time, this is displayed as a strain percentage or applied force in Newtons. The frequency (of which the unit is often in Hertz) indicates how many load cycles are performed every second. The loading duration represents the time frame in which the loading is applied, either the number of cycles or the number of hours a day. Mechanical loading is often alternated with rest periods in which the constructs are not experiencing mechanical load, called intermittent loading. The loading cycle can be applied following a (co)sine, square, triangle, sawtooth, etc. waveform. Lastly, the total culture time is the time a construct is cultured in the bioreactor and thus experiencing the specified mechanical loading regime.

11.3.2 2D and 2.5D Tendon Bioreactors with Mechanical Stimulation

The first bioreactors that could apply mechanical load were designed to apply in-plane, two-dimensional (2D), load to cultured cells. These '2D' bioreactors can be used to study cellular responses to mechanical loading [8]. These bioreactors deform the flexible substrate that contains an attached monolayer of cells [55] (Figure 11.4a). Back in 1985, Banes et al. developed an instrument that applied cyclic or static strain to cells *in vitro*, based on a vacuum that deforms the flexible wells of a Petri dish [56]. A few years later, Banes founded the Flexcell® International Corporation and their bioreactors have been used in numerous studies since [26,57–62]. For example, Riboh et al. aimed to find a favorable mechanical loading protocol for cell proliferation and collagen production [26]. They plated cells (rabbit tenocytes, fibroblasts, BMSCs, or ASCs) on fibronectin-coated silicone UniFlex culture membranes, placed them in a Flexcell® system (Flexcell® International Corporation, Burlington, NC), and showed that intermittent cyclic strain of 4% at 0.1 Hz increased cell proliferation and collagen type I production. Moreover, they showed that cell morphology is regulated by this mechanical strain [26]. Many other (custom-made) '2D' bioreactors

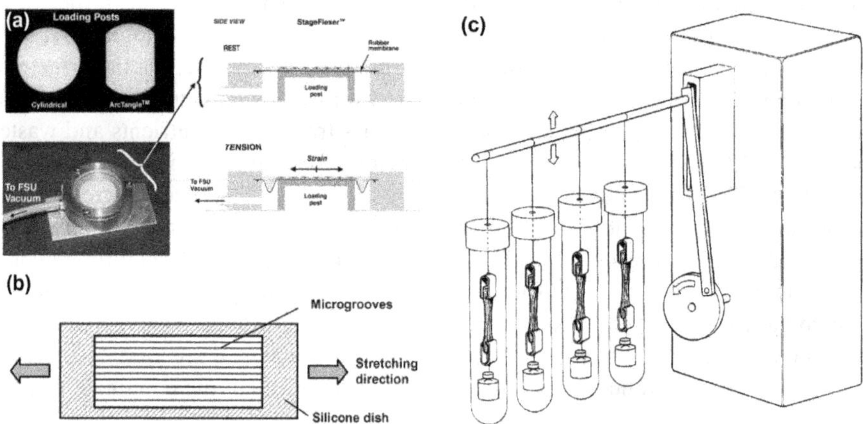

FIGURE 11.4 Examples of '2D', '2.5D', and '3D' tendon bioreactors. (a) '2D' tendon bioreactor. Strain is applied via a vacuum, when the vacuum is applied, the membrane is deformed, and the cells will experience strain. Modified from: Wall 2007, with permission. (b) '2.5D' tendon bioreactor. Using a vacuum, microgrooved substrates plated with cells are strained. Modified from: Wang 2005, with permission. (c) First '3D' tendon bioreactor with mechanical stimulation. To cyclically load the tendon, a weight was attached to the distal clamp and the other end of the tendon was raised and lowered using the arm of a rotating cam. Modified from Hannafin (1994), with permission.

have since been developed [39,63–66]. Zhang and coworkers used a custom-made device to apply uniaxial cyclic strain to rat BMSCs seeded on gelatin-coated elastic silicone membranes [67]. Stimulation with 10% strain at 1 Hz for 24 hours resulted in elongated cells with a significant upregulation of tendon-specific genes, such as COL I, COL III, and TNC, compared to the non-stimulated BMSCs, indicating tendon-like behavior of these BMSCs under mechanical loading [67].

These ‘2D’ bioreactors, however, reveal cellular responses to mechanical loading through cytoskeletal deformation and not through 3D cell–matrix interactions [55]. Therefore, as a next step, researchers started plating cells on patterned surfaces, for example, aligned surfaces, or onto fibrous scaffolds to study the effects of surface geometry and scaffold surface organization in combination with mechanical loading on cell behavior [8] (Figure 11.4b). This ‘2.5D’ environment is used in several studies [68–75], for example, by Zhang et al., who studied the effects of mechanical loading on rabbit tendon stem cells (TSCs) seeded on silicone surfaces fabricated with microgrooves [75]. Their results showed that the TSCs elongated, proliferated, aligned along the microgrooves, and differentiated toward tenocytes in response to 4% mechanical cyclic stretch, while on non-stretched surfaces fewer TSCs were elongated and the total cell number was lower [75]. However, high-magnitude stretching of 8% induced TSC differentiation into adipogenic, chondrogenic, and osteogenic lineages [73,75]. This demonstrates that there is an optimal loading regime for tenogenic differentiation of stem cells.

While these 2D and 2.5D devices are highly useful to study cellular responses to mechanical loading, a three-dimensional (3D) environment remains physiologically more relevant [8]. Therefore, the development and use of ‘3D’ bioreactors became more and more popular.

11.3.3 3D Bioreactors with Mechanical Stimulation

‘3D’ bioreactors allow for testing of constructs that contain cells embedded in a (3D) scaffold while mimicking specific aspects of the *in vivo* environment. Moreover, ‘3D’ bioreactors can be used to create tendon-like tissues via organized ECM production by cells in response to mechanical loading [8]. The more simple ‘3D’ bioreactors were designed to geometrically constrain constructs, for example, in well plates, in a way that the cells, for example, in a collagen matrix, could contract and constrain the scaffold material toward a uniaxially oriented matrix [8]. For this, researchers suspend cells in a gel mixture provided with geometrical constraints, such as posts or anchors, resulting in cell-induced contraction of the gel around the constraint. Hereby, bioartificial tendons were created to study cellular responses to mechanical stimulation and the mechanisms thereof [40,76,77]. Using native tendon cells (from avian flexor tendons) resuspended in a collagen type I matrix, Garvin et al. aimed to create tissue-engineered tendons [76]. They mechanically stimulated these constructs (for 1 hour a day at 1% elongation and 1 Hz) and showed that mechanically loaded constructs had homogeneously distributed and elongated cells similar to native tendon tissue after 2 weeks of culture. The elastic modulus increased with mechanical loading, however, still far from native tendon tissue [76]. Besides, Kuo et al. used the same system to study the mechanism of tenogenesis of human BMSCs in a collagen type I gel [40]. They mechanically stimulated the gels for 7 days (30 minutes a day at 1% strain) and found that cyclic loading maintained the expression of SCX over time, whereas the SCX gene expression level in statically cultured samples decreased over time [40]. This, again, highlights the need for dynamic mechanical stimulation for tenocytic differentiation of BMSCs.

Researchers also aimed to apply mechanical loading to large-size constructs or even whole tendons. The first '3D' tendon bioreactor for these large-size specimens was developed by Arnockzy's group [78]. Using small clamps, they applied cyclic tensile load to canine flexor tendons [78] (Figure 11.4c). Using this device, they found that canine flexor tendons could maintain their mechanical properties and structure for 4 weeks *ex vivo*, whereas stress-deprived tendons displayed decreased mechanical properties [79].

The use of these bioreactors for larger constructs has gained popularity over the last decades. Nowadays, several '3D' bioreactors are commercially available (e.g., the LigaGen Tension Bioreactor Systems from BISS TGT; the ElectroForce 5200 BioDynamic from TA Instruments; the TC-3 from EBERS Medical Technology SL; and the MechanoCulture J1 from CellScale [80–83]). These commercial bioreactors are used in several studies, often to investigate the behavior of new tendon grafts [18,27,46,47,84–92]. Still, many research groups develop their custom-made bioreactors [9], likely to keep full control over the desired possibilities.

11.4 BIOREACTOR DESIGN AND CHARACTERISTICS

11.4.1 Actuator

All (custom-made) bioreactors need some specific components in order to work properly, most importantly, the actuator. This is the element that produces the motion initiating the mechanical loading to the constructs. This can either be done with a linear motor, a pneumatic actuator, or a step motor [9,93]. Electrical-driven linear motors [94,95] have a high accuracy and can be used to apply uniaxial strains [9,93]. Pneumatic motors, as exploited in the following references [24,96,97], use air as an actuating medium and can generate biaxial strains. They are, however, subject to friction and, therefore, generally have a lower accuracy [9,93]. Step motors [98–100], based on a ball–screw linkage and slider–crank mechanism, are mostly used to generate rotational strains. The accuracy of step motors is in between that of linear and pneumatic motors. Multiple actuators can be combined to create multi-dimensional strains [9,93].

Bioreactors can operate in either a force- or displacement-controlled manner. If a bioreactor uses a force-controlled mechanism, the constructs will experience a force, whereas in displacement-controlled bioreactors, the constructs experience a strain. Force control is used in, for example, the bioreactor used in the study of Pedaprolu et al. [101] and displacement control in, for example, the bioreactor of Wang et al. [21]. Even though tendons function in a load-controlled fashion in the body [101], most of the bioreactors used in research are displacement-controlled [102]. One of the disadvantages of a displacement-controlled bioreactor is the occurrence of stress relaxation in tendon tissue [103], that is, lengthening

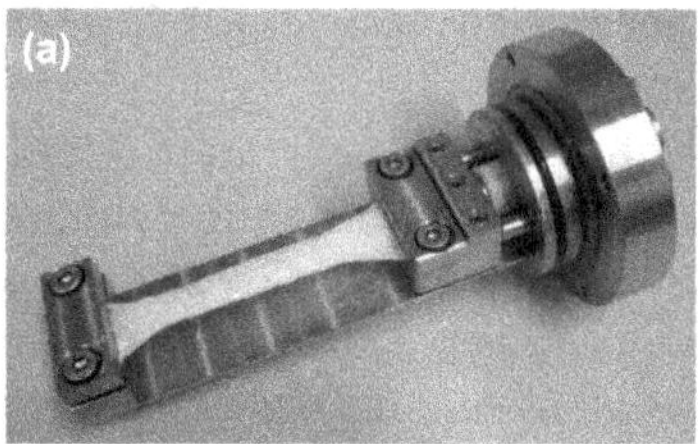

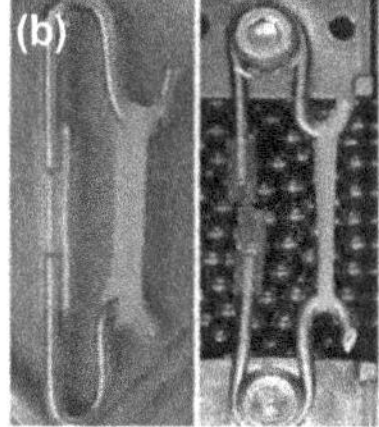

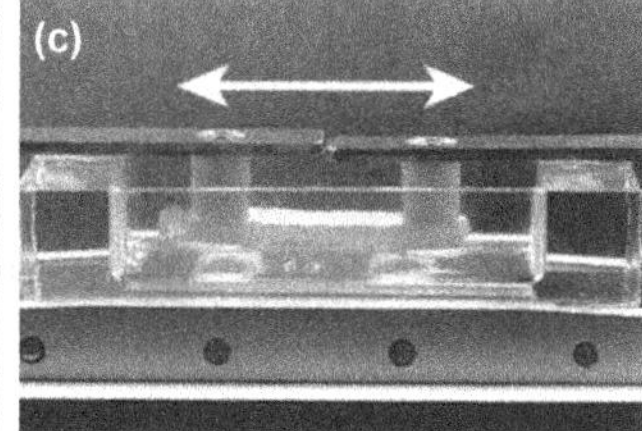

FIGURE 11.5 Different connection types between the actuator and a tendon construct. (a) Decellularized tendons are pressed between the surfaces of clamps. Modified from: Burk 2016. (b) 3D tendon cell constructs are wrapped around hooks. Modified from: Wang 2018, with permission. (c) PLA construct is placed between two movable posts. Modified from Kreja (2012), with permission.

of the construct while the applied strain remains equal. As a consequence, the tendon constructs become lax over time and the mechanical loading or stimulation becomes almost negligible [104]. Load-controlled bioreactors can of course also result in tissue lengthening and associated issues, however, do not risk stress-deprivation problems.

11.4.2 Connection between Actuator and Construct

In order to transmit the mechanical load initiated by the actuator toward the constructs, a connection is needed. Such connections often come with issues, for example, sample slippage at the interface and local tissue weakening due to tissue damage [9,105]. Clamps are mostly used in tendon bioreactors, where the tissue is pressed in between two rough surfaces. For example, the bioreactor of Burk and colleagues uses clamps to fix decellularized tendons [31] (Figure 11.5a). Such connections, unfortunately, associate with cell death in the squeezed tissue [9,105]. Alternatively, Wang and colleagues wrapped their 3D tendon-derived stem cell constructs around hooks [55,106] (Figure 11.5b) and Kreja et al. fixed their poly(L-lactide) (PLA) construct between two movable posts in order to mechanically condition them [107] (Figure 11.5c), a system similar to that is used by others [95,108–111].

11.4.3 Culture Chamber

The next important element of a bioreactor is the culture chamber. The culture chamber is a sterile container that holds the media in which the construct is cultured [9,105]. The culture medium within the culture chamber can be controlled to create the optimal conditions for the constructs [105]. In integrated culture chambers, multiple samples are cultured in the same culture chamber and thus share the same culture medium and conditions. An example of this is the bioreactor created by Brandt et al. who used their bioreactor to dynamically load three decellularized tendon constructs in the same culture chamber, resulting in three technical replicates [112]. Contrarily, separate culture chambers can provide different independent culture environments for each construct without cross-contamination [9]. For example, the custom-developed bioreactors of Wang et al., Wunderli et al., and

Talo et al. all have separate culture chambers for independent samples [21,22,113], allowing to test multiple conditions at the same time.

Constructs are often cultured under controlled humidity and temperature (~99% humidity and 37°C). This combined with the fact that chemicals in the culture media may be corrosive to materials, which in turn can be toxic to cells, illustrates the importance of material choices for the culture chamber. Ideal materials are non-corrosive, non-degradable, non-porous, non-protein binding, biocompatible or bioinert, easy to clean, and sterilizable (preferably in an autoclave). Popular choices are polyoxymethylene (POM), polyetherimide (PEI), polysulfone (PSF), polytetrafluoroethylene (PTFE), and polyether ether ketone (PEEK). If optical transparency is preferred, transparent polymethylmethacrylate (PMMA), polycarbonate (PC), polydimethylsiloxane (PDMS), glass, or silicon rubber are most commonly used, and for load-bearing parts inside the chamber, corrosion-resistant stainless steel, titanium, aluminum, and nylon are good options [9,105,114,115]. Moreover, with the rise of 3D-printing technologies, culture chambers have also been fabricated using printing techniques [115]. Within the culture chamber, like in standard culture flasks, adequate gas exchange is vital [9]. This can be obtained through a permeable membrane to prevent infections or, as the bioreactor is often placed inside a standard incubator, a venting system that forms an open channel between the environment in the incubator and the sample, in analogy to the lid of a well plate [105].

11.4.4 Monitoring Mechanical Properties Using Sensors

In particular for tendon tissue engineering for *in vivo* applications, the mechanical properties of tendon constructs are crucial [8]. Often, mechanical tests to quantify tissue mechanical properties are performed after culturing, as destructive tests require a more robust system with strong actuators and load cells that can cope with maximum tissue stresses. Real-time monitoring of the mechanical properties can give useful information about the development of mechanics within the tissue. Even though the price of the bioreactor will increase, this can be achieved by connecting the constructs to load cells that record the force during culturing [8,116]. Load cells are often placed between the actuating device and the point where the construct is fixed in the bioreactor and should be placed opposite to the actuating rod to avoid interference during movement [115–117]. It should also be considered that friction is minimized to overcome errors, in particular when using force-controlled tissue loading. Especially when handling soft biological materials, the induced friction can easily exceed the applied load [9]. Next to force monitoring, tissue strain can be measured using several types of sensors, for example, using strain gauges or inductive displacement transducers. These sensors must be coupled to the moving parts whose displacement is being monitored, which complicates the bioreactor design as it can induce friction [115]. Non-contact sensors, such as laser-based micrometers, optical encoders, or inductive displacement sensors are therefore preferred since they do not require direct contact and thus eliminate friction [115]. Within the tendon bioreactor field, several displacement sensors are being used. For example, the bioreactor of David Butler's laboratory makes use of linear differential transducers to monitor the end-to-end displacement of their collagen sponges [96,108,109], and Parent and colleagues used optical encoders to measure the distance between both ends of tendon explants [118]. Together, load and displacement sensors give real-time information about construct maturation, that is, the development of mechanical properties [8]. On the other hand, these sensors can also be used to provide feedback to the actuating system, both in force- and displacement-controlled bioreactors [9] to apply a known load to the constructs, correcting for creep and stress relaxation effects that can reduce the applied load over time, as discussed earlier.

11.4.5 Media Circulation System and Environmental Control

Next, a medium circulation system can be included in the bioreactor to avoid depletion of nutrients and accumulation of waste products [9,105,114]. This can be achieved by implementing a port through which 'old' medium can exit and a second port where 'new' medium can enter the culture chamber [114]. This also enables adding a medium analysis system for real-time monitoring and even controlling or changing medium conditions real time (O_2, pH, temperature, metabolites, waste products) [114]. As mentioned earlier, bioreactors are often placed inside a culture incubator to control, for example, CO_2 and O_2 levels, humidity, and temperature. For benchtop incubators, these levels can be controlled using air valves [100]. Both have up- and downsides. The major downsides of placing bioreactors in an incubator include size restrictions (the bioreactor needs to fit in the incubator), and the limited selection of actuators and sensors as they need to be incubator-proof (IP67), making them more expensive [105]. The major downside of a benchtop version is the challenging necessity to control the environment.

11.5 APPLICATIONS OF TENDON BIOREACTORS

Bioreactors can be used in multiple ways and for different purposes. In this paragraph, we define four different applications for tendon bioreactors: (i) tendon homeostasis and tendon pathology; (ii) tissue engineering and maturation of tendon constructs; (iii) disease modeling, diagnostics, and drug screening; and (iv) replacement of animal experimentation.

11.5.1 Tendon Homeostasis and Tendon Pathology

Bioreactors can assist in unraveling the different aspects of tendon biology in the context of health and homeostasis and tendon pathology [8]. For instance, Jones et al. used a bioreactor to investigate the mechanism behind the response of MMPs and their relation to tendon homeostasis [77]. By embedding human Achilles' tenocytes in type I rat tail collagen gels, anchored to constraining posts, and applying mechanical load (5% cyclic uniaxial strain at 1 Hz for 48 hours), they showed that mechanical strain regulated the expression of several proteases and matrix genes. When adding TGFβ to the culture medium at static mechanical loading conditions, similar gene expression levels were found compared to mechanically stimulated constructs. In turn, inhibition of the TGFβ pathway abrogated the strain-induced changes. Therefore, they concluded that TGFβ activation plays a key role in mechanotransduction [77], and possibly, targeting the TGFβ pathway presents an interesting treatment option for treating tendinopathy. Next to that, multiple researchers have cultured whole tendons or tendon fascicles *ex vivo* in a bioreactor to explore tendon homeostasis and/or pathology [21,22,106,119–122]. Tempfer and Spitzer et al. used an *ex vivo* setup to examine vascular endothelial growth factor (VEGF) signaling in tendon pathology [120]. Using a bioreactor to *ex vivo* overload rat flexor tendons for 72 hours (150 cycles of 8% strain followed by 8 hours of rest), they observed nuclear rounding and collagen degradation. However, when they inhibited VEGF receptor 3 with SAR131675, both the shape of the cell nuclei and the collagen degradation were similar to freshly isolated tendons [120]. This shows that VEGF signaling affects the degenerative processes in these tendons. Besides, Wang et al. cultured rabbit Achilles' tendons in a bioreactor to investigate the effects of mechanical underloading (3% strain at 0.25 Hz for 8 hours followed by 16 hours rest) on tendon ossification and the molecular mechanisms behind this [106]. After 20 days, they found multiple ossification sites within the tendon tissue cultured at underloading conditions. Moreover, the maximum load and stiffness were significantly lower than that of native Achilles' tendons [106].

Another option is to explore the effect of growth factors in combination with mechanical stimulation on cell-populating constructs in bioreactors, which has been done extensively [44,85,90,123,124]. By doing so, a synergistic effect between biochemical and mechanical stimuli was found, which can accelerate the differentiation of stem cells into the tendon lineage [123,124] and potentially accelerates tendon healing [90]. Govoni et al. used fibrin as a carrier to embed human BMSCs in a scaffold of hyaluronate braided fibers with poly-lactic-co-glycolic acid (PLGA) microcarriers that were loaded with human growth differentiation factor 5 (hGDF-5). These constructs were subsequently subjected to mechanical loading (10% strain at 1 Hz for 3 days). An increased tenogenic gene expression was found, but only when both cyclic strain and locally released hGDF-5 were exposed to the cells. mRNA levels of COL1A1, COL1A3, DCN, SCX, and TNC were significantly upregulated, whereas in absence of the biochemical stimuli, only SCX levels were found to be significantly higher than statically cultured samples [123]. Similarly, Rinoldi and coworkers [124] showed a significant increase in the expression of tendon markers after 7 days when electrospun PCL fibers, coated with an hBMSC-laden hydrogel, were treated with bone morphogenetic protein 12 (BMP-12). When a mechanical stimulus of 10% strain at 1 Hz for 4 hours a day was added to the constructs, gene expression levels of TNMD, DCN, and TNC were significantly higher compared to unloaded controls. Next to that, cyclic strain and BMP-12 treatment synergistically increased cell viability, proliferation, and alignment [124]. Furthermore, Barber et al. [85] used a bioreactor to show that mechanical stimulation of human BMSCs in a braided poly(L-lactic acid) (PLLA) nanofiber construct can halt osteogenesis, which was induced via supplementation of a differentiation medium containing BMP-2, GDF-5, and fibroblast growth factor 2 (FGF-2). With the addition of mechanical load (10% strain at 1 Hz for 2 hours a day, for 10 days), the gene expression level of runt-related transcription factor 2 (RUNX2), a bone-specific differentiation marker, was significantly downregulated. Moreover, tendon-specific markers such as SCX, COL I, and COL III were upregulated with mechanical stimulation [85]. This indicates that mechanical stimulation of stem cells can induce tenogenesis even when the culture medium steers the cells to differentiate into another cell lineage.

Additionally, with a bioreactor it is possible to examine the response of cells, embedded inside a scaffold, to different loading regimes [18,21,23–34,106,119]. One of these studies is by Engebretson et al. [32]. They studied the effect of varying frequency and duration of mechanical stimulation on tissue-engineered tendon constructs. Rat BMSCs were cultured on human decellularized umbilical veins for 7 days strained at 2% at different frequencies (0.5, 1, or 2 cycles per minute) and duration (0.5, 1, or 2 hours a day). Based on their outcomes, the slower frequencies and shorter durations, such as 0.5 cycles per minute and 0.5 hours a day, were the most favorable for construct quality in the first week of culture, as cellular proliferation increased and tenogenesis of the BMSCs was detected [32]. Subramanian et al. concluded that the lowest percentual strain at the lowest frequency tested (2% strain at 0.1 Hz, compared to 4% and 6% at 1 Hz) was optimal for tenogenic differentiation of human ASCs inside a reconstituted 3D rat tail collagen matrix [34]. However, Scott and colleagues found that increasing strain levels up to 10% resulted in increased COL1A1 and SCX levels and a cell morphology more similar to tenocytes of C3H10T1/2 cells cultured in a reconstituted 3D collagen matrix [35]. Moreover, they found an increased SCX expression with the highest number of cycles tested (1,000 cycles, compared to 10 or 100 cycles), which suggests that relatively few repetitions are insufficient to induce tenogenesis and that mechanical stimulation for a longer period can improve differentiation [35]. Although these results seem contradictory, it should be noted that the cell type and scaffold material differ between the studies.

11.5.2 Tissue Engineering and Maturation of Tendon Constructs

Bioreactors are important in tissue-engineering strategies aiming at neo-tissue formation. In a bioreactor, tissue-engineered constructs can be exposed to mechanical stimuli that facilitate tissue maturation by accelerating the formation of appropriate tissue composition, morphology, and architecture [2,14,114]. This can aid in the development of constructs with mechanical properties similar to that of native tendon tissue [14]. Multiple researchers found increased mechanical properties of tissue-engineered tendon constructs after *in vitro* mechanical conditioning [16,27,28,44–47,76,86,96,97,99,108,125–129]. Consequently, several studies used *in vitro* mechanical conditioning of tissue-engineered constructs in bioreactors before *in vivo* implantation [84,90,96,130].

In 2012, Thorfinn et al. used *in vitro* mechanical conditioning to improve tissue strength before *in vivo* implantation [84]. Applying cyclic strain (1.25 N at 1 Hz, alternating 1 hour of load and 1 hour of rest, for 5 days) to tenocyte-reseeded acellular rabbit flexor tendons, increased both the ultimate tensile strength and the elastic modulus [46]. When implanting these tendons in tendon defects in rabbits for 4 weeks and performing biomechanical tests afterward, they found superior strength and elastic modulus for the *in vitro* bioreactor-conditioned constructs compared to constructs that did not undergo preoperative *in vitro* mechanical conditioning [84]. Next to that,

Juncosa-Melvin and colleagues aimed to repair patellar tendon defects in rabbits by seeding type I collagen sponges with rabbit BMSCs and mechanically conditioning the constructs (2.4% strain at 0.2 Hz for 8 hours a day for 2 weeks). Mechanical stimulation increased the mechanical properties, such as maximum stress and elastic modulus [96,109]. Afterward, they implanted the collagen sponges in a rabbit central tendon defect model. After 12 weeks, the *in vitro* conditioned constructs had significantly higher mechanical properties than the non-conditioned ones, although still being significantly lower than a native patellar tendon [96]. Hereby, the mechanical properties after *in vitro* mechanical stimulation turned out to be a good predictor for the corresponding mechanical properties, 12 weeks after implantation [96].

If tissue maturation is the goal of using a bioreactor, it can be of great value to monitor tissue maturation during culture [8]. This can be obtained by recording the force and the displacement over time using sensors (see paragraph 6.4.4).

11.5.3 Disease Modeling, Diagnostics, and Drug Screening

Bioreactors enable mimicking various clinically relevant types of environment that cells or tissues are exposed to *in vivo* [8]. For instance, bioreactors can be used to examine the effects of external influences such as pharmaceuticals or non-physiological external loads. They can also be used to model diseases or simulate controlled drug delivery [15]. To examine the responses to drugs, bioreactors can be exploited to increase model complexity and more closely mimic the *in vivo* situation. This can increase the success of clinical translation in the development and testing of new therapies and drugs [48,131]. Both '2D' and '3D' bioreactors with mechanical stimulation are used to examine external influences on tendon cells or (tissue-engineered) tendon constructs [33,112,132,133].

In 2018, Brandt and colleagues created an inflammatory environment, by means of a bioreactor system. They supplemented decellularized equine tendon constructs, reseeded with equine ASCs *in vitro*, with pro-inflammatory cytokines, such as interleukin 1 beta (IL-1β) and tumor necrosis factor-alpha (TNF-α), or by co-culture with allogeneic peripheral blood leukocytes [112]. When they cultured the tendons under uniaxial strain (intermittent loading of 2% at 1 Hz for 3 days), they found that the inflammatory conditions resulted in an increased number of dead cells. Besides, with the high cytokine concentration or with the leukocyte co-culture, the viable ACSs integration in the construct was lower [112].

A bioreactor for 2D culture with mechanical stimulation was used by Hsiao et al. to model the pathophysiology of tendinopathy to examine the effect of different treatment options on tendon-derived cells [33]. They studied the effect of epigallocatechin (EGCG), which has antioxidant and anti-inflammatory properties, and piracetam, which is a neuroprotective drug, on tendon-derived cells. The tendon-derived cells were seeded on culture plates made of polydimethylsiloxane (PDMS) and subjected to excessive mechanical loading (8% strain at a frequency of 0.5 Hz for 8 hours). This loading regime increased the gene expression of non-tenocyte lineage genes such as peroxisome proliferator-activated receptor gamma (PPAR-γ), RUNX2, and SOX9 and increased the ratio of collagen type III/I, indicative of tendon pathophysiology. However, when the cells were supplied with EGCG or piracetam, these increased gene expressions were diminished, indicating that EGCG and piracetam can reduce gene expression toward the non-tenogenic lineage in tendon-derived cells [33]. Proposedly, eliminating oxidative stress can contribute to the treatment of tendinopathy.

In a slightly different way, Triantafillopoulos [133] used a 3D model to investigate the effect of an anabolic steroid (nandrolone decanoate) on tenocytes [133]. They stretched cells, isolated from human supraspinatus tendons, in a 3D collagen matrix (1% strain at 1 Hz for 1 hour a day for 7 days in total). With the addition of the steroid, the cytoskeleton of the cells was better organized, and the addition of mechanical load enhanced this effect. The MMP3 gene expression level increased transiently with time in constructs where steroid was added, and mechanical stimulation was applied. Next to that, the addition of steroid and mechanical load synergistically increased the ultimate tensile stress and strain of the constructs [133]. Together this indicates that the addition of an anabolic steroid can accelerate matrix remodeling and stimulate the development of bioartificial tendons.

11.5.4 Replacement of Animal Experimentation

Finally, bioreactors can be exploited in the replacement of animal experimentation [15], that is, minimizing the use of animals in experiments [134]. In 1959, Russell and Burch introduced the concept of the Three Rs (replacement, reduction, and refinement) [135], which was seen as a breakthrough in the more humane use of animals for scientific purposes. In short, replacement refers to all strategies that avoid or replace the use of animals. Reduction denotes all methods that result in fewer animals being used to obtain sufficient data, for example, maximizing the information that can be obtained from one animal and limiting or avoiding the need for subsequent animal experiments. Lastly, refinement is modifying the experimental procedures to minimize animal pain and distress to ensure animal welfare [134].

Especially regarding replacement and reduction, bioreactors can play a major role. So far, bioreactors cannot completely mimic the *in vivo* environment; however, they can provide an attractive alternative. Next to the ethical and welfare issues regarding the use of animals in research, the main advantages of using bioreactors are the option to investigate more technical replicates, lower costs, better control of environmental cues (such as mechanical and chemical inputs and local drug delivery), and the possibility for real-time data collection [8,15]. Bioreactors can be used as an *in vitro* testing and screening platform that can predict the response of an isolated tissue [96]. Thereby, they can be used as a tool to study, test, and predict clinical scenarios in a physiologically relevant environment before continuing with animal models or (pre)clinical trials [136]. On the other hand, when developing different novel tendon constructs, for example, 3D-printed constructs with a variation in mechanical and/or biochemical properties, bioreactors can provide a preclinical *in vitro* mechanobiological validation tool in which the most promising constructs can be selected before *in vivo* testing. As is schematically represented in Figure 11.6, the number of different constructs, which might be suitable for *in vivo* applications, decreases after bioreactor studies, resulting in fewer constructs being interesting to test *in vivo*. That

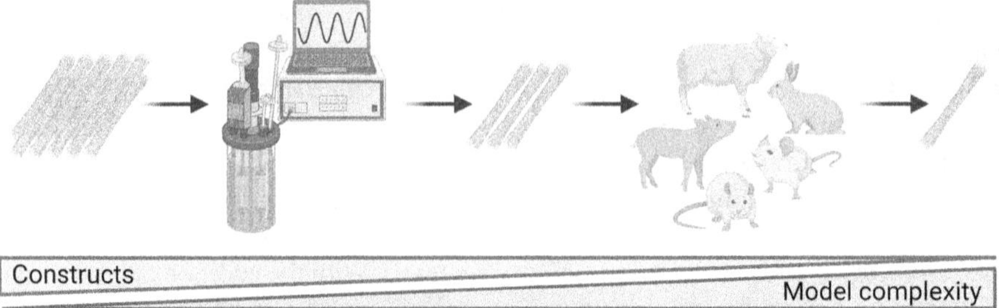

FIGURE 11.6 Schematic overview of replacing and reducing animal experimentation with bioreactor studies. Bioreactor studies can provide a preclinical validation tool in which the most promising constructs for animal experimentation can be selected, resulting in fewer animals needed. Created with BioRender.com.

way, the use of animals can be reduced, and, in some cases, it might even be possible to completely replace animal experiments with bioreactor studies. However, fully replacing animal experiments with bioreactor studies might be hard, for example, because vascularization remains an experimentally challenging feature to add to a bioreactor system.

11.6 FUTURE DIRECTIONS

Since the development of the first (3D) bioreactor by Arnockzy's group [78], bioreactors have been more commonly used for various purposes, and this use is expected to only increase in the future [114]. The major limitations that still need to be overcome in future bioreactor experiments are the short duration of culture time and the lack of standardized loading regimes [54]. Up to now, the longest bioreactor cultures are performed by Wang et al. [130] and Jiang et al. [137]. Both studies dynamically cultured constructs for 10 weeks, whereas the culture time in most studies varies from a few days up to 2 weeks only. This, of course, pales compared to the follow-up time the constructs need to endure in *in vivo* studies. Next to that, the optimal *in vitro* conditions for tendon homeostasis and tendon construct maturation have not yet been established, while there is a clear need to standardize these loading regimes. Even though it might be hard to standardize these loading regimes since they are cell type and scaffold dependent, standardized versions will aid in comparing the results of different studies. Finally, for future clinical use, bioreactors need to be further refined, considering ease of handling, safety, cost-effectiveness, scalability, and regulatory compliant manufacturing processes [114].

These optimized bioreactors can in addition to the different ways in which bioreactors are currently being used, as outlined in this chapter, be useful in other future applications. For example, culturing (stem) cells without a scaffold inside bioreactors with the addition of complex mechanical stimuli to encourage organoid formation and mimic embryonic development [1]. Another option is the validation of complex computer models using bioreactor experiments [138]. Particularly with the rise in the use of computer models, this can become an interesting possibility.

11.7 CONCLUDING REMARKS

Multiple bioreactors have been developed over the past decades, and they are being increasingly used in research. As mentioned in this chapter, bioreactors can be used for different useful applications, for example, to unravel (mechano)biological mechanisms or replace and reduce animal experimentation. They can improve and assist the development of new tissue-engineered tendon constructs that more closely resemble native tendon tissue and help us in the understanding of fundamental cellular mechanisms. Additionally, they have the potential toward scale-up strategies, with vascularization as an experimentally challenging hurdle to overcome. Although up till now the use of bioreactors for developing tendon constructs is still in preclinical studies and has not yet been used in clinical trials, this can change in the forthcoming years. Especially if bioreactor designs will be further optimized in a way that they fully comprise the biological and biomechanical demands of tendon tissue, then, possibly, the use of bioreactors will result in better and more beneficial treatment options for patients, either by aiding in the screening of different pharmaceuticals or by the development and maturation of constructs that closely resemble native tendon properties.

REFERENCES

1. Lim WL, Liau LL, Ng MH, Chowdhury SR, Law JX. Current progress in tendon and ligament tissue engineering. *Tissue Eng Regen Med.* 2019;16(6):549–71. Available from: https://pubmed.ncbi.nlm.nih.gov/31824819/.
2. Rodrigues MT, Reis RL, Gomes ME. Engineering tendon and ligament tissues: Present developments towards successful clinical products. *J Tissue Eng Regen Med.* 2013;7(9):673–86. Available from: https://pubmed.ncbi.nlm.nih.gov/22499564/.
3. Steinmann S, Pfeifer CG, Brochhausen C, Docheva D. Spectrum of tendon pathologies: Triggers, trails and end-state. *Int J Mol Sci.* 2020;21(3):844. Available from: https://www.mdpi.com/1422-0067/21/3/844.
4. Ruiz-Alonso S, Lafuente-Merchan M, Ciriza J, Saenz-del-Burgo L, Pedraz JL. Tendon tissue engineering: Cells, growth factors, scaffolds and production techniques. *J Controlled Release.* 2021;333(September 2020):448–86.
5. Benhardt HA, Cosgriff-Hernandez EM. The role of mechanical loading in ligament tissue engineering. *Tissue Eng Part B Rev.* 2009;15(4):467–75. Available from: https://www.liebertpub.com/doi/10.1089/ten.teb.2008.0687.
6. Wang JHC, Guo Q, Li B. Tendon biomechanics and mechanobiology—A minireview of basic concepts and recent advancements. *J Hand Ther.* 2012;25(2):133–41. Available from: /pmc/articles/PMC3244520/.
7. Wang JHC, Jia F, Gilbert TW, Woo SLY. Cell orientation determines the alignment of cell-produced collagenous matrix. *J Biomech.* 2003;36(1):97–102. Available from: https://linkinghub.elsevier.com/retrieve/pii/S0021929002002336.
8. Dyment NA, Barrett JG, Awad HA, Bautista CA, Banes AJ, Butler DL. A brief history of tendon and ligament bioreactors: Impact and future prospects. *J Orthop Res.* 2020 Nov 1 [cited 2022 Jan 19];38(11):2318–30. Available from: https://onlinelibrary.wiley.com/doi/full/10.1002/jor.24784.
9. Wang T, Gardiner BS, Lin Z, Rubenson J, Kirk TB, Wang A, et al. Bioreactor design for tendon/ligament engineering. *Tissue Eng Part B Rev.* 2013;19(2):133–46. Available from: /pmc/articles/PMC3589869/.

10. Martin I, Wendt D, Heberer M. The role of bioreactors in tissue engineering. *Trends Biotechnol.* 2004;22(2):80–6.
11. Correia SI, Pereira H, Silva-Correia J, van Dijk CN, Espregueira-Mendes J, Oliveira JM, et al. Current concepts: Tissue engineering and regenerative medicine applications in the ankle joint. *J R Soc Interface.* 2014 Dec 18;11(92):20130784. Available from: http://doi.org/10.1098/rsif.2013.0784. PMID: 24352667; PMCID: PMC3899856.
12. Galloway MT, Lalley AL, Shearn JT. The role of mechanical loading in tendon development, maintenance, injury, and repair. *J Bone Joint Surg.* 2013;95(17):1620–8. Available from: /pmc/articles/PMC3748997/.
13. Gracey E, Burssens A, Cambré I, Schett G, Lories R, McInnes IB, et al. Tendon and ligament mechanical loading in the pathogenesis of inflammatory arthritis. *Nat Rev Rheumatol.* 2020;16(4):193–207. Available from: /pmc/articles/PMC7815340/.
14. Abousleiman RI, Sikavitsas VI. Bioreactors for tissues of the musculoskeletal system. In: *Tissue Eng.* Boston, MA: Springer US; 2006. pp. 243–59. Available from: https://link.springer.com/chapter/10.1007/978-0-387-34133-0_17.
15. Ravichandran A, Liu Y, Teoh SH. Review: Bioreactor design towards generation of relevant engineered tissues: Focus on clinical translation. *J Tissue Eng Regen Med.* 2018;12(1):e7–22. Available from: https://onlinelibrary.wiley.com/doi/10.1002/term.2270.
16. Abousleiman RI, Reyes Y, McFetridge P, Sikavitsas V. Tendon tissue engineering using cell-seeded umbilical veins cultured in a mechanical stimulator. *Tissue Eng Part A.* 2009;15(4):787–95.
17. Liu Q, Hatta T, Qi J, Liu H, Thoreson AR, Amadio PC, et al. Novel engineered tendon–fibrocartilage–bone composite with cyclic tension for rotator cuff repair. *J Tissue Eng Regen Med.* 2018;12(7):1690–701. Available from: https://doi.org/10.1002/term.2696.
18. Deniz P, Guler S, Çelik E, Hosseinian P, Aydin HM. Use of cyclic strain bioreactor for the upregulation of key tenocyte gene expression on Poly(glycerol-sebacate) (PGS) sheets. *Mater Sci Eng C.* 2020;106(August 2018):110293. Available from: https://doi.org/10.1016/j.msec.2019.110293.
19. Subramony SD, Su A, Yeager K, Lu HH. Combined effects of chemical priming and mechanical stimulation on mesenchymal stem cell differentiation on nanofiber scaffolds. *J Biomech.* 2014;47(9):2189–96. Available from: https://pubmed.ncbi.nlm.nih.gov/24267271/.
20. Wang T, Lin Z, Ni M, Thien C, Day RE, Gardiner B, et al. Cyclic mechanical stimulation rescues achilles tendon from degeneration in a bioreactor system. *J Orthop Res.* 2015;33(12):1888–96. Available from: https://onlinelibrary.wiley.com/doi/10.1002/jor.22960.
21. Wang T, Lin Z, Day RE, Gardiner B, Landao-Bassonga E, Rubenson J, et al. Programmable mechanical stimulation influences tendon homeostasis in a bioreactor system. *Biotechnol Bioeng.* 2013;110(5):1495–507. Available from: https://onlinelibrary.wiley.com/doi/10.1002/bit.24809.
22. Wunderli SL, Widmer J, Amrein N, Foolen J, Silvan U, Leupin O, et al. Minimal mechanical load and tissue culture conditions preserve native cell phenotype and morphology in tendon-a novel ex vivo mouse explant model. *J Orthop Res.* 2018;36(5):1383–90. Available from: https://onlinelibrary.wiley.com/doi/10.1002/jor.23769.
23. Gilbert TW, Stewart-Akers AM, Sydeski J, Nguyen TD, Badylak SF, Woo SLY. Gene expression by fibroblasts seeded on small intestinal submucosa and subjected to cyclic stretching. *Tissue Eng.* 2007;13(6):1313–23. Available from: https://www.liebertpub.com/doi/10.1089/ten.2006.0318.
24. Nirmalanandhan VS, Shearn JT, Juncosa-Melvin N, Rao M, Gooch C, Jain A, et al. Improving linear stiffness of the cell-seeded collagen sponge constructs by varying the

components of the mechanical stimulus. *Tissue Eng Part A*. 2008 Nov;14(11):1883–91. Available from: https://www.liebertpub.com/doi/10.1089/ten.tea.2007.0125.

25. Kinneberg KRC, Nirmalanandhan VS, Juncosa-Melvin N, Powell HM, Boyce ST, Shearn JT, et al. Chondroitin-6-sulfate incorporation and mechanical stimulation increase MSC-collagen sponge construct stiffness. *J Orthop Res*. 2010;28(8):1092–9. Available from: /pmc/articles/PMC3123395/.
26. Riboh J, Chong AKS, Pham H, Longaker M, Jacobs C, Chang J. Optimization of flexor tendon tissue engineering with a cyclic strain bioreactor. *J Hand Surg Am*. 2008;33(8):1388–96. Available from: https://linkinghub.elsevier.com/retrieve/pii/S0363502308003924.
27. Woon CYL, Kraus A, Raghavan SS, Pridgen BC, Megerle K, Pham H, et al. Three-dimensional-construct bioreactor conditioning in human tendon tissue engineering. *Tissue Eng Part A*. 2011;17(19–20):2561–72. Available from: https://www.liebertpub.com/doi/10.1089/ten.tea.2010.0701.
28. Joshi SD, Webb K. Variation of cyclic strain parameters regulates development of elastic modulus in fibroblast/substrate constructs. *J Orthop Res*. 2008;26(8):1105–13. Available from: https://onlinelibrary.wiley.com/doi/10.1002/jor.20626.
29. Paxton JZ, Hagerty P, Andrick JJ, Baar K. Optimizing an intermittent stretch paradigm using ERK1/2 phosphorylation results in increased collagen synthesis in engineered ligaments. *Tissue Eng Part A*. 2012 Feb;18(3–4):277–84. Available from: https://www.liebertpub.com/doi/10.1089/ten.tea.2011.0336.
30. Youngstrom DW, Rajpar I, Kaplan DL, Barrett JG. A bioreactor system for in vitro tendon differentiation and tendon tissue engineering. *J Orthop Res*. 2015;33(6):911–8. Available from: https://onlinelibrary.wiley.com/doi/10.1002/jor.22848.
31. Burk J, Plenge A, Brehm W, Heller S, Pfeiffer B, Kasper C. Induction of tenogenic differentiation mediated by extracellular tendon matrix and short-term cyclic stretching. *Stem Cells Int*. 2016;2016:1–11. Available from: http://www.hindawi.com/journals/sci/2016/7342379/.
32. Engebretson B, Mussett ZR, Sikavitsas VI. The effects of varying frequency and duration of mechanical stimulation on a tissue-engineered tendon construct. *Connect Tissue Res*. 2018;59(2):167–77. Available from: https://www.tandfonline.com/doi/full/10.1080/03008207.2017.1324431.
33. Hsiao MY, Lin PC, Liao WH, Chen WS, Hsu CH, He CK, et al. The effect of the repression of oxidative stress on tenocyte differentiation: A preliminary study of a rat cell model using a novel differential tensile strain bioreactor. *Int J Mol Sci*. 2019;20(14):3437. Available from: https://www.mdpi.com/1422-0067/20/14/3437.
34. Subramanian G, Stasuk A, Elsaadany M, Yildirim-Ayan E. Effect of uniaxial tensile cyclic loading regimes on matrix organization and tenogenic differentiation of adipose-derived stem cells encapsulated within 3D collagen scaffolds. *Stem Cells Int*. 2017;2017:1–16. Available from: https://www.hindawi.com/journals/sci/2017/6072406/.
35. Scott A, Danielson P, Abraham. T, Fong G, Sampaio Av, Underhill TM. Mechanical force and expression of tenocyte-related genes. *J Musculoskelet Neuronal Interact*. 2011;11(2):124–32.
36. Liu Y, Ramanath HS, Wang DA. Tendon tissue engineering using scaffold enhancing strategies. *Trends Biotechnol*. 2008;26(4):201–9. Available from: https://linkinghub.elsevier.com/retrieve/pii/S0167779908000553.
37. Youngstrom DW, LaDow JE, Barrett JG. Tenogenesis of bone marrow-, adipose-, and tendon-derived stem cells in a dynamic bioreactor. *Connect Tissue Res*. 2016;57(6):454–65. Available from: https://www.tandfonline.com/doi/full/10.3109/03008207.2015.1117458.
38. Plunkett N, O'Brien FJ. Bioreactors in tissue engineering. *Tech Health Care*. 2011;19(1):55–69. Available from: https://www.medra.org/servlet/aliasResolver?alias=iospress&doi=10.3233/THC-2011-0605.

39. Nam HY, Pingguan-Murphy B, Abbas AA, Merican AM, Kamarul T. Uniaxial cyclic tensile stretching at 8% strain exclusively promotes tenogenic differentiation of human bone marrow-derived mesenchymal stromal cells. *Stem Cells Int.* 2019;2019:1–16.
40. Kuo CK, Tuan RS. Mechanoactive tenogenic differentiation of human mesenchymal stem cells. *Tissue Eng Part A.* 2008;14(10):1615–27. Available from: https://www.liebertpub.com/doi/abs/10.1089/ten.tea.2006.0415.
41. Vindigni V, Tonello C, Lancerotto L, Abatangelo G, Cortivo R, Zavan B, et al. Preliminary report of in vitro reconstruction of a vascularized tendonlike structure. *Ann Plast Surg.* 2013;71(6):664–70. Available from: https://journals.lww.com/00000637-201312000-00011.
42. Lee KI, Lee JS, Kim JG, Kang KT, Jang JW, Shim YB, et al. Mechanical properties of decellularized tendon cultured by cyclic straining bioreactor. *J Biomed Mater Res A.* 2013;101(11). Available from: https://onlinelibrary.wiley.com/doi/10.1002/jbm.a.34624.
43. Raimondi MT, Laganà M, Conci C, Crestani M, di Giancamillo A, Gervaso F, et al. Development and biological validation of a cyclic stretch culture system for the ex vivo engineering of tendons. *Int J Artif Organs.* 2018;41(7):400–12. Available from: https://doi.org/10.1177/0391398818774496.
44. Testa S, Costantini M, Fornetti E, Bernardini S, Trombetta M, Seliktar D, et al. Combination of biochemical and mechanical cues for tendon tissue engineering. *J Cell Mol Med.* 2017;21(11):2711–9. Available from: https://onlinelibrary.wiley.com/doi/10.1111/jcmm.13186.
45. Banik BL, Brown JL. 3D-printed bioreactor enhances potential for tendon tissue engineering. *Regen Eng Transl Med.* 2020;6(4):419–28. Available from: https://link.springer.com/10.1007/s40883-019-00145-y.
46. Saber S, Zhang AY, Ki SH, Lindsey DP, Smith RL, Riboh J, et al. Flexor tendon tissue engineering: Bioreactor cyclic strain increases construct strength. *Tissue Eng Part A.* 2010;16(6):2085–90. Available from: https://www.liebertpub.com/doi/10.1089/ten.tea.2010.0032.
47. Angelidis IK, Thorfinn J, Connolly ID, Lindsey D, Pham HM, Chang J. Tissue engineering of flexor tendons: The effect of a tissue bioreactor on adipoderived stem cell–seeded and fibroblast-seeded tendon constructs. *J Hand Surg Am.* 2010;35(9):1466–72. Available from: https://linkinghub.elsevier.com/retrieve/pii/S0363502310007550.
48. Selden C, Fuller B. Role of bioreactor technology in tissue engineering for clinical use and therapeutic target design. *Bioengineering.* 2018;5(2):32. Available from: http://www.mdpi.com/2306-5354/5/2/32.
49. Drapal V, Gamble JM, Robinson JL, Tamerler C, Arnold PM, Friis EA. Integration of clinical perspective into biomimetic bioreactor design for orthopedics. *J Biomed Mater Res B Appl Biomater.* 2022;110(2):321–37. Available from: https://onlinelibrary.wiley.com/doi/full/10.1002/jbm.b.34929.
50. Vunjak-Novakovic G, Meinel L, Altman G, Kaplan D. Bioreactor cultivation of osteochondral grafts. *Orthod Craniofac Res.* 2005;8(3):209–18. Available from: https://pubmed.ncbi.nlm.nih.gov/16022723/.
51. Talukdar S, Kundu SC. Silk scaffolds for three-dimensional (3D) tumor modeling. In: *Silk Biomaterials for Tissue Engineering and Regenerative Medicine.* Elsevier; 2014. pp. 472–502. Available from: https://linkinghub.elsevier.com/retrieve/pii/B9780857096999500185.
52. Schwarz RP, Goodwin TJ, Wolf DA. Cell culture for three-dimensional modeling in rotating-wall vessels: An application of simulated microgravity. Vol. 14, *J Tiss Cult Meth.* 1992.
53. Radtke AL, Herbst-Kralovetz MM. Culturing and applications of rotating wall vessel bioreactor derived 3D epithelial cell models. *J Visualized Exp.* 2012 Apr 3;(62):3868. doi:10.3791/3868.

54. Mace J, Wheelton A, Khan WS, Anand S. The role of bioreactors in ligament and tendon tissue engineering. *Curr Stem Cell Res Ther.* 2016;11(1):35–40. Available from: http://www.eurekaselect.com/openurl/content.php?genre=article&issn=1574-888X&volume=11&issue=1&spage=35.
55. Wang T, Chen P, Zheng M, Wang A, Lloyd D, Leys T, et al. In vitro loading models for tendon mechanobiology. *J Orthop Res.* 2017;36(2):566–75. Available from: https://onlinelibrary.wiley.com/doi/10.1002/jor.23752.
56. Banes AJ, Gilbert J, Taylor D, Monbureau O. A new vacuum-operated stress-providing instrument that applies static or variable duration cyclic tension or compression to cells in vitro. *J Cell Sci.* 1985;75(1):35–42. Available from: https://journals.biologists.com/jcs/article/75/1/35/59723/A-new-vacuum-operated-stress-providing-instrument.
57. Arnoczky SP, Tian T, Lavagnino M, Gardner K, Schuler P, Morse P. Activation of stress-activated protein kinases (SAPK) in tendon cells following cyclic strain: The effects of strain frequency, strain magnitude, and cytosolic calcium. *J Orthop Res.* 2002;20(5):947–52. Available from: http://doi.wiley.com/10.1016/S0736-0266%2802%2900038-4.
58. Ralphs JR, Waggett AD, Benjamin M. Actin stress fibres and cell–cell adhesion molecules in tendons: Organisation in vivo and response to mechanical loading of tendon cells in vitro. *Matrix Biol.* 2002;21(1):67–74. Available from: https://linkinghub.elsevier.com/retrieve/pii/S0945053X01001792.
59. Goodman SA, May SA, Heinegård D, Smith RKW. Tenocyte response to cyclical strain and transforming growth factor beta is dependent upon age and site of origin. *Biorheology.* 2004;41(5):613–28. Available from: http://www.ncbi.nlm.nih.gov/pubmed/15477668.
60. Wall ME, Weinhold PS, Siu T, Brown TD, Banes AJ. Comparison of cellular strain with applied substrate strain in vitro. *J Biomech.* 2007;40(1):173–81. Available from: https://linkinghub.elsevier.com/retrieve/pii/S0021929005004999.
61. Crockett RJ, Centrella M, McCarthy TL, Grant Thomson J. Effects of cyclic strain on rat tail tenocytes. *Mol Biol Rep.* 2010 Jul 15;37(6):2629–34. Available from: http://link.springer.com/10.1007/s11033-009-9788-8.
62. Shi Y, Fu Y, Tong W, Geng Y, Lui PPY, Tang T, et al. Uniaxial mechanical tension promoted osteogenic differentiation of rat tendon-derived stem cells (rTDSCs) via the Wnt5a-RhoA pathway. *J Cell Biochem.* 2012;113(10):3133–42. Available from: https://onlinelibrary.wiley.com/doi/10.1002/jcb.24190.
63. Zeichen J, van Griensven M, Bosch U. The proliferative response of isolated human tendon fibroblasts to cyclic biaxial mechanical strain. *Am J Sports Med.* 2000;28(6):888–92. Available from: http://journals.sagepub.com/doi/10.1177/03635465000280061901.
64. Barkhausen T, van Griensven M, Zeichen J, Bosch U. Modulation of cell functions of human tendon fibroblasts by different repetitive cyclic mechanical stress patterns. *Exp Toxicol Pathol.* 2003;55(2–3):153–8. Available from: https://linkinghub.elsevier.com/retrieve/pii/S0940299304701542.
65. Rui YF, Lui PPY, Ni M, Chan LS, Lee YW, Chan KM. Mechanical loading increased BMP-2 expression which promoted osteogenic differentiation of tendon-derived stem cells. *J Orthop Res.* 2011;29(3):390–6.
66. Nam HY, Pingguan-Murphy B, Amir Abbas A, Mahmood Merican A, Kamarul T. The proliferation and tenogenic differentiation potential of bone marrow-derived mesenchymal stromal cell are influenced by specific uniaxial cyclic tensile loading conditions. *Biomech Model Mechanobiol.* 2015;14(3):649–63. Available from: http://doi.org/10.1007/s10237-014-0628-y.
67. Zhang L, Kahn CJF, Chen HQ, Tran N, Wang X. Effect of uniaxial stretching on rat bone mesenchymal stem cell: Orientation and expressions of collagen types I and III and tenascin-C. *Cell Biol Int.* 2008;32(3):344–52. Available from: http://doi.wiley.com/10.1016/j.cellbi.2007.12.018.

68. Wang JHC, Jia F, Yang G, Yang S, Campbell BH, Stone D, et al. Cyclic mechanical stretching of human tendon fibroblasts increases the production of prostaglandin E 2 and levels of cyclooxygenase expression: A novel in vitro model study. *Connect Tissue Res.* 2003;44(3–4):128–33. Available from: http://www.tandfonline.com/doi/full/10.1080/03008200390223909.
69. Wang JHC, Yang G, Li Z, Shen W. Fibroblast responses to cyclic mechanical stretching depend on cell orientation to the stretching direction. *J Biomech.* 2004;37(4):573–6. Available from: https://linkinghub.elsevier.com/retrieve/pii/S0021929003003452.
70. Wang JHC, Yang G, Li Z. Controlling cell responses to cyclic mechanical stretching. *Ann Biomed Eng.* 2005;33(3):337–42. Available from: http://link.springer.com/10.1007/s10439-005-1736-8.
71. Yang G, Crawford RC, Wang JHC. Proliferation and collagen production of human patellar tendon fibroblasts in response to cyclic uniaxial stretching in serum-free conditions. *J Biomech.* 2004;37(10):1543–50. Available from: https://linkinghub.elsevier.com/retrieve/pii/S002192900400034X.
72. Yang G, Im HJ, Wang JHC. Repetitive mechanical stretching modulates IL-1β induced COX-2, MMP-1 expression, and PGE2 production in human patellar tendon fibroblasts. *Gene.* 2005;363(1–2):166–72. Available from: /pmc/articles/PMC2901527/.
73. Zhang J, Wang JHC. The effects of mechanical loading on tendons - An in vivo and in vitro model study. Roeder RK, editor. *PLoS One.* 2013;8(8):e71740. Available from: https://dx.plos.org/10.1371/journal.pone.0071740.
74. Chen W, Deng Y, Zhang J, Tang K. Uniaxial repetitive mechanical overloading induces influx of extracellular calcium and cytoskeleton disruption in human tenocytes. *Cell Tissue Res.* 2015;359(2):577–87.
75. Zhang J, Wang JHC. Mechanobiological response of tendon stem cells: Implications of tendon homeostasis and pathogenesis of tendinopathy. *J Orthop Res.* 2010;28(5):639–43. Available from: https://onlinelibrary.wiley.com/doi/10.1002/jor.21046.
76. Garvin J, Qi J, Maloney M, Banes AJ. Novel system for engineering bioartificial tendons and application of mechanical load. *Tissue Eng.* 2003;9(5):967–79. Available from: https://www.liebertpub.com/doi/10.1089/107632703322495619.
77. Jones ER, Jones GC, Legerlotz K, Riley GP. Cyclical strain modulates metalloprotease and matrix gene expression in human tenocytes via activation of TGFβ. *Biochim Biophys Acta Mol Cell Res.* 2013;1833(12):2596–607. Available from: https://linkinghub.elsevier.com/retrieve/pii/S0167488913002425.
78. Hannafin JA, Arnoczky SP. Effect of cyclic and static tensile loading on water content and solute diffusion in canine flexor tendons: An in vitro study. *J Orthop Res.* 1994;12(3):350–6. Available from: https://pubmed.ncbi.nlm.nih.gov/8207588/.
79. Hannafin JA, Arnoczky SP, Hoonjan A, Torzilli PA. Effect of stress deprivation and cyclic tensile loading on the material and morphologic properties of canine flexor digitorum profundus tendon: An in vitro study. *J Orthop Res.* 1995;13(6):907–14.
80. Bangalore Integrated System Solutions Pvt Ltd. LigaGen: Tension Bioreactor Systems. 2015 [cited 2022 Apr 25]. Available from: http://www.tissuegrowth.com/prod_ligament.cfm.
81. TA Instruments. BioDynamic 5200. 2016 [cited 2022 Apr 25]. Available from: https://tainstruments.com.cn/5200-products/?lang=en.
82. EBERS Medical Technology SL. TC-3 Bioreactor. [cited 2022 Apr 25]. Available from: https://ebersmedical.com/tissue-engineering/bioreactors/load-culture/tc-3.
83. CellScale. MechanoCulture J1. [cited 2022 Apr 25]. Available from: https://www.cellscale.com/products/mcj1/.
84. Thorfinn J, Angelidis IK, Gigliello L, Pham HM, Lindsey D, Chang J. Bioreactor optimization of tissue engineered rabbit flexor tendons in vivo. *J Hand Surg*

(European Volume). 2012;37(2):109–14. Available from: http://journals.sagepub.com/doi/10.1177/1753193411419439.

85. Barber JG, Handorf AM, Allee TJ, Li WJ. Braided nanofibrous scaffold for tendon and ligament tissue engineering. *Tissue Eng Part A*. 2013;19(11–12):1265–74. Available from: https://www.liebertpub.com/doi/10.1089/ten.tea.2010.0538.
86. Bosworth LA, Rathbone SR, Bradley RS, Cartmell SH. Dynamic loading of electrospun yarns guides mesenchymal stem cells towards a tendon lineage. *J Mech Behav Biomed Mater.* 2014;39:175–83. Available from: http://doi.org/10.1016/j.jmbbm.2014.07.009.
87. Bourdón-Santoyo M, Quiñones-Uriostegui I, Martínez-López V, Sánchez-Arévalo F, Alessi-Montero A, Velasquillo C, et al. Preliminary study of an in vitro development of new tissue applying mechanical stimulation with a bioreactor as an alternative for ligament reconstruction. *Rev Invest Clin.* 2014;66 Suppl 1(August 2020):S100–10. Available from: http://www.ncbi.nlm.nih.gov/pubmed/25264790.
88. Wu S, Wang Y, Streubel PN, Duan B. Living nanofiber yarn-based woven biotextiles for tendon tissue engineering using cell tri-culture and mechanical stimulation. *Acta Biomater.* 2017;62:102–15. Available from: https://doi.org/10.1016/j.actbio.2017.08.043.
89. Sensini A, Cristofolini L, Zucchelli A, Focarete ML, Gualandi C, de Mori A, et al. Hierarchical electrospun tendon-ligament bioinspired scaffolds induce changes in fibroblasts morphology under static and dynamic conditions. *J Microsc.* 2020;277(3):160–9. Available from: https://onlinelibrary.wiley.com/doi/10.1111/jmi.12827.
90. Jayasree A, Kottappally Thankappan S, Ramachandran R, Sundaram MN, Chen CH, Mony U, et al. Bioengineered braided micro–nano (multiscale) fibrous scaffolds for tendon reconstruction. *ACS Biomater Sci Eng.* 2019;5(3):1476–86. Available from: https://pubs.acs.org/doi/10.1021/acsbiomaterials.8b01328.
91. Chen CH, Li DL, Chuang ADC, Dash BS, Chen JP. Tension stimulation of tenocytes in aligned hyaluronic acid/platelet-rich plasma-polycaprolactone core-sheath nanofiber membrane scaffold for tendon tissue engineering. *Int J Mol Sci.* 2021;22(20):11215. Available from: https://www.mdpi.com/1422-0067/22/20/11215.
92. Baumgartner W, Wolint P, Hofmann S, Nüesch C, Calcagni M, Brunelli M, et al. Impact of electrospun piezoelectric core–shell PVDFhfp/PDMS mesh on tenogenic and inflammatory gene expression in human adipose-derived stem cells: Comparison of static cultivation with uniaxial cyclic tensile stretching. *Bioengineering.* 2022;9(1):21. Available from: https://www.mdpi.com/2306-5354/9/1/21.
93. Govoni M, Muscari C, Lovecchio J, Guarnieri C, Giordano E. Mechanical actuation systems for the phenotype commitment of stem cell-based tendon and ligament tissue substitutes. *Stem Cell Rev Rep.* 2016;12(2):189–201. Available from: http://link.springer.com/10.1007/s12015-015-9640-6.
94. Nguyen TD, Liang R, Woo SLY, Burton SD, Wu C, Almarza A, et al. Effects of cell seeding and cyclic stretch on the fiber remodeling in an extracellular matrix–derived bioscaffold. *Tissue Eng Part A.* 2009;15(4):957–63. Available from: https://www.liebertpub.com/doi/10.1089/ten.tea.2007.0384.
95. Doroski DM, Levenston ME, Temenoff JS. Cyclic tensile culture promotes fibroblastic differentiation of marrow stromal cells encapsulated in poly(ethylene glycol)-based hydrogels. *Tissue Eng Part A.* 2010;16(11):3457–66. Available from: https://www.liebertpub.com/doi/10.1089/ten.tea.2010.0233.
96. Juncosa-Melvin N, Shearn JT, Boivin GP, Gooch C, Galloway MT, West JR, et al. Effects of mechanical stimulation on the biomechanics and histology of stem cell–collagen sponge constructs for rabbit patellar tendon repair. *Tissue Eng.* 2006;12(8):2291–300. Available from: https://www.liebertpub.com/doi/10.1089/ten.2006.12.2291.
97. Nirmalanandhan VS, Rao M, Shearn JT, Juncosa-Melvin N, Gooch C, Butler DL. Effect of scaffold material, construct length and mechanical stimulation on the in vitro

stiffness of the engineered tendon construct. *J Biomech.* 2008;41(4):822–8. Available from: https://linkinghub.elsevier.com/retrieve/pii/S0021929007004794.

98. Chen JL, Yin Z, Shen WL, Chen X, Heng BC, Zou XH, et al. Efficacy of hESC-MSCs in knitted silk-collagen scaffold for tendon tissue engineering and their roles. *Biomaterials.* 2010;31(36):9438–51. Available from: http://doi.org/10.1016/j.biomaterials.2010.08.011.
99. Webb K, Hitchcock RW, Smeal RM, Li W, Gray SD, Tresco PA. Cyclic strain increases fibroblast proliferation, matrix accumulation, and elastic modulus of fibroblast-seeded polyurethane constructs. *J Biomech.* 2006;39(6):1136–44.
100. Altman GH, Lu HH, Horan RL, Calabro T, Ryder D, Kaplan DL, et al. Advanced bioreactor with controlled application of multi-dimensional strain for tissue engineering. *J Biomech Eng.* 2002;124(6):742–9. Available from: https://asmedigitalcollection.asme.org/biomechanical/article/124/6/742/450706/Advanced-Bioreactor-with-Controlled-Application-of.
101. Pedaprolu K, Szczesny SE. A novel, open-source, low-cost bioreactor for load-controlled cyclic loading of tendon explants. *J Biomech Eng.* 2022;144(8):1–8. Available from: https://asmedigitalcollection.asme.org/biomechanical/article/144/8/084505/1135618/A-Novel-Open-Source-Low-Cost-Bioreactor-for-Load.
102. Devkota AC, Weinhold PS. A tissue explant system for assessing tendon overuse injury. *Med Eng Phys.* 2005;27(9):803–8. Available from: http://doi.org/10.1016/j.medengphy.2005.02.008.
103. Asundi KR, Kursa K, Lotz J, Rempel DM. In vitro system for applying cyclic loads to connective tissues under displacement or force control. *Ann Biomed Eng.* 2007;35(7):1188–95.
104. Viens M, Chauvette G, Langelier È. A roadmap for the design of bioreactors in mechanobiological research and engineering of load-bearing tissues. *J Med Device.* 2011;5(4). Available from: https://asmedigitalcollection.asme.org/medicaldevices/article/5/4/041006/477562/A-Roadmap-for-the-Design-of-Bioreactors-in.
105. Walser J, Ferguson SJ, Gantenbein-Ritter B. Design of a mechanical loading device to culture intact bovine spinal motion segments under multiaxial motion. In: *Replacing Animal Models.* Wiley; 2012. pp. 89–105. Available from: https://onlinelibrary.wiley.com/doi/10.1002/9781119940685.ch9.
106. Wang T, Chen P, Chen L, Zhou Y, Wang A, Zheng Q, et al. Reduction of mechanical loading in tendons induces heterotopic ossification and activation of the β-catenin signaling pathway. *J Orthop Translat.* 2021;29(March):42–50. Available from: https://linkinghub.elsevier.com/retrieve/pii/S2214031X21000206.
107. Kreja L, Liedert A, Schlenker H, Brenner RE, Fiedler J, Friemert B, et al. Effects of mechanical strain on human mesenchymal stem cells and ligament fibroblasts in a textured poly(l-lactide) scaffold for ligament tissue engineering. *J Mater Sci Mater Med.* 2012;23(10):2575–82. Available from: http://link.springer.com/10.1007/s10856-012-4710-7.
108. Nirmalanandhan VS, Dressler MR, Shearn JT, Juncosa-Melvin N, Rao M, Gooch C, et al. Mechanical stimulation of tissue engineered tendon constructs: Effect of scaffold materials. *J Biomech Eng.* 2007;129(6):919–23.
109. Juncosa-Melvin N, Matlin KS, Holdcraft RW, Nirmalanandhan VS, Butler DL. Mechanical stimulation increases collagen type I and collagen type III gene expression of stem cell–collagen sponge constructs for patellar tendon repair. *Tissue Eng.* 2007;13(6):1219–26. Available from: https://www.liebertpub.com/doi/10.1089/ten.2006.0339.
110. Breidenbach AP, Dyment NA, Lu Y, Rao M, Shearn JT, Rowe DW, et al. Fibrin gels exhibit improved biological, structural, and mechanical properties compared with collagen gels in cell-based tendon tissue-engineered constructs. *Tissue Eng Part A.* 2015;21(3–4):438–50. Available from: https://www.liebertpub.com/doi/10.1089/ten.tea.2013.0768.

111. Grier W, Moy A, Harley B. Cyclic tensile strain enhances human mesenchymal stem cell Smad 2/3 activation and tenogenic differentiation in anisotropic collagen-glycosaminoglycan scaffolds. *Eur Cell Mater.* 2017;33:227–39. Available from: http://ecmjournal.org/journal/papers/vol033/pdf/v033a17.pdf.
112. Brandt L, Schubert S, Scheibe P, Brehm W, Franzen J, Gross C, et al. Tenogenic properties of mesenchymal progenitor cells are compromised in an inflammatory environment. *Int J Mol Sci.* 2018;19(9):2549. Available from: http://www.mdpi.com/1422-0067/19/9/2549.
113. Talò G, D'Arrigo D, Lorenzi S, Moretti M, Lovati AB. Independent, controllable stretch-perfusion bioreactor chambers to functionalize cell-seeded decellularized tendons. *Ann Biomed Eng.* 2020 Mar 8;48(3):1112–26. Available from: http://link.springer.com/10.1007/s10439-019-02257-6.
114. Lim D, Renteria ES, Sime DS, Ju YM, Kim JH, Criswell T, et al. Bioreactor design and validation for manufacturing strategies in tissue engineering. *Biodes Manuf.* 2022;5(1):43–63. Available from: https://doi.org/10.1007/s42242-021-00154-3.
115. Lei Y, Ferdous Z. Design considerations and challenges for mechanical stretch bioreactors in tissue engineering. *Biotechnol Prog.* 2016;32(3):543–53. Available from: https://onlinelibrary.wiley.com/doi/10.1002/btpr.2256.
116. Butler DL, Hunter SA, Chokalingam K, Cordray MJ, Shearn J, Juncosa-Melvin N, et al. Using functional tissue engineering and bioreactors to mechanically stimulate tissue-engineered constructs. *Tissue Eng Part A.* 2009;15(4):741–9. Available from: /pmc/articles/PMC2792090/.
117. Hohlrieder M, Teuschl AH, Cicha K, van Griensven M, Redl H, Stampfl J. Bioreactor and scaffold design for the mechanical stimulation of anterior cruciate ligament grafts. *Biomed Mater Eng.* 2013;23(3):225–37.
118. Parent G, Huppé N, Langelier E. Low stress tendon fatigue is a relatively rapid process in the context of overuse injuries. *Ann Biomed Eng.* 2011;39(5):1535–45. Available from: http://link.springer.com/10.1007/s10439-011-0254-0.
119. Xu Y, Wang Q, Li Y, Gan Y, Li P, Li S, et al. Cyclic tensile strain induces tenogenic differentiation of tendon-derived stem cells in bioreactor culture. *Biomed Res Int.* 2015;2015:1–13. Available from: http://www.hindawi.com/journals/bmri/2015/790804/.
120. Tempfer H, Spitzer G, Lehner C, Wagner A, Gehwolf R, Fierlbeck J, et al. VEGF-D-mediated signaling in tendon cells is involved in degenerative processes. *Faseb J.* 2022;36(2):1–13. Available from: https://onlinelibrary.wiley.com/doi/10.1096/fj.202100773RRR.
121. Tohidnezhad M, Zander J, Slowik A, Kubo Y, Dursun G, Willenberg W, et al. Impact of uniaxial stretching on both gliding and traction areas of tendon explants in a novel bioreactor. *Int J Mol Sci.* 2020;21(8):2925. Available from: https://www.mdpi.com/1422-0067/21/8/2925.
122. Jafari L, Lemieux-LaNeuville Y, Gagnon D, Langelier E. Low amplitude characterization tests conducted at regular intervals can affect tendon mechanobiological response. *Ann Biomed Eng.* 2014;42(3):589–99. Available from: http://link.springer.com/10.1007/s10439-013-0916-1.
123. Govoni M, Berardi AC, Muscari C, Campardelli R, Bonafè F, Guarnieri C, et al. An engineered multiphase three-dimensional microenvironment to ensure the controlled delivery of cyclic strain and human growth differentiation factor 5 for the tenogenic commitment of human bone marrow mesenchymal stem cells. *Tissue Eng Part A.* 2017;23(15–16):811–22. Available from: https://www.liebertpub.com/doi/10.1089/ten.tea.2016.0407.
124. Rinoldi C, Fallahi A, Yazdi IK, Campos Paras J, Kijeńska-Gawrońska E, Trujillo-de Santiago G, et al. Mechanical and biochemical stimulation of 3D multilayered scaffolds for tendon tissue engineering. *ACS Biomater Sci Eng.* 2019 Jun 10;5(6):2953–64. Available from: https://pubs.acs.org/doi/10.1021/acsbiomaterials.8b01647.

125. Shearn JT, Juncosa-Melvin N, Boivin GP, Galloway MT, Goodwin W, Gooch C, et al. Mechanical stimulation of tendon tissue engineered constructs: Effects on construct stiffness, repair biomechanics, and their correlation. *J Biomech Eng.* 2007;129(6):848–54. Available from: https://pubmed.ncbi.nlm.nih.gov/18067388/.
126. Androjna C, Spragg RK, Derwin KA. Mechanical conditioning of cell-seeded small intestine submucosa: A potential tissue-engineering strategy for tendon repair. *Tissue Eng.* 2007;13(2):233–43. Available from: https://www.liebertpub.com/doi/10.1089/ten.2006.0050.
127. Engebretson B, Mussett ZR, Sikavitsas VI. Tenocytic extract and mechanical stimulation in a tissue-engineered tendon construct increases cellular proliferation and ECM deposition. *Biotechnol J.* 2017;12(3):1600595. Available from: https://onlinelibrary.wiley.com/doi/10.1002/biot.201600595.
128. Lee J, Guarino V, Gloria A, Ambrosio L, Tae G, Kim YH, et al. Regeneration of Achilles' tendon: the role of dynamic stimulation for enhanced cell proliferation and mechanical properties. *J Biomater Sci Polym Ed.* 2010;21(8–9):1173–90. Available from: https://www.tandfonline.com/doi/full/10.1163/092050609X12471222313524.
129. Issa RI, Engebretson B, Rustom L, McFetridge PS, Sikavitsas VI. The effect of cell seeding density on the cellular and mechanical properties of a mechanostimulated tissue-engineered tendon. *Tissue Eng Part A.* 2011;17(11–12):1479–87. Available from: https://www.liebertpub.com/doi/10.1089/ten.tea.2010.0484.
130. Wang B, Liu W, Zhang Y, Jiang Y, Zhang WJ, Zhou G, et al. Engineering of extensor tendon complex by an ex vivo approach. *Biomaterials.* 2008 Jul;29(20):2954–61. Available from: https://linkinghub.elsevier.com/retrieve/pii/S0142961208002081.
131. Peroglio M, Gaspar D, Zeugolis DI, Alini M. Relevance of bioreactors and whole tissue cultures for the translation of new therapies to humans. *J Orthop Res.* 2017;36(1):10–21. Available from: https://pubmed.ncbi.nlm.nih.gov/28718947/.
132. Hsiao MY, Lin PC, Lin AC, Wu YW, Chen WS, Lin FH. Oxidized hyaluronic acid/adipic acid dihydrazide hydrogel as drug-carrier for cytoprotective medications—Preliminary results. *Biomed Eng* (Singapore). 2019;31(05):1950036. Available from: https://www.worldscientific.com/doi/abs/10.4015/S1016237219500364.
133. Triantafillopoulos IK, Banes AJ, Bowman KF, Maloney M, Garrett WE, Karas SG. Nandrolone Decanoate and load increase remodeling and strength in human supraspinatus bioartificial tendons. *Am J Sports Med.* 2004;32(4):934–43. Available from: http://journals.sagepub.com/doi/10.1177/0363546503261700.
134. Fenwick N, Griffin G, Gauthier C. The welfare of animals used in science: How the "Three Rs" ethic guides improvements. *Can Vet J.* 2009;50(5):523–30. Available from: /pmc/articles/PMC2671878/.
135. Russell WMS, Burch RL. The principles of humane experimental technique. *Med J Aust.* 1960;1(13):500–500. Available from: https://onlinelibrary.wiley.com/doi/abs/10.5694/j.1326-5377.1960.tb73127.x.
136. Gantenbein B, Frauchiger DA, May RD, Bakirci E, Rohrer U, Grad S. Developing bioreactors to host joint-derived tissues that require mechanical stimulation. In: *Reference Module in Biomedical Sciences.* Elsevier; 2019. pp. 261–80. Available from: http://doi.org/10.1016/B978-0-12-801238-3.65611-8.
137. Jiang Y, Liu H, Li H, Wang F, Cheng K, Zhou G, et al. A proteomic analysis of engineered tendon formation under dynamic mechanical loading in vitro. *Biomaterials.* 2011;32(17):4085–95. Available from: https://linkinghub.elsevier.com/retrieve/pii/S0142961211001852.
138. Castro APG, Paul CPL, Detiger SEL, Smit TH, van Royen BJ, Pimenta Claro JC, et al. Long-term creep behavior of the intervertebral disk: comparison between bioreactor data and numerical results. *Front Bioeng Biotechnol.* 2014;2(NOV):56. Available from: http://journal.frontiersin.org/article/10.3389/fbioe.2014.00056/abstract.

12 Bioprinted Combined Medicinal Products

Regulatory Challenges for Their Authorization and Commercialization

Eva Martín-Becerra, Rossana García-Castro, and Ana Torres-García
Gradocell

CONTENTS

12.1 INTRODUCTION

Products that affect human health are heavily regulated to guarantee the quality of their production, as well as their safety and efficacy, which must be demonstrated in non-clinical and clinical studies, prior to their authorization and marketing.

Regulations and standards are set by individual governments and the regulatory agencies and/or other competent authorities are responsible for oversight to ensure that health risks are minimized, and compliance is achieved in each territory.

The regulatory framework of the different countries or regions may contemplate some differences in the regulatory definitions, but in general, we can classify the products into medicinal products for human use, medical devices, food and food supplements, herbal medicinal products, cosmetics, tissue transplants, biocides, and hygiene products.

Among medicinal products for human use, according to the origin of their active pharmaceutical ingredients (API), we distinguish between chemical-based drugs and biological medicinal products, which are in turn classified into vaccines, biotechnological products, blood products, and advanced therapy medicinal products (ATMPs), which are therapies based on genes, tissues, or cells.

DOI: 10.1201/9781003274568-12

The legislation in force in each territory will define the requirements to be met by products used for human or animal health, food, or hygiene. However, as Figure 12.1 shows, this classification is not entirely obvious, and it is not uncommon to find borderline products that are difficult to classify under a single regulatory framework. This is more complex in the case of products containing components classified as different from a regulatory point of view, known as *combined products.*

The boundaries between the different types of products are not always clearly defined, and when it comes to determining which regulatory framework should be applied to their marketing, difficulties can arise, and it depends directly on the legislation applicable in each territory. The same product may, for example, be defined as a drug in one country but considered a cosmetic product in another.

Moreover, even when considering a single legislation, we may encounter borderline products, which will be difficult to classify. In case of doubt, it will be up to the regulatory agencies to decide, on a case-by-case basis, which regulatory framework is applicable to a specific product.

In addition, regulatory classification can change significantly between different territories and due to the entry into force of new regulations or standards.

Taking into account the classification of the product, we have to comply with specific requirements according to the applicable regulatory framework, and different

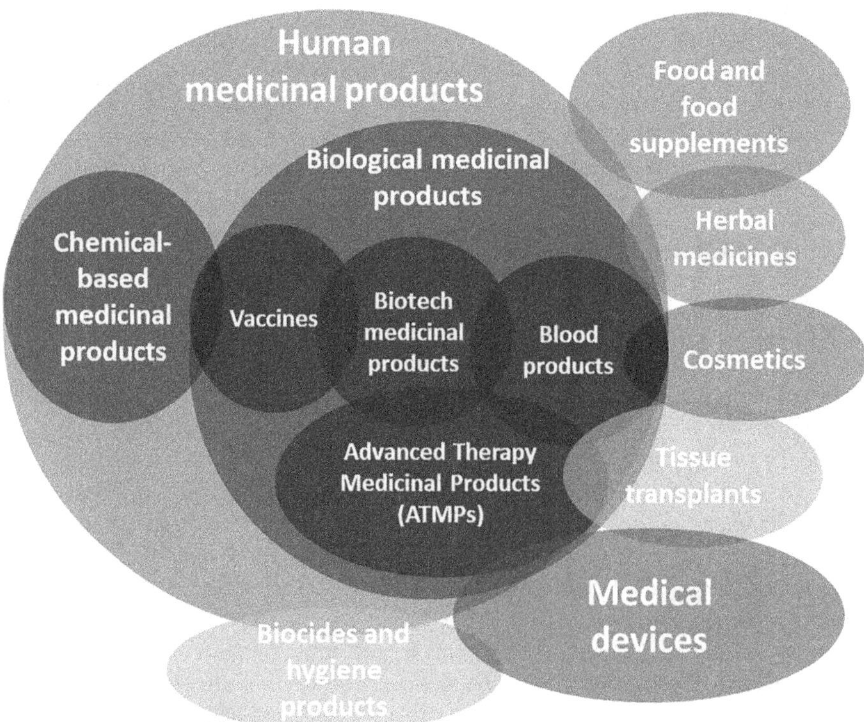

FIGURE 12.1 Classification of different products according to their regulatory definition.

competent authorities will oversee the evaluation and authorization, depending on the territory where the product intends to be launched (Figure 12.2).

Therefore, the product classification will have a significant impact on the timing and costs of the product development plan, as well as on the steps to be taken to obtain marketing authorization.

The legislation applicable to a type of product in a specific territory will mark different key aspects that we will have to take into account in our commercialization strategy, such as:

- Will we need to adapt our facilities to manufacture the product under a specific quality system? Will we need to obtain a specific International Standard Organization (ISO) certification or good manufacturing practices (GMP) accreditation?
- Is animal and/or human testing necessary to demonstrate the safety and efficacy of the product?
- Which regulatory agencies and/or public or private institutions will be responsible for granting marketing authorization or authorizing clinical trials, if necessary?

For instance, the commercialization of medicinal products for human use will require the involvement of a medicine's agency in most territories in order to obtain a marketing authorization.

In the case of the European Union (EU), there is a national medicines agency in each Member State, and a regional medicines agency, the European Medicines Agency (EMA). The EMA is responsible for assessing the quality, safety, and efficacy of marketing authorization applications evaluated through the centralized procedure. In the event of a positive scientific opinion, the European Commission (EC) will grant a marketing authorization valid throughout the EU. On the other side, in the United States, the Food and Drug Administration (FDA) is the competent authority for the evaluation of drugs for human use.

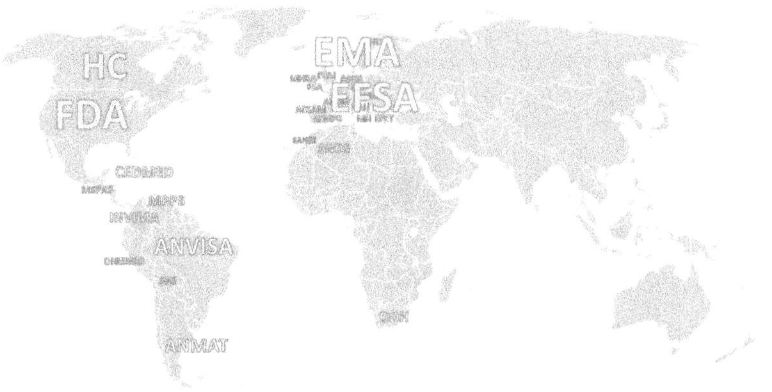

FIGURE 12.2 Examples of regulatory agencies from different countries and regions.

In the case of other health products, such as medical devices, cosmetics, or food supplements, there are different formulas in each territory: sometimes the regulatory agency holds competencies in most of the regulatory issues, as in the case of the FDA, but in other regions, there are specific agencies.

In the EU, some competences are held by the national agencies, as in the case of cosmetics of biocides, while they have a specific regional body for establishing regulations related to food safety, the European Food Safety Agency (EFSA).

Furthermore, all medical devices placed on the EU market must undergo a conformity assessment to demonstrate that they meet the legal requirements to ensure that they are safe and perform as intended, and for this purpose Member States can appoint accredited Notified Bodies to carry out conformity assessments.

Conformity assessment usually involves an audit of the manufacturer's quality system and, depending on the type of device, a review of the manufacturer's technical documentation on the safety and performance of the product.

Once this assessment has been successfully passed, manufacturers can affix the *Conformité Européenne* (CE) marking to the medical device, complying with several requirements (Figure 12.3):

- If the CE marking is reduced or enlarged, the proportions must be respected.
- The various elements of the CE marking shall have substantially the same vertical dimension, which may not be less than 5 mm. Exceptions to the minimum dimension are allowed for small products.
- It shall be affixed visibly, legibly, and indelibly on the product or on its sterile packaging. If this is not possible, it shall be placed on the container. In addition, it should appear on all instructions for use and on all sales packaging.
- It shall be followed by the identification number of the notified body responsible for the conformity assessment procedure (four digits). In the case of self-marking products, the CE marking shall not be followed by the digits.

At the European level, the authorization of medical devices is excluded from the centralized authorization procedure, although the EMA can provide scientific advice and prepare guidelines related to the regulation of certain medical devices.

This is the case for medical devices that are used in combination with medicinal products or are manufactured with substances that are absorbed by the human body

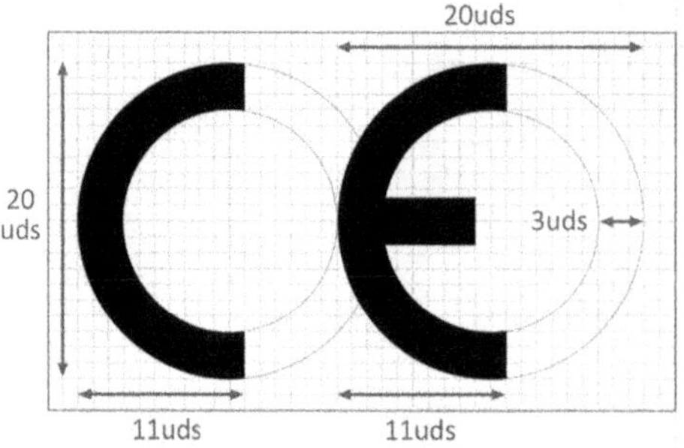

CE
0318

FIGURE 12.3 CE marking and CE marking assessed by Notified Body 0318 (AEMPS).

to achieve their intended purpose. It will be necessary to assess the safety and performance of the device in relation to its use with the medicinal product or with its different components.

Similarly, for in vitro diagnostic medical devices that are used for therapeutic decision making, identifying patients who are suitable or unsuitable for a specific treatment, it will be necessary to obtain a scientific opinion on the suitability of the companion diagnostic.

The evaluation and issuing of these scientific reports will be the responsibility of the EMA if the medicinal product has been authorized by the centralized procedure; otherwise, the Notified Body may request the opinion of a national competent authority or the EMA.

In any case, the authorization of clinical trials with medical devices, the granting of manufacturer's licences, the certification of facilities, and the granting of the CE marking of conformity, among other activities related to medical devices, are the responsibility of the national regulatory agencies and/or the Notified Bodies.

12.2 COMBINATION OF MEDICAL DEVICES AND MEDICINAL PRODUCTS

Combinations of medical devices and medicinal products are known as *combined medicinal* products and are generally regulated as human medicinal products.

For the classification of this complex products, it has to be determined whether the main intended action is achieved by the medicinal component or by the medical device. Typically, the function of the medical device in combination with medicinal products is to enable the administration of the medicinal product and/or to provide a mechanical or supportive function.

In these cases, it is considered a medicinal product that includes a medical device (combined medicinal product), and the entire combined medicinal product is regulated by EU pharmaceutical legislation (Directive 2001/83/EC and EMA/CHMP/QWP/BWP/259165/2019) and an integral medicinal product marketing authorization must be obtained.

In the EU, this marketing authorization can be obtained through the national competent authorities of the different members, known as the national procedure, or through the centralized procedure, with evaluation by the EMA.

It is important to note that when the active therapeutic components are based on genes, tissues, or cells, they are classified as ATMPs, and therefore, according to EU pharmaceutical legislation (EU Regulation 1394/2007), all ATMPs are authorized centrally through the EMA, in a single evaluation and authorization procedure.

The ATMPs that contain one or more medical devices as an integral part of the medicine, are classified as *combined ATMPs*, and these products must comply with the Directive 2001/83/EC (consolidated version 16/11/2012) of November 2001 relating to medicinal products for human use; Regulation (EC) No. 1394/2007, which provides the overall framework for ATMPs; the Directive 2009/120/EC (amending Directive 2001/83/EC), which updated the definitions and detailed scientific and technical requirements for gene therapy medicinal products and somatic cell therapy medicinal products, and include detailed scientific and technical requirements for tissue-engineered products, as well as for ATMPs containing devices and combined

ATMPs; and Regulation (EC) No. 726/2004 (consolidated version 5/6/2013) of March 2004 on procedures for the authorization and supervision of medicines for human and veterinary use and establishing the EMA.

As established in the Regulation EU 1394/2007, a *Combined advanced therapy medicinal product* means an advanced therapy medicinal product that fulfils the following conditions:

- it must incorporate, as an integral part of the product, one or more medical devices within the meaning of Article 1(2)(a) of Directive 93/42/EEC or one or more active implantable medical devices within the meaning of Article 1(2)(c) of Directive 90/385/EEC, and
- its cellular or tissue part must contain viable cells or tissues, or
- its cellular or tissue part containing non-viable cells or tissues must be liable to act upon the human body with action that can be considered as primary to that of the devices referred to

Nevertheless, we must consider specific requirements for the medical device, as established in the he Regulation on Medical Devices in the EU (Regulation EU 2017/745 of 5 April 2017):

1. A medical device which forms part of a combined advanced therapy medicinal product shall meet the essential requirements laid down in Annex I to Directive 93/42/EEC.
2. An active implantable medical device which forms part of a combined advanced therapy medicinal product shall meet the essential requirements laid down in Annex 1 to Directive 90/385/EEC.

In addition, Regulation EU 2017/745 defines that all medical devices must undergo a conformity assessment to demonstrate they meet legal requirements to ensure they are safe and perform as intended.

The Certification of UNE-EN ISO 13485:2016 Standard about quality management systems for medical devices is required for regulatory purposes related to conformity assessment CE. As mentioned in the previous section, the CE marking of conformity or CE marking is issued once a medical device has passed a conformity assessment by Notified Body (at least, assessment of technical documentation with essential requirements compliance and manufacturer ISO 13485:2016 certification).

The conformity assessment involves an audit of the manufacturer's quality system and, depending on the type of device, a review of technical documentation from the manufacturer on the safety and performance of the device. This assessment is carried out by accredited Notified Bodies.

Nevertheless, this is only mandatory when the devices are intended to commercialize alone, and this requirement will not be applicable when combined with medicinal products.

In addition to the requirements laid down in Article 6(1) of Regulation (EC) No. 726/2004, applications for the authorization of an advanced therapy medicinal product containing medical devices, biomaterials, scaffolds, or matrices shall include a description of the physical characteristics and performance of the product and a description of the product design methods, in accordance with Annex I to Directive 2001/83/EC.

The legal framework in force (Regulation EU 2017/745) introduces new responsibilities for EMA and national competent authorities in the assessment of certain categories of medical device (among them, the medical device in combination with a medicinal product).

The regulation establishes that if the principal intended action of the product is achieved by the medicine (not by the medical device); the product is considered a medicinal product that includes a medical device, and therefore, the entire product is regulated under EU pharmaceutical legislation (Directive 2001/83/EC) and must obtain a marketing authorization for a medicinal product.

However, the marketing authorization application should include a CE certificate for the device or, if not CE marked but would need to be certified if marketed separately, applicant must include an opinion from a Notified Body on conformity of device.

In the Article 9 of the Regulation EU 1394/2007 for ATMPs, the following is specified regarding the evaluation procedure of combined ATMPs:

1. Where a combined advanced therapy medicinal product is concerned, the whole product shall be subject to final evaluation by the Agency.
2. The application for a marketing authorisation for a combined advanced therapy medicinal product shall include evidence of conformity with the essential requirements referred to in Article 6.
3. The application for a marketing authorisation for a combined advanced therapy medicinal product shall include, where available, the results of the assessment by a notified body in accordance with Directive 93/42/EEC or Directive 90/385/EEC of the medical device part or active implantable medical device part.

   The Agency shall recognise the results of that assessment in its evaluation of the medicinal product concerned.

   The Agency may request the relevant notified body to transmit any information related to the results of its assessment. The notified body shall transmit the information within a period of 1 month.

   If the application does not include the results of the assessment, the Agency shall seek an opinion on the conformity of the device part with Annex I to Directive 93/42/EEC or Annex 1 to Directive 90/385/EEC from a notified body identified in conjunction with the applicant, unless the Committee for Advanced Therapies advised by its experts for medical devices decides that involvement of a notified body is not required.

In conclusion, the EMA will be responsible for evaluating the quality, safety, and efficacy of marketing authorization applications assessed through the centralized procedure, including the safety and performance of a medical device in relation to its use with a medicinal product.

All advanced therapy medicines and biotechnological medicinal products are authorized centrally, via EMA (single evaluation and authorization procedure).

As with all medicines, the Agency continues to monitor the safety and efficacy of advanced therapy medicines after they are approved and marketed.

In July 2021, the EMA issued a final guideline on quality documentation for medicinal products that include a medical device (EMA/CHMP/QWP/BWP/259165/2019). This guideline clarifies expectations laid down in Directive 2001/83/EC and addresses obligations in the Medical Devices Regulation, establishing the roles and responsibilities of both the EMA and the Notified Bodies in the assessment and authorization of these complex products.

12.3 BIOPRINTERS FOR THE MANUFACTURING OF MEDICINAL PRODUCTS

Bioprinting, also known as three-dimensional (3D) bioprinting, combines the 3D printing technology with biomaterials to replicate parts of the human body, such as tissue, cartilage, bone, blood vessels, and even an entire organ.

In the field of regenerative medicine, it is common to combine biomaterials with drugs, for example, to produce cellular scaffolds to repair damaged ligaments and joints.

A 3D bioprinter can add depth to the final product, which is very useful for recreating human tissues, as the bioprinter can distribute different biomaterials such as living cells, synthetic glue, or collagen scaffolds in layers, creating an object very similar to a natural part of the human body.

This process is called additive manufacturing and allows the materials fed into the printer to solidify into a 3D object. Previously, the bioprinter needs to receive a computer-generated image of the final product, known as *blueprint*, which can be based on a scan of the patient, to make a customized implant.

There are already 3D bioprinters available on the market for biomedical research, as is the case of the bioprinters marketed by the company CELLINK Bioprinting AB, one of the consortium members of the TriAnkle project (developed as a practical example in the following section) (Figure 12.4).

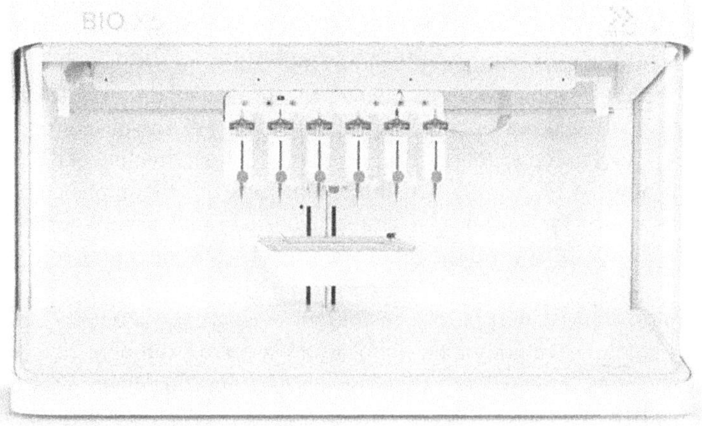

FIGURE 12.4 BIO X6™ bioprinter, CELLINK.

The materials used to produce these artificial live tissues are mostly composed of living cells and additional biomaterials, forming a composition called *bioink*, that will be fed into the bioprinter. The printer will read the digital file (*blueprint*) while printing out the materials in layers, creating one solid, stable piece.

The disruptive nature of 3D bioprinting technologies not only poses technical issues to become a truly effective tool for tissue engineering and regenerative medicine in clinical practice, but also challenges the current regulatory framework.

From the regulatory point of view to date there is not specific regulation for the bioprinting process. However, the use of 3D bioprinters to produce regenerative products containing cell or tissue engineering is considered under the European Commission (EC) Regulation on ATMPs, and therefore the principles applicable to the manufacturing of ATMPs are applicable to 3D bioprinting, as well as the EC Tissues and Cells Directive, the pharmaceutical regulations, or the new Medical Device Regulation, when combined medicinal products are manufactured using 3D bioprinters.

Specific elements of the 3D bioprinter must be considered to guarantee the quality of the final product among all the production processes, for instance the qualification equipment, including software information, and the location in a GMP/ISO-certified clean room, as well as the sterile or aseptic compliance. All these regulations will be applicable at different stages of production, affecting all the instruments (hardware and software) involved in the pre-printing, printing, and post-printing phases.

Therefore, 3D bioprinters will be considered a critical manufacturing equipment, and it must be ensured that the final product is obtained under aseptic process and according to the GMP or the applicable manufacturing standards.

When the 3D bioprinter is involved in the manufacturing of human medicinal products, they must comply with all the manufacturing requirements to ensure that the final product is safe and performs as intended.

Since GMP guidelines are also applicable to innovative automated manufacturing technologies (including 3D bioprinting) and ultimately applicable to all EU manufacturers or marketing authorization holders, these standards should be taken into account in the specific design and performance requirements of the 3D printer.

Special attention should be paid to automated aseptic manufacturing as described in the EU GMP Guidelines (EudraLex Volume 4, GMP Guidelines). In addition, it is important to consider specific aspects in the case of ATMP manufacturing (EudraLex Volume 4, GMP Guidelines, Part IV) when including live cells in the *bioink* (see Figure 12.5).

In addition, it should detail the relevant aspects in the combined ATMP manufacturing process, such as critical parameters in the 3D printing technology, in-process controls, and aseptic compliance.

To ensure that the 3D bioprinter is suitable for aseptic manufacturing, it has to be located in a GMP-certificated clean room. Also, the 3D bioprinter must be used, cleaned, maintained, and qualified in classified areas, and the 3D bioprinter software must be used in compliance with Design Qualification, Installation Qualification, Operational Qualification, and Performance Qualification and must be fully traceable.

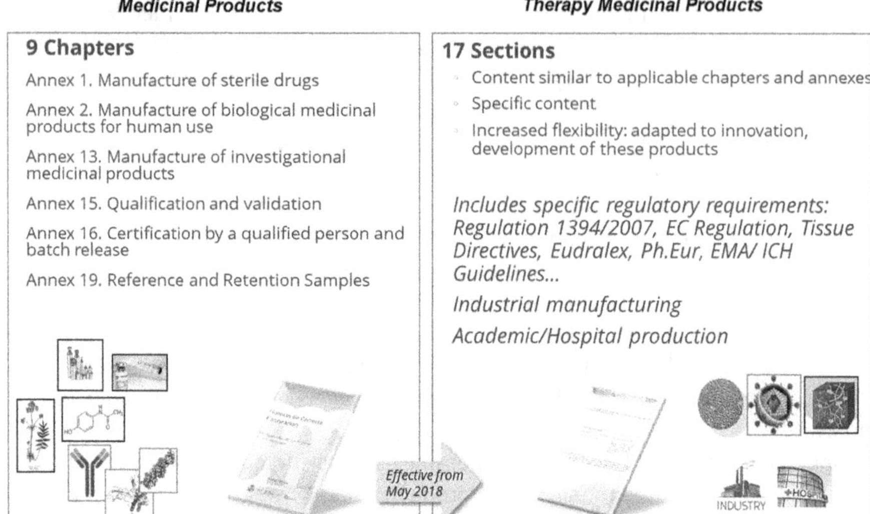

FIGURE 12.5 EudraLex Volume 4, GMP guidelines, part IV specific requirements for ATMPs.

Therefore, the aseptic processes will be carried out using 3D printing technology to demonstrate repeatability, reproducibility, homogeneity, and uniformity of the manufactured and final product, as well as the full validation of the GMP.

Moreover, although the 3D printer equipment is not classified as a medical device according to definitions of Regulation EU 2017/745, it also requires the CE conformity marking for marketing authorization.

The European regulatory framework (Directive 2006/42/EC) related to machinery, equipment, and components requires the CE conformity marking for ensuring the health and safety of persons, in particular workers and consumers. As we previously described, the CE marking is the certification which guarantees that machinery conforms with the essential health and safety requirements covered by the harmonized standards.

In conclusion, the manufacturer of 3D printing equipment bears full responsibility for the conformity of the machinery, as well as its compliance with all applicable regulations related to the classification of the final product and its intended use.

12.4 TRIANKLE: A PRACTICAL EXAMPLE OF BIOPRINTED COMBINED MEDICINAL PRODUCT

The TriAnkle project will provide patients with tendinopathies such as Achilles tendon partial ruptures and cartilage injuries a suitable therapy, based on an innovative personalized collagen- and gelatine-based implants manufactured with 3D bioprinting technology.

The TriAnkle consortium consists of a team of 12 leading international organizations that cover the complete spectrum from advanced research to the market, including industry partners, non-profit organizations, small and medium-sized enterprises (SME), research development centres, healthcare institutions, and academic partners.

Throughout this project, different candidates are being evaluated to define a final TriAnkle product. All potential candidates are based on a customized implant manufactured with 3D bioprinting technology (Figure 12.6).

The final project results developed by all TriAnkle consortium partners will allow the definition and selection of a preferred candidate for the final TriAnkle product. At the moment, the TriAnkle consortium is evaluating the following potential candidates:

1. Collagen-based scaffolds (Colma)
2. Gelatine-based scaffolds (GelMa)
3. Nano-encapsulated active factors combined with collagen scaffold
4. Nano-encapsulated active factors combined with gelatine scaffold
5. Human stem cells (ASCs), combined with collagen scaffold
6. Human stem cells (ASCs), combined with gelatine scaffold

According to the EU regulation, the potential candidates based on collagen and gelatine scaffolds (products 1 and 2) could be classified as a medical device; and the rest of the candidates (3–6) could be classified as human medicinal products that include a medical device (combined medicinal products).

These 3D bioprinted implant candidates are considered as *combined medicinal products* as the main intended action is achieved by the medicinal component, and the function of the medical device is to enable the drug delivery and/or has a mechanical or supporting function.

As described in the section 9.2, in these cases, it is considered as a medicinal product that includes a medical device, and the entire combined medicinal product is regulated under EU pharmaceutical legislation (Directive 2001/83/EC and EMA/CHMP/QWP/BWP/259165/2019) and must obtain a marketing authorization for an integral medicinal product.

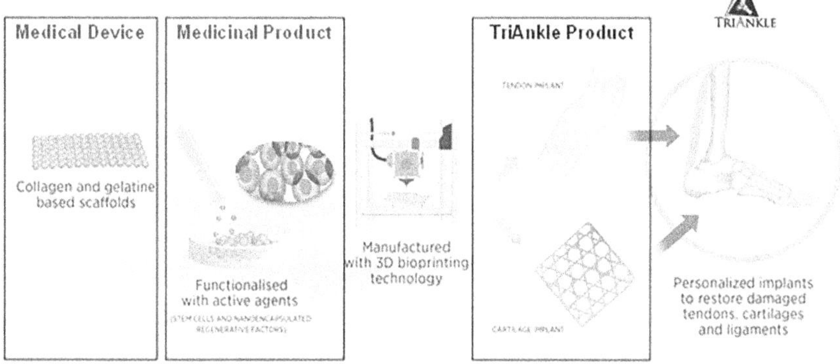

FIGURE 12.6 3D bioprinted implant candidates, under development by the TriAnkle consortium.

The nano-encapsulated active factors are produced by recombinant DNA technology and classified as a biotechnological medicinal product for human use. Therefore, when combined with a collagen scaffold or gelatine-based scaffold (products 3 and 4) the combined product must comply the specific EU regulation for biotechnological medicines.

These products must be evaluated using the EMA centralized procedure and manufactured according to GMP standards.

In the case of the 3D bioprinted implant candidates 5 and 6, the active therapeutic components are human adipose-derived stem cells (ADSCs). The ADSCs are somatic cells that have been manipulated to change their biological characteristics and are used for the treatment of a human disease (tendinopathies such as Achilles tendon partial ruptures and cartilage injuries).

TriAnkle Product Potential Candidates (3D bioprinted implants)	**Activity or function**	**Product Classification and applicable Regulation**	**Competent Authority**	**Authorization for use and / or commercialization**
Colma 3D bioprinted implant, containing: collagen hydrogel- scaffold	Mechanical or physical function.	Medical device **Regulation (EU) 2017/745**	Notified Body	Conformity assessment: CE mark
GelMa 3D bioprinted implant, containing gelatine scaffold	Mechanical or physical function.	Medical device **Regulation (EU) 2017/745**	Notified Body	Conformity assessment: CE mark
3D bioprinted implant, containing: Human Allogenic Adipose Stem cells (ADSCs) and Collagen or gelatine scaffold TENDON IMPLANT CARTILAGE IMPLANT	ADSC Active Substance: Pharmacological/ immunological or metabolic action to regenerate, restore or replace a human tissue. Collagen or gelatine scaffold: Mechanical or physical function. Support, scaffold Medicinal product: regenerate, restore or replace a human tissue	Combined Advanced Therapy Medicinal Product with a medical device. **Regulation (EC) No 1394/2007** **Directive 2001/83/EC** **Regulation (EU) 2017/745**	EMA (CAT) (European Medicines Agency – Committee for Advanced Therapies CAT) and Notified Body evaluation / opinion NBOp (conformity assessment: CE mark or NBOp)	Marketing authorization (centralized procedure)
3D bioprinted implant, containing: Nanoparticules of active agents (regenerative factors) and Collagen or gelatine scaffold TENDON IMPLANT Functionalised with active agents CARTILAGE IMPLANT	Active Substance: component with pharmacological, immunological, or metabolic action. The product contains a mixture of different regenerative factors produced by recombinant DNA technology, so they could be classified as biotechnological medicinal products. Collagen or gelatine scaffold: Mechanical or physical function. Support, scaffold Medicinal product: regenerate, restore or replace a human tissue	Biotechnological Medicinal Product combined with a medical device: **Directive 2001/83/EC.** **Regulation (EU) 2017/745** ***EMA/CHMP/QWP/ BWP/259165/2019***	EMA (European Medicines Agency) and Notified Body evaluation/ opinion NBOp (conformity assessment: CE mark or NBOp)	Marketing authorization (centralized procedure)

FIGURE 12.7 Summary of the regulation and authorization requirements for the 3D bioprinted implants under development by TriAnkle consortium.

Medicinal products for human use that are based on genes, tissues, or cells are classified as ATMPs. According to the EU pharmaceutical legislation (Regulation EU 1394/2007), all advanced therapy medicines are authorized centrally via the EMA, in a single evaluation and authorization procedure.

The ATMPs that contain one or more medical devices as an integral part of the medicine are referred to or classified as combined ATMPs. These candidates will be classified as a combined medicinal product, specifically combined advanced therapy medicinal product with a medical device.

As discussed above, according to EU legislation, 3D bioprinted implant candidates 1 and 2, collagen-based scaffolds (Colma) and gelatine-based scaffolds (GelMa), are considered medical devices, as they do not contain an active medicinal component with pharmacological, immunological, or metabolic activity.

If these products are intended to be marketed alone (not combined with medicinal products), they must comply with Regulation (EU) 2017/745 on medical devices and CE marking for marketing must be obtained.

Figure 12.7 shows an overview of the classification of all 3D bioprinted implant candidates according to the applicable EU regulation, as well as the competent authorities for evaluation and the applicable authorization procedure.

REFERENCES

1. REGULATION (EC) No. 1394/2007 of the European Parliament and of the Council of 13 November 2007 on advanced therapy medicinal products and amending Directive 2001/83/EC and Regulation (EC) No. 726/2004.
2. DIRECTIVE 2001/83/EC of the European Parliament and of the Council of 6 November 2001 on the Community code relating to medicinal products for human use.
3. DIRECTIVE 2009/120/EC of 14 September 2009 amending Directive 2001/83/EC of the European Parliament and of the Council on the Community code relating to medicinal products for human use as regards advanced therapy medicinal products.
4. Regulation (EC) No. 726/2004 of the European Parliament and of the Council of 31 March 2004 laying down Community procedures for the authorisation and supervision of medicinal products for human and veterinary use and establishing a European Medicines Agency.
5. REGULATION (EU) No. 536/2014 of the European Parliament and of the Council of 16 April 2014 on clinical trials on medicinal products for human use, and repealing Directive 2001/20/EC Text with EEA relevance.
6. Guideline on quality documentation for medicinal products when used with a medical device. EMA/CHMP/QWP/BWP/259165/2019 (22 July 2021).
7. Good Laboratory Practice (GLP) principles in relation to ATMPS 26 January 2017. https://www.ema.europa.eu/en/documents/other/good-laboratory-practice-glp-principles-relation-advanced-therapy-medicinal-products-atmps_en.pdf.
8. Guidelines on Good Clinical Practice specific to Advanced Therapy Medicinal Products. Brussels, 10.10.2019 C(2019) 7140. https://health.ec.europa.eu/system/files/2019-10/atmp_guidelines_en_0.pdf.
9. Good manufacturing practice specific to Advanced Therapy Medicinal Products (EudraLex Volume 4, GMP part IV. https://ec.europa.eu/health/sites/default/files/files/eudralex/vol-4/2017_11_22_guidelines_gmp_for_atmps.pdf.

10. REGULATION (EU) 2017/745 of the European Parliament and of the Council of 5 April 2017 on medical devices, amending Directive 2001/83/EC, Regulation (EC) No. 178/2002 and Regulation (EC) No. 1223/2009 and repealing Council Directives 90/385/EEC and 93/42/EEC.
11. MDCG 2021-6. Regulation (EU) 2017/745 – Questions & Answers regarding clinical investigation. Medical Device Coordination Group Document, European Commission. April 2021.
12. Directive 2006/42/EC of the European Parliament and of the Council of 17 May 2006 on machinery, and amending Directive 95/16/EC (recast).

13 3D-Bioprinted Scaffold Technology to Promote Articular Cartilage Regeneration in Osteoarthritis

An Example of Challenges of 3D Bioprinting

A. Mallick
University of Galway

V. Ward
University of Galway
and
Trinity College Dublin & University of Galway

M. B. O'Reilly
University of Galway

G. P. Duffy
University of Galway
and
Trinity College Dublin & University of Galway

T. Mitra
University of Galway

CONTENTS

DOI: 10.1201/9781003274568-13

13.1 INTRODUCTION

Osteoarthritis (OA) is the most common form of arthritis, affecting 300 million people worldwide. OA is a complex degenerative disease affecting joints, which is characterised by cartilage degeneration, subchondral bone thickening, osteophyte formation, synovial inflammation, and structural changes in the joint capsule, ligaments, and associated muscles [1,2]. The tibiofemoral joint in the knee is most commonly affected, followed by the joints of the hands and hips. OA is a leading cause of disability worldwide, with the characteristic symptom being chronic pain [3]. The prevalence of OA increases with age; approximately 14% of adults aged 25 years and older have clinical OA in at least one joint, while approximately 34% of adults aged 65 years and older have OA [4]. By 2032, OA prevalence is estimated to increase from 26.6% to 29.5% in the population aged 45 years and older in all locations around the world, with the prevalence increasing from 13.8% to 15.7% in the knee joint and from 5.8% to 6.9% in the hip joint [2,5]. Research suggests that OA of the knee or hand is more common in women than in men, particularly symptomatic OA attributable to genetic, hormonal, environmental, and social factors [6,7].

The key pathological feature of OA is the degeneration of articular cartilage, which is present at joint surfaces [8]. The primary function of articular cartilage is to provide a smooth, frictionless, and lubricated surface between the two articulating bones at a joint, thereby facilitating the transmission of loads to the underlying subchondral bone [9]. Obesity, excessive exercise, improper diet, and accidental injuries can all cause degeneration of the articular cartilage [10]. This causes extreme pain and slowly inhibits movements of the joint. The repair process is slow, as the articular cartilage is avascular and lacks nerves and lymphatics [11]. Therefore, novel treatments for articular cartilage degeneration in OA have become a major research focus.

The first line of treatment for OA consists of lifestyle adjustments, including weight loss and regular exercise, and nonsurgical interventions, such as pain relief medications and physiotherapy [12]. For patients with chronic pain, surgical intervention may be necessary. These include knee arthroplasty, bone marrow stimulation (BMS), osteochondral autografts and allografts, autologous chondrocyte implantation (ACI), and matrix-assisted ACI [13]. However, due to a variety of factors including immunogenic responses, insufficient donor availability, and lack of long-term efficacy, these treatments often do not progress to clinical use [14]. In recent years, cartilage regeneration by tissue engineering has been introduced as a new therapeutic approach for the treatment of OA [15]. It involves the use of cell-based scaffolds, which are cultured in an *in vitro* 3D environment and then implanted into the affected joint to promote faster regeneration of the damaged cartilage [16]. The advantages of this method are less concern for donor deficiency and less risk of rejection by the immune system in the articular cartilage–based regeneration technique [17–19]. 3D bioprinting has evolved as a revolutionary scaffold-based technology for articular cartilage regeneration by tissue engineering. 3D bioprinting is a computer-aided technology that involves layer-by-layer deposition of a bioink to form a 3D structure that mimics the living tissue [20]. Bioinks typically consist of natural or synthetic polymers called biomaterials, which can have therapeutic drugs, cells, and growth factors integrated into them. As bioprinting is a computer-assisted process, it can be uniquely programmed to position cells and growth factors at specific locations and within specific matrix layers. As a result, bioprinting can mimic complex biological structures by a controlled layering process making it an attractive solution for articular cartilage development [21].

In this chapter, we mainly focus on the techniques and bioinks used for the development of 3D-bioprinted articular cartilage and provide examples of *in vitro* and *in vivo* studies of bioprinted structures for the treatment of OA.

13.2 TREATMENTS FOR OSTEOARTHRITIS

Treatments for OA can be categorised into nonsurgical, surgical, and cartilage regeneration-based techniques. The treatment chosen for each individual case of OA depends on the severity of the disease.

13.2.1 Nonsurgical Interventions

Typically, nonsurgical interventions comprise the first line of treatment for OA. Lifestyle adjustments, namely exercise and weight loss, are commonly recommended in the early stages of OA, as they help reduce the stress on the weight-bearing joints, including those in the hip, knee, and lower back [22]. Pain relief medications may also be prescribed to help control the patient's pain levels. These include paracetamol, nonsteroidal anti-inflammatory drugs, opioids, capsaicin cream, and steroid injections [23]. Intra-articular viscosupplementation may also be used, which involves injecting hyaluronic acid (HA) into the joint to stimulate cartilage repair [24]. Other nonsurgical therapies include transcutaneous electrical nerve stimulation, applying a hot or cold pack to the affected joint(s), and physiotherapy.

13.2.2 Surgical Interventions

In cases where nonsurgical interventions fail, surgery may be required. There are several common surgical methods to treat OA, including arthroplasty (joint replacement), arthrodesis (joint fusion), and osteotomy (bone remodelling). Other surgical interventions include BMS, osteochondral autografts or allografts, and ACI [13].

13.2.2.1 Arthroplasty

Arthroplasty involves replacing the natural articulating surfaces in a joint with plastic or metal prostheses to re-establish joint function [25]. Arthroplasty is often performed on hip or knee joints affected by OA. Although arthroplasty can improve a patient's quality of life by alleviating pain and increasing mobility, a prosthesis can often fail due to mechanical issues, joint infection, poor bone fixation, improper alignment, and instability due to soft tissue laxity around the joint [26]. When knee replacement complications arise, a second surgery is often required [27]. Chronic pain is often associated with arthroplasty surgery leading to a demand for alternative cartilage replacement options.

13.2.2.2 Bone Marrow Stimulation (BMS)

This is a technique that promotes cartilage formation by inducing mesenchymal cells in the underlying bone marrow to differentiate into fibrous cartilage [28]. Microfracture surgery, abrasion arthroplasty, and subchondral drilling are the most common techniques to activate the underlying bone marrow [29]. However, stimulating underlying bone marrow often drives tissue differentiation towards biomechanically inferior fibrocartilage forming instead of native hyaline cartilage [30]. Therefore, while BMS techniques are effective in small lesions, with fibrocartilage acting as a soft tissue filler, severe cases of OA that require bulk cartilage replacement do not benefit from this technique [31].

13.2.2.3 Osteochondral Implantation (Autografting or Allografting)

It can be defined as the restoration of articular cartilage by transferring healthy cartilage tissue into the site of damage. In autografting, the cartilage is extracted from the low load-bearing zones around the joints in the patient's own body and transferred into the diseased site [32]. Autografting is a cost-effective and simple surgical procedure and does not require immunosuppression as it uses the patient's own tissue [33]. Limitations of autografting include enhanced risk of infection, additional surgical procedures, enhanced blood loss, and donor-site morbidity [34]. Under these circumstances, allografting is considered the next alternative. Allografting involves extracting the tissue from cadaveric donors for implantation. This technique has a larger yield due to whole cartilage extraction as opposed to selective extraction in autografting. However, potential disease transmission, histocompatibility issues, suitable donor matching, and high cost are the limiting factors for this technique [35].

13.2.2.4 ACI

ACI is an FDA-approved two-step cell-based therapy to treat articular cartilage defects. In the first step, a small amount of cartilage is surgically removed from a low weight-bearing area of the patient's joint. In the second step, chondrocytes are enzymatically extracted from the extracellular matrix (ECM), cultured *in vitro* for several weeks, and injected back into the damaged cartilage site through a periosteal flap. The disadvantage of ACI is the inhomogeneous distribution of the chondrocytes [36]. To achieve homogeneous chondrocyte distribution, chondrocyte-based scaffolds (collagen I/III as scaffolds) are implanted in a technique called matrix-assisted ACI [37]. However, the major disadvantage of this technique is the loss of the chondrocyte phenotype when the cells expand on 2D cell culture surfaces. The cell expansion results in the formation of nonspecific ECM-based proteins instead of cartilage-specific proteins such as proteoglycan and collagen type II. Therefore, ACI is not suitable for patients with advanced OA [36]. Other disadvantages of these techniques include the high cost and the complicated surgical procedures involved.

13.2.3 Cartilage Regeneration Strategies

Both nonsurgical and surgical interventions discussed above can help alleviate the pain and symptoms of OA patients. However, these treatments fail to prevent disease progression. Tissue engineering has evolved in recent years, with scaffold-based approaches for cartilage regeneration emerging as potential solutions for the treatment of OA [38].

13.2.3.1 Scaffold-Based Approaches

Scaffold-based approaches are tissue engineering processes which involve developing new tissues in a 3D microenvironment, where cell attachment, proliferation, and differentiation are supported by scaffolds [39]. Scaffolds are porous materials usually made up of biocompatible and biodegradable polymers [40]. The porous nature of the scaffold makes the 3D microenvironment suitable for cell migration, growth, and transport of wastes and nutrients [41,42]. 3D bioprinting has emerged as a promising scaffold-based technology with the potential to develop cell-loaded biomaterials in a 3D environment, where the spatial distribution of the cells can be controlled [20]. In the following sections, the complex anatomy of the articular cartilage will be discussed, along with recent research which demonstrates that bioprinting is a promising medical solution for cartilage regeneration in the treatment of OA.

13.3 ANATOMY OF THE ARTICULAR CARTILAGE

As mentioned earlier, degeneration of the articular cartilage is the main pathological feature of OA. Thus, it is very important to understand the anatomy of the articular cartilage. Cartilage is an elastic, avascular connective tissue in the body that resists compressive forces in joints and provides structural support. The cartilage that surrounds freely moving diarthrodial joints is called articular cartilage. Articular cartilage is a hyaline form of cartilage composed of water and ECM components, aggrecan (ACAN), and other proteoglycans. A key ECM component, collagen type

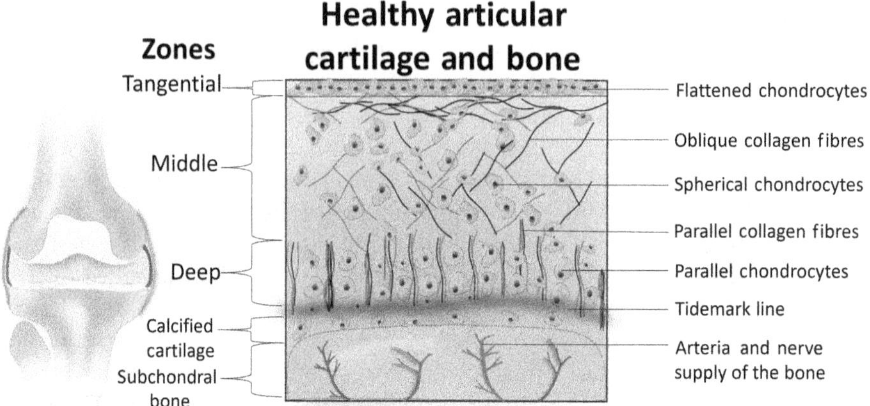

FIGURE 13.1 Schematic representation of the knee joint, highlighting the articular cartilage zonal layers and their interaction with the underlying bone.

II, found in the articular cartilage, forms an interconnecting network that provides tensile strength to the cartilage [43]. Chondrocytes are highly specialised and metabolically active cells embedded in the cartilage layers. Chondrocytes are mechanosensitive and play unique roles in the zonal environment of the cartilage to ensure the development, maintenance, and repair of the ECM [44].

The zonal layers in the articular cartilage contribute to the overall protection of bone against sustained compressive forces (Figure 13.1). The superficial layer, called the tangential zone, protects the deeper layers from shear forces, and its collagen fibres are densely packed and oriented parallel to the articular surface [42]. The middle transition zone accounts for the largest tissue volume and is composed primarily of proteoglycans and collagen fibrils [42]. The deep zone provides the greatest resistance to compressive forces, with the collagen fibres arranged perpendicular to the articular surface. In addition, this deep zone has the thickest diameter of collagen fibres, the highest proteoglycan content, and the lowest water content [42]. The deep zone transitions from noncalcified, avascular zonal regions proximally to a vascular and nerve-rich network of the calcified cartilage distally. The calcified cartilage is permeable and facilitates biochemical interactions between the noncalcified cartilage and the subchondral bone while resisting shear deformation. The subchondral bone is the proximal part of the bone involved in the initial load bearing and transmission of mechanical forces [42].

13.4 BIOPRINTING

13.4.1 3D Bioprinting

3D bioprinting is a computer-assisted technology in which a 3D scaffold of living tissue–like structures is formed in a layer-by-layer pattern using a bioink [20]. Bioinks typically consist of living cells or growth factors combined with natural or synthetic biomaterials (Figure 13.2). Since it is a computer-assisted process, cells can be positioned at specific locations in the 3D-bioprinted structures [45]. Moreover,

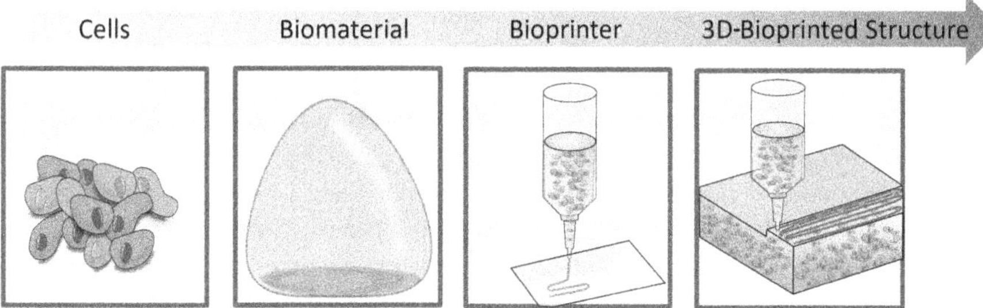

FIGURE 13.2 Schematic representation of step-by-step process of 3D bioprinting: deposition of cells and biomaterials in a layer-by-layer pattern using a 3D bioprinter.

complicated biological structures can be fabricated in a controlled manner by 3D bioprinting, with high reproducibility [45]. Bioprinting allows users to produce customised cell-laden hydrogels, with controlled shape, size, and porosity, and homogeneous distribution of cells and growth factors [20]. 3D bioprinting has attracted increasing attention worldwide and is being used for a wide range of applications in regenerative medicine, tissue engineering, pharmaceuticals, and cancer therapeutics [46].

13.4.2 Types of Bioprinting

There are three different types of bioprinting: extrusion, inkjet, and laser-assisted bioprinting (LAB). *Extrusion bioprinting* is a cost-effective and widely used high-throughput bioprinting technique, in which a bioink is extruded from a nozzle by pneumatics and deposited on the bioprinter platform as a tissue-like 3D structure [47]. The major drawback of extrusion-based bioprinting is the low resolution of the bioprinted structure. Moreover, during extrusion-based bioprinting, cells are subjected to mechanical constraints that may affect cell viability. Therefore, it is essential to optimise the printing parameters for good cell viability during extrusion-based bioprinting [48]. The principle of *inkjet bioprinting* is like that of a normal inkjet modified to print 3D structures with bioinks. Inkjet bioprinting has advantages such as high printing speed and low cost, which makes it accessible [49]. However, this technique can lead to cell damage and cell aggregation due to the high shear stress on the nozzle, which is caused by clogging [49]. *Laser-assisted bioprinting (LAB)* is a nozzle-free bioprinting method based on the technique of laser-induced forward transfer. The energy source used is a laser that deposits the bioink dropwise on the printing substrate to form a 3D-bioprinted structure [50]. The main advantage of using LAB is that the viability of the cells in the 3D-bioprinted structure is quite high. The high cost and complicated operating procedure of LAB are the reasons for its infrequent use [50].

13.4.3 Bioink

Bioink is the most important factor in bioprinting, which consists of cells, biomaterials, and growth factors. An ideal bioink should be injectable/extrudable from a thin needle and have excellent shear-thinning properties and suitable elasticity to obtain highly cross-linked, porous, 3D structures with good shape fidelity [51]. Bioink should also allow diffusion of nutrients and oxygen in the scaffold and be biocompatible, cytocompatible, and biodegradable [52]. It should also support cell growth and be printable at optimal temperatures and pressures [53]. However, low-viscosity bioinks support cellular growth but have poor mechanical properties, whereas high-viscosity bioinks have good printability but show low cellular viability. Therefore, the bioink used must provide synergy between biomechanical properties and high cellular activity [54]. Furthermore, the bioinks are designed in such a manner that after bioprinting, the 3D scaffolds can be cross-linked by physical or chemical methods for enhanced rheological properties [55]. The most commonly used chemical methods include methacrylation of biomaterials followed by cross-linking with a photoinitiator such as Irgacure and lithium phenyl-2,4,6-trimethylbenzoyl phosphinate using UV and visible light, respectively [56]. Physical methods include the use of calcium ions, which exhibit excellent cross-linking properties when used with sodium alginate [57].

13.4.4 Biomaterials

Biomaterials used in bioinks are generally natural or artificial polymer-based hydrogels. Naturally occurring polymers include collagen, gelatin, alginate, HA, cellulose, chitosan, and silk, while artificial polymers include polyvinyl alcohol, polycaprolactone (PCL), and polyethylene glycol (PEG). The naturally occurring polymers are generally biocompatible, biodegradable, hydrophilic, and cytocompatible but have poor biomechanical properties. In contrast, artificial polymers have distinct biomechanical properties but are less hydrophilic and cytocompatible than natural polymers [58].

13.4.5 Cells

Cells used in bioinks also play a very important role in mimicking native 3D tissues after bioprinting, and they should also proliferate to maintain tissue viability [59]. The primary source of cells is commercially available cell lines from humans or animals. Primary cell lines derived from animal tissues and organs can also be an option. However, loss of cell phenotype during expansion *in vitro* and formation of mixed populations during isolation are the two limitations of primary cells [60]. Alternative cell sources such as stem cells may overcome the problem associated with phenotype differentiation. There are three types of stem cells typically used in bioprinting: mesenchymal stem cells (MSCs), embryonic stem cells (ESCs), and induced pluripotent stem cells (iPSCs) [61]. MSCs are multipotent meaning that they can form all cell types within a certain lineage, such as osteoblasts [62]. ESCs and iPSCs are pluripotent, meaning that they can form any cell type in the human body, but they may cause tumorigenesis [63]. The cell source is an important factor to consider for biomaterial applications and bioprinting purposes.

13.5 BIOPRINTING ARTICULAR CARTILAGE

As discussed earlier, articular cartilage exhibits a complex zonal organisation with specific cell densities and ECM components that can be mimicked by bioprinting [64]. Extrusion-based bioprinting is the most widely used technique for bioprinting articular cartilage [65]. Articular cartilage of human adults has a dynamic modulus of 0.1–1.3 MPa to accommodate *in vivo* load bearing and shear forces [66]. Therefore, the bioprinted scaffold required for articular cartilage regeneration must achieve the mechanical properties of the natural cartilage and provide abundant oxygen and nutrients for chondrocyte proliferation and maturation.

13.5.1 Cells Used in Bioprinting Articular Cartilage

Chondrocytes are specialised cells involved in cartilage formation and are mainly responsible for the production and regulation of cartilage ECM. However, because chondrocyte yields can be low and are often associated with loss of phenotype, morphology, and cell expression, alternative sources are often considered [44]. MSCs are commonly used as an alternative source of chondrocytes because of their capacity for self-renewal, multipotency, and chondrogenic properties [62]. Bone marrow-derived stem cells (BM-MSCs) have good proliferation abilities and can be differentiated into a chondrogenic lineage with the help of differentiation factors such as TGF-β1 and TGF-β3 [63]. Adipose-derived stem cells (ADSCs) are also used for cartilage bioprinting due to their chondrogenic properties, particularly in the synthesis of collagen type II [63].

Chondrocytes and MSCs are most commonly used for bioprinting of the articular cartilage [63]. They are usually used with either natural polymers such as gelatin, alginate, HA, and decellularised ECM (dECM) or a mixture of natural and synthetic polymers to produce the bioink [64]. The 3D cell-loaded cartilage scaffolds are usually fabricated by extrusion-based bioprinting. The bioprinted structures are then evaluated for chondrogenesis by measuring gene expression and matrix synthesis [65]. However, due to their good accessibility and availability after *in vitro* expansion, MSCs are often used for translational application of 3D bioprinting of the articular cartilage [66].

13.5.2 Biomaterials Used in Articular Cartilage Bioprinting

Naturally occurring biomaterials provide oxygen and nutrients to chondrocytes for chondrogenesis because they can mimic the ECM of native cartilage. However, their low mechanical strength and rapid biodegradability can challenge long-term cartilage regeneration [67]. Therefore, artificial polymers have advantages such as tuneable mechanical properties, a controlled degradation rate, and ease of printability, which make them suitable for cartilage tissue engineering. However, their lower cytocompatibility makes them difficult to be used as bioink [68]. In recent research, there have been several suitable biomaterials identified for cartilage regeneration in OA, including alginate, collagen, gelatin, HA, dECM, nanofibrillated cellulose (NC), silk protein, and PCL [69] (Table 13.1).

Collagen is the principal component of the ECM of articular cartilage, providing its structural framework and biomechanical properties [70]. Therefore, it is extensively used in bioprinting articular cartilage. Studies have shown that porous collagen, using the cross-linker genipin, has excellent biomechanical properties, printability, and cell viability when used with chondrocytes. When this cell-laden collagen structure was implanted *in vivo* in a rabbit model of OA, newly formed

TABLE 13.1
3D Bioprinting for Articular Cartilage Regeneration

			In Vitro								
					Immunohistochemistry/PCR						
Biomaterial	**Modification**	**Cells**	**Cell Viability**	**Histological Analysis**	**Col2a1**	**ACAN**	**SOX9**	**Col1a1**	**DNA and GAG**	***In Vivo* (Model of OA)**	**References**
Collagen	Collagen–Alginate	Chondrocytes	+	+	++	++	++	--	+	NA	Yang [71]
	Collagen Type I	Articular chondrocytes	+	NA	NA	NA	Na	NA	+	Rabbit	Koo [70]
	Atelocollagen + hyaluronic acid	hTMSCs	+	+	++	++	++	--	+	Rabbit	Shim [91]
	Collagen Type II	Chondrocytes	+	+	++	NA	NA	--	+	NA	Ren [92]
Gelatin	Gelatin methacryalate (GelMA)	ACPCs, BM-MSCs, Chondrocytes	NA	+	++	++	NA	--	+	NA	Levato [93]
	GelMA+ chondroitin sulphate amino ethyl methacrylate	BM-MSCs	+	NA	++	++	NA	--	NA	NA	Costantini [74]
	GelMA + alginate + polycaprolactone (PCL)	Chondrocytes, BM-MSCs	+	+	++	NA	NA	--	+	NA	Schipani [73]
	GelMA+ methacrylated poly (vinyl alcohol)	ACPCs	+	+	NA	NA	NA	NA	NA	NA	Lim [94]
Hyaluronic acid (HA)	Norbornene-modified hyaluronic acid	MSCs	+	+	++	NA	NA	--	+	NA	Galarraga [76]
	HA-biotin-streptavidin	hADSCs	+	+	++	++	++	--	+	NA	Nedunchezian [78]
	Methacrylated hyaluronic acid (HAMA)	Chondrocytes	+	+	NA	NA	NA	NA	NA	NA	Kessel [95]
	HAMA-GelMA	ADMSCs	NA	+	++	NA	NA	--	NA	Sheep	Bella [89]
	HA+ alginate + polylactic acid	Chondrocytes	+	NA	++	++	++	--	+	NA	Antich [77]

(Continued)

TABLE 13.1 (*Continued*)
3D Bioprinting for Articular Cartilage Regeneration

			In Vitro							*In Vivo*	
					Immunohistochemistry/PCR						
Biomaterial	**Modification**	**Cells**	**Cell Viability**	**Histological Analysis**	**Col2a1**	**ACAN**	**SOX9**	**Col1a1**	**DNA and GAG**	**(Model of OA)**	**References**
Decellularised ECM (dECM)	dECM-Silk-PEG	BM-MSCs	+	+	++	++	++	--	+	NA	Zhang [81]
	Methacrylated dECM + gelatin	BM-MSCs	+	+	NA	NA	NA	NA	+	NA	Behan [80]
	dECM-alginate	BM-MSCs	+	+	++	++	+	NA	+	NA	Rathan [96]
Nonofibrillated cellulose (NC)	NC+ alginate	iPSCs	+	+	++	++	NA	--	NA	NA	Nguyen [83]
	NC+ alginate	Chondrocytes	+	-	++	++	NA	--	NA	NA	Gatenholm [84]
Silk protein	Silk methacrylate + polyethylene glycol diacrylate	Chondrocytes	+	NA	++	++	NA	NA	+	NA	Bandyopadhyay [85]
	Silk+ gellan gum+ alginate	BM-MSCs	NA	+	++	++	NA	NA	NA	NA	Chakraborty [86]
	Silk–gelatin	BM-MSCs	+	NA	++	++	++	NA	+	NA	Chawla [97]
Polycaprolactone (PCL)	Poly (L-lactide-co-caprolactone)-aggrecan	hMSCs	NA	NA	NA	NA	NA	NA	NA	Rabbit	Guo [98]
	PCL+ HAMA+ kartogenin+ diclofenac sodium	BM-MSCs	+	+	++	++	++	NA	NA	Rat	Liu [90]
	PCL + alginate	BM-MSCs, chondrocytes, FPSCs	NA	+	++	NA	NA	--	+	Mouse, Caprine	Critchley [87]

BM-MSCs, bone marrow stem cells; ADMSCs, adipose-derived marrow stem cells; ACPCs, articular cartilage progenitor cells; iPSCs, human-derived induced pluripotent stem cell; hADSCs, human-derived adipose-derived marrow stem cells; hTMSCs, human turbinate-derived mesenchymal stromal cells; FPSCs, fat pad-derived stem cells.
+ denotes successful completion of the experiment, ++ denotes enhancement of the gene expression, -- denotes lowering of the gene expression, NA denotes experiment not done.

hyaline cartilage was identified through immunohistochemistry and histological analysis [70]. However, collagen has poor biomechanical properties and high solubility in water at 37°C, which limits its applications in bioprinting. Therefore, collagen can be paired with different polymers to further improve its biomechanical properties and post-printing stability. This has been studied by Yang et al. using a collagen–alginate biomaterial which shows variable biomechanical strength while facilitating cell adhesion and proliferation of chondrocytes embedded within the biomaterial matrix. Through this research, they highlighted enhanced gene expression associated with correct phenotype formation, including increased SOX-9, COL2A1, and ACAN expression, while lowering markers associated with the formation of fibrocartilage such as Col1a1 [71].

Gelatin is derived from the hydrolytic degradation of collagen. The amphoteric nature of the amino acid (arginine-glycine-aspartate) present within gelatin further enhances its suitability as a biomaterial for 3D bioprinting articular cartilage [72]. However, gelatin displays excellent swelling capabilities at 37°C and thus is either methacrylated to form gelatin methacrylate (GelMA) or combined with other biomaterials for post-bioprinting curing purposes. In a study by Schipani et al., 3D-bioprinted scaffolds were developed using a combination of interpenetrating network hydrogels such as GelMA and alginate and PCL fibres in a co-culture with BM-MSCs and chondrocytes. The bioprinted structure induced chondrogenesis and the formation of articular cartilage, which was confirmed by staining that showed the presence of sulphated glycosaminoglycans (sGAGs) and collagen type II and the absence of collagen type X [73]. Costantini et al. developed a bioink comprising GelMA, chondroitin sulphate, amino ethyl methacrylate, and alginate in combination with BM-MSCs. The 3D-bioprinted scaffolds promoted the formation of neocartilage with the highest collagen type II/collagen type I and collagen type II/collagen type X ratios. These ratios were confirmed qualitatively by means of fluorescence immunocytochemistry and quantitatively by means of reverse transcription quantitative real-time PCR (RT-qPCR) [74].

Hyaluronic acid (HA) is a major component of the ECM of the articular cartilage making it an excellent choice of biomaterial in articular cartilage regeneration. However, due to its hydrophilic nature, it has lower mechanical strength and stability, which limits its use as a bioink. HA is usually modified into hyaluronic acid methacrylate (HAMA) to improve mechanical stability for bioprinting [75]. Galarraga et al. reported that norbornene-modified HA with curing agents such as thiol-ene is suitable for bioprinting with MSCs. In this study, the 3D-bioprinted constructs had an enhanced expression of sGAG and collagen, which was confirmed by histological staining of the cartilage tissue matrix [76]. Antich et al. showed that HA-based alginate co-printed with polylactic acid using chondrocytes as bioink exhibited improved mechanical properties and printability. The 3D-bioprinted scaffold in this study promoted chondrogenesis, as shown by an increase in the expression of articular cartilage-specific markers such as SOX-9, COL2A1, and ACAN, suggesting the regeneration of articular cartilage [77]. Nedunchezian et al. used HA-biotin-streptavidin hydrogel in combination with sodium alginate and ADSCs as a bioink to obtain 3D-bioprinted structures that can induce chondrogenesis. This was confirmed by the enhanced expression of chondrogenic marker genes such as SOX-9, COL2A1, and ACAN [78].

Decellularised extracellular matrix (dECM) is obtained by the removal of the cellular components of native ECM tissue, leaving an intact dECM scaffold for tissue and organ regeneration [79]. The presence of proteins and bioactive molecules that replicate the environment of the native tissues is the main advantage of dECM [79]. Therefore, dECM has emerged as a potential bioink with tissue-specific composition for articular cartilage bioprinting [79]. A study by Behan et al. showed that methacrylated cartilage-derived dECM with gelatin as a viscosity enhancer has excellent shear-thinning properties and formed 3D-bioprinted structures when cross-linked with a photoinitiator in the presence of UV light. Post-bioprinting analysis showed that BM-MSCs had high cell viability, while sGAGs and collagens were overexpressed suggesting that chondrogenesis had occurred. Therefore, this makes this dECM structure suitable for articular cartilage regeneration [80]. Another study by Zhang et al. showed that silk fibroin along with cartilage-derived dECM and PEG increases the mechanical properties, biodegradability, and porosity of the bioink. TGF-β3 released from 3D-bioprinted structures facilitated chondrogenic differentiation of BM-MSCs, thereby making it excellent for articular cartilage repair [81].

Nanofibrillated cellulose (NC) is widely used for articular cartilage bioprinting due to its structural similarity to the ECM and shear-thinning properties. However, due to its poor biodegradability, NC is usually combined with other natural polymers for cartilage bioprinting [82]. Nguyen et al. found that 3D-bioprinted structures using NC/alginate (60:40) and iPSCs could fabricate articular-like cartilaginous tissue with collagen type II expression, lacking tumorigenic Oct4 expression [83]. Gatenholm et al. used NC in combination with alginate (80:20) and human chondrocytes as a bioink in the development of a 3D-bioprinted structure. This structure was able to produce native articular cartilage fragments in 2 weeks characterised by the high level of production of Col IIA and ACAN analysed by RT-PCR [84].

Silk protein is a biomaterial widely used in tissue engineering because of its structural resemblance to collagen. However, silk protein has poor printability and slow gelation kinetics, restricting its application in 3D bioprinting. It can be used with other biomaterials to form a bioink for use in articular cartilage bioprinting. Bandyopadhyay et al. developed a photo-cross-linkable bioink containing silk methacrylate and polyethylene glycol diacrylate in combination with chondrocytes. The 3D-bioprinted constructs were cytocompatible and produced neocartilage. This was confirmed by increased deposition of articular cartilage-specific ECM sGAG and collagen type II in the biochemical evaluation and enhanced expression of collagen type II and ACAN in the immunohistochemical analysis [85]. Chakraborty et al. designed a bioink comprised of alginate, gellan gum, and silk nanoparticles with BM-MSCs for enhanced printability and biomechanical and biological properties. Interestingly, 3D-bioprinted structures with alginate, gellan gum, and silk fibrin solution with BM-MSCs induced chondrogenesis with enhanced expression of SOX-9, COL2A1, and ACAN and diminished expression of the hypertrophic markers (COL X) in comparison to bioink with silk nanoparticles [86].

Polycaprolactone (PCL) is an FDA-approved thermoplastic polyester used in implantable devices. It has excellent mechanical properties and thus is mainly used for structural reinforcement of natural hydrogels for articular cartilage bioprinting. Critchley et al. engineered a biphasic construct having MSC-laden alginate hydrogel reinforced throughout with a PCL fibre network. The 3D-printed fibre-reinforced cartilaginous template was able to repair osteochondral defects by regenerating both the articular cartilage and subchondral bone within the defective area in caprine joints [87].

13.5.3 Recent Developments on Articular Cartilage Regeneration Using 3D Bioprinting

Bioprinting is an important tool for designing a zonally stratified arrangement in articular cartilage. Mouser et al. developed gelatin methacryloyl, gellan gum, and HAMA hydrogels (GGH) along with chondrocytes, articular cartilage progenitor cells (ACPCs), and MSCs to mimic a zonal-specific articular cartilage model. GGH with ACPCs showed high proteoglycan IV mRNA levels, which is a characteristic feature of the superficial zone, while GGH with MSCs showed the highest chondrogenic potential, which is a characteristic feature of the middle and deep zones. Thus, a two-zone bioprinting scaffold was fabricated with zone-specific matrix production, using different bioinks in each layer to build the superficial zone and the middle/deep zone of articular cartilage [88].

Another important feature of 3D bioprinting in articular cartilage regeneration is *in situ* printing, which allows researchers to apply tissue engineering techniques specifically to the defective articular surface. Bella et al. successfully developed a handheld 3D extrusion printing tool called BioPen using the biomaterials GelMA and HAMA to successfully print scaffolds with ADSCs. The aim of this biofabrication design was to determine the surgical applicability of this tool for the regeneration of full-thickness cartilage defects, using an ovine model. The regenerated cartilage at early time points showed better overall macroscopic and microscopic characteristics when compared with pre-constructed 3D bioscaffolds and untreated controls [89] (Figure 13.3).

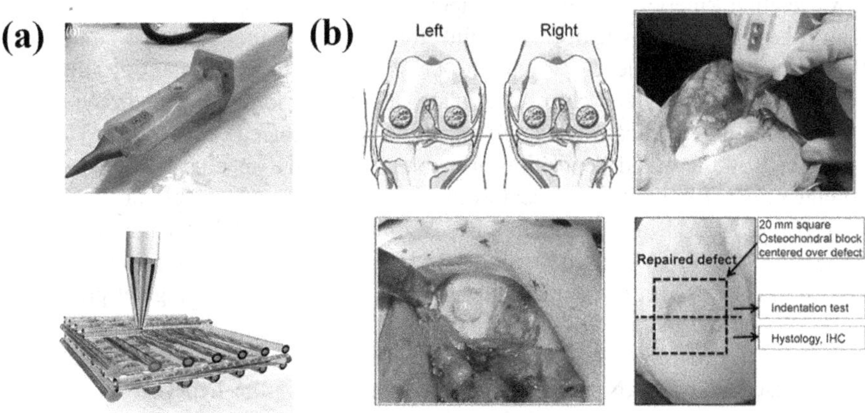

FIGURE 13.3 Schematic representation of the use of a BioPen for the *in situ* regeneration of cartilage bioprinting. (a) A BioPen containing two different chambers for the coaxial printing of two different bioinks HAMA and GelMA controlled by a motor. (b) The chondral defect area in the weight-bearing region of the medial and lateral femoral condyles of both knee joints is filled with the handheld scaffold by a BioPen. Adapted from Ref. [89].

Another major progression in 3D bioprinting-based articular cartilage regeneration is the development of 3D-printed scaffolds having therapeutic and regenerative properties for the treatment of OA joints. Yanzhi Liu et al. reported their research results describing the repair of osteochondral defects in a severe joint injury rat model. They designed a 3D-bioprinted multiphasic scaffold containing a subchondral layer, a bone-forming layer, a cartilage-forming layer, and an anti-inflammatory layer. The bioink used for the subchondral bone region was PCL with β-tricalcium phosphate, while the cartilage-forming layer had a combination of two different bioinks: HAMA with BM-MSCs and PCL with kartogenin. The third anti-inflammatory layer contained diclofenac sodium–incorporated matrix metalloproteinase-sensitive peptide-modified HAMA. After 12 weeks of scaffold implantation, they confirmed that the scaffold treatment provided functional recovery of the injured joint, effective osteochondral repair, and inflammatory management *in vivo* through the mechanism of cartilage protection and inflammatory modulation [90] (Figure 13.4).

13.6 CONCLUSION

OA remains the leading cause of disability and represents a significant burden on healthcare systems worldwide. The fact that conventional treatments for OA fail clinically in most patients opens the window for new research strategies in this area. Cartilage regeneration therapy using 3D bioprinting is a new therapeutic approach, which involves development of complicated 3D living tissue–like structures using biomaterials, cells, and growth factors. In this chapter, we have mainly focussed on the recent developments in bioprinting of articular cartilage with emphasis on the different types of biomaterials and cells in the process. We have also focussed on the current development in the field of 3D bioprinting including designing the complicated zonally stratified layer of articular cartilage, *in situ* bioprinting in defective joint sites, and therapeutic and regenerative properties of 3D-bioprinted articular cartilage. Although bioprinting articular cartilage is still in a very early stage of research where the focus is mainly to optimise the bioink for *in vitro* chondrogenesis, there have been many reports of the *in vivo* study in a smaller animal model which has been discussed in this chapter. However, there are still many hurdles in bioprinting articular cartilage for clinical translation. First, the optimum mechanical properties of the 3D-bioprinted scaffolds to withstand the large load-bearing capability of articular cartilage is still under investigation. Second, although the development of stratified zonal articular cartilage has been attempted by a number of investigators, there was an insignificant zonal difference obtained after culture. Third, the *in vivo* study of 3D-bioprinted scaffolds for articular cartilage regeneration is restricted to smaller animal models. The articular cartilage in larger animals is thicker with major differences in biomechanical properties and repair abilities which limits the use of 3D-bioprinted scaffolds in human clinical trials. Finally, the stringent regulatory challenges faced to develop bioprinted 3D scaffolds like articular cartilage are a major limitation in terms of cost effectivity. Overcoming these challenges will add a new dimension to 3D bioprinting of articular cartilage, creating a paradigm shift in the treatment of OA.

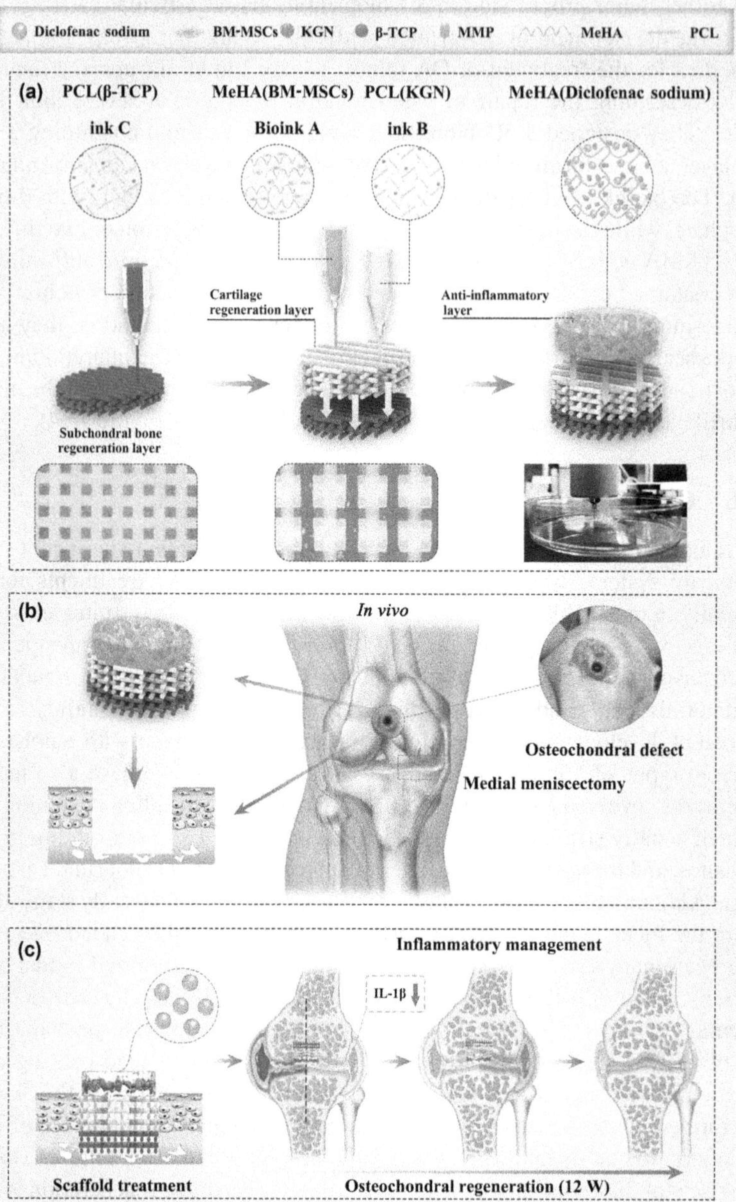

FIGURE 13.4 Schematic representation of bioprinted scaffold fabrication and treatment in osteoarthritic joints. (a) 3D-bioprinted multilayer scaffold was fabricated containing a bone-forming layer of PCL with β-tricalcium phosphate at the bottom and a cartilage-forming layer of HAMA with BM-MSCs and PCL with kartogenin in the middle. Finally, an anti-inflammatory layer of diclofenac sodium–incorporated matrix metalloproteinase-sensitive peptide-modified HAMA was printed at the top. (b) The evaluation of the 3D multi-layered scaffold was done by implanting it into a severe joint injury rat model with osteochondral defect and medial meniscectomy. (c) The implanted multilayer 3D scaffold resulted in the efficient treatment of osteochondral defects in osteoarthritic joints, preventing the development of OA in the rat model. Adapted from Ref. [90].

REFERENCES

1. Prieto-Alhambra D, Judge A, Javaid MK, Cooper C, Diez-Perez A, Arden NK. Incidence and risk factors for clinically diagnosed knee, hip and hand osteoarthritis: influences of age, gender and osteoarthritis affecting other joints. *Annals of the Rheumatic Diseases*. 2014;73(9):1659–64.
2. Turkiewicz A, Petersson IF, Björk J, Hawker G, Dahlberg LE, Lohmander LS, et al. Current and future impact of osteoarthritis on health care: a population-based study with projections to year 2032. *Osteoarthritis and Cartilage*. 2014;22(11):1826–32.
3. Hunter DJ, Bierma-Zeinstra S. Osteoarthritis. *The Lancet*. 2019;393(10182):1745–59.
4. Neogi T. The epidemiology and impact of pain in osteoarthritis. *Osteoarthritis and Cartilage*. 2013;21(9):1145–53.
5. Boer CG, Hatzikotoulas K, Southam L, Stefánsdóttir L, Zhang Y, Coutinho de Almeida R, et al. Deciphering osteoarthritis genetics across 826,690 individuals from 9 populations. *Cell*. 2021;184(18):4784–818.e17.
6. Wolf JM, Cannada L, Van Heest AE, O'Connor MI, Ladd AL. Male and female differences in musculoskeletal disease. *Journal of the American Academy of Orthopaedic Surgeons*. 2015;23(6):339–47.
7. Pinn VW. Past and future: sex and gender in health research, the aging experience, and implications for musculoskeletal health. *Orthopedic Clinics of North America*. 2006;37(4):513–21.
8. He Y, Li Z, Alexander PG, Ocasio-Nieves BD, Yocum L, Lin H, et al. Pathogenesis of osteoarthritis: risk factors, regulatory pathways in chondrocytes, and experimental models. *Biology*. 2020;9(8):194. Published 2020 Jul 29. DOI:10.3390/biology9080194.
9. Sophia Fox AJ, Bedi A, Rodeo SA. The basic science of articular cartilage: structure, composition, and function. *Sports Health: A Multidisciplinary Approach*. 2009;1(6):461–8.
10. Jevotovsky DS, Alfonso AR, Einhorn TA, Chiu ES. Osteoarthritis and stem cell therapy in humans: a systematic review. *Osteoarthritis and Cartilage*. 2018;26(6):711–29.
11. Buckwalter JA, Mankin HJ, Grodzinsky AJ. Articular cartilage and osteoarthritis. *Instructional Course Lectures*. 2005;54:465–80.
12. Geba GP, Weaver AL, Polis AB, Dixon ME, Schnitzer TJ. Efficacy of rofecoxib, celecoxib, and acetaminophen in osteoarthritis of the knee. *JAMA*. 2002 Feb 27;287(1):64–71. DOI:10.1001/jama.287.1.64.
13. Zhu W, Niu T, Wei Z, Yang B, Weng X. Advances in biomaterial-mediated gene therapy for articular cartilage repair. *Bioengineering*. 2022;9(10):502. Published 2022 Sep 24. DOI:10.3390/bioengineering9100502.
14. Huey DJ, Hu JC, Athanasiou KA. Unlike bone, cartilage regeneration remains elusive. *Science*. 2012;338(6109):917–21.
15. Vacanti JP, Langer R. Tissue engineering: the design and fabrication of living replacement devices for surgical reconstruction and transplantation. *The Lancet*. 1999;354:S32–S4.
16. Wasyłeczko M, Sikorska W, Chwojnowski A. Review of synthetic and hybrid scaffolds in cartilage tissue engineering. *Membranes*. 2020;10(11):348. Published 2020 Nov 17. DOI:10.3390/membranes10110348.
17. Cao Z, Dou C, Dong S. Scaffolding biomaterials for cartilage regeneration. *Journal of Nanomaterials*. 2014;2014:1–8.
18. Bhosale AM, Richardson JB. Articular cartilage: structure, injuries and review of management. *British Medical Bulletin*. 2008;87(1):77–95.
19. Bernhard JC, Vunjak-Novakovic G. Should we use cells, biomaterials, or tissue engineering for cartilage regeneration? *Stem Cell Research & Therapy*. 2016;7(1):56.

20. Murphy SV, Atala A. 3D bioprinting of tissues and organs. *Nature Biotechnology.* 2014;32(8):773–85.
21. Agarwal S, Saha S, Balla VK, Pal A, Barui A, Bodhak S. Current developments in 3D bioprinting for tissue and organ regeneration–a review. *Frontiers in Mechanical Engineering.* 2020;6:589171.
22. Walker-Bone K. Regular review: medical management of osteoarthritis. *BMJ.* 2000;321(7266):936–40.
23. Zhang W, Robertson WB, Zhao J, Chen W, Xu J. Emerging trend in the pharmacotherapy of osteoarthritis. *Frontiers in Endocrinology.* 2019;10:431.
24. Arrich J. Intra-articular hyaluronic acid for the treatment of osteoarthritis of the knee: systematic review and meta-analysis. *Canadian Medical Association Journal.* 2005;172(8):1039–43.
25. Madry H. Surgical therapy in osteoarthritis. *Osteoarthritis and Cartilage.* 2022;30(8):1019–34.
26. Portillo ME, Salvadó M, Alier A, Sorli L, Martínez S, Horcajada JP, et al. Prosthesis failure within 2 years of implantation is highly predictive of infection. *Clinical Orthopaedics & Related Research.* 2013;471(11):3672–8.
27. Simmen H-P, Palmer CK, Gooberman-Hill R, Blom AW, Whitehouse MR, Moore AJ. Post-surgery and recovery experiences following one- and two-stage revision for prosthetic joint infection—A qualitative study of patients' experiences. *PLoS ONE.* 2020;15(8): e0237047.
28. Murawski CD, Foo LF, Kennedy JG. A review of arthroscopic bone marrow stimulation techniques of the talus. *Cartilage.* 2010;1(2):137–44.
29. Gill TJ, Steadman JR. Bone marrow stimulation techniques: microfracture, drilling, and abrasion. In: Cole BJ and Malek MM (Eds.), *Articular Cartilage Lesions.* 2004. pp. 63–72. Springer, New York, NY.
30. Nehrer S, Spector M, Minas T. Histologic analysis of tissue after failed cartilage repair procedures. *Clinical Orthopaedics and Related Research.* 1999;365:149–62.
31. Tang QO, Shakib K, Heliotis M, Tsiridis E, Mantalaris A, Ripamonti U, et al. TGF-β3: a potential biological therapy for enhancing chondrogenesis. *Expert Opinion on Biological Therapy.* 2009;9(6):689–701.
32. Ng A, Bernhard K. Osteochondral autograft and allograft transplantation in the talus. *Clinics in Podiatric Medicine and Surgery.* 2017;34(4):461–9.
33. Inderhaug E, Solheim E. Osteochondral autograft transplant (mosaicplasty) for knee articular cartilage defects. *JBJS Essential Surgical Techniques.* 2019;9(4):e34.1–2.
34. Tahmasebi Birgani Z, Malhotra A, Yang L, Harink B, Habibovic P. 1.19 Calcium phosphate ceramics with inorganic additives ☆. In: Ducheyne P (Editor in Chief), *Comprehensive Biomaterials II.* 2017. pp. 406–27. Elsevier.
35. Torrie AM, Kesler WW, Elkin J, Gallo RA. Osteochondral allograft. *Current Reviews in Musculoskeletal Medicine.* 2015;8(4):413–22.
36. Minas T, Ogura T, Bryant T. Autologous chondrocyte implantation. *JBJS Essential Surgical Techniques.* 2016;6(2):e24.
37. Gille J, Behrens P, Schulz AP, Oheim R, Kienast B. Matrix-associated autologous chondrocyte implantation. *Cartilage.* 2016;7(4):309–15.
38. Fu J-N, Wang X, Yang M, Chen Y-R, Zhang J-Y, Deng R-H, et al. Scaffold-based tissue engineering strategies for osteochondral repair. *Frontiers in Bioengineering and Biotechnology.* 2022;9: 812383. Published 2022 Jan 11. DOI:10.3389/fbioe.2021.812383.
39. Sun AX, Numpaisal P-O, Gottardi R, Shen H, Yang G, Tuan RS. Cell and biomimetic scaffold-based approaches for cartilage regeneration. *Operative Techniques in Orthopaedics.* 2016;26(3):135–46.
40. Chan BP, Leong KW. Scaffolding in tissue engineering: general approaches and tissue-specific considerations. *European Spine Journal.* 2008;17(S4):467–79.

41. Adel IM, ElMeligy MF, Elkasabgy NA. Conventional and recent trends of scaffolds fabrication: a superior mode for tissue engineering. *Pharmaceutics.* 2022;14(2):306. Published 2022 Jan 27. DOI:10.3390/pharmaceutics14020306.
42. Wei W, Dai H. Articular cartilage and osteochondral tissue engineering techniques: recent advances and challenges. *Bioactive Materials.* 2021;6(12):4830–55.
43. Wang C, Brisson BK, Terajima M, Li Q, Hoxha Kh, Han B, et al. Type III collagen is a key regulator of the collagen fibrillar structure and biomechanics of articular cartilage and meniscus. *Matrix Biology.* 2020;85–86:47–67.
44. Zhao Z, Li Y, Wang M, Zhao S, Zhao Z, Fang J. Mechanotransduction pathways in the regulation of cartilage chondrocyte homoeostasis. *Journal of Cellular and Molecular Medicine.* 2020;24(10):5408–19.
45. Mota C, Camarero-Espinosa S, Baker MB, Wieringa P, Moroni L. Bioprinting: from tissue and organ development to in vitro models. *Chemical Reviews.* 2020;120(19):10547–607.
46. Saini G, Segaran N, Mayer J, Saini A, Albadawi H, Oklu R. Applications of 3D bioprinting in tissue engineering and regenerative medicine. *Journal of Clinical Medicine.* 2021;10(21):4966. Published 2021 Oct 26. DOI:10.3390/jcm10214966.
47. Ramesh S, Harrysson OLA, Rao PK, Tamayol A, Cormier DR, Zhang Y, et al. Extrusion bioprinting: recent progress, challenges, and future opportunities. *Bioprinting.* 2021;21:e00116. ISSN 2405-8866, DOI:10.1016/j.bprint.2020.e00116.
48. Zhang YS, Haghiashtiani G, Hübscher T, Kelly DJ, Lee JM, Lutolf M, et al. 3D extrusion bioprinting. *Nature Reviews Methods Primers.* 2021;1(1):76. DOI:10.1038/s43586-021-00078-3.
49. Li X, Liu B, Pei B, Chen J, Zhou D, Peng J, et al. Inkjet bioprinting of biomaterials. Chemical Reviews. 2020;120(19):10793–833.
50. Ventura RD. An overview of laser-assisted bioprinting (LAB) in tissue engineering applications. *Medical Lasers.* 2021;10(2):76–81.
51. Gungor-Ozkerim PS, Inci I, Zhang YS, Khademhosseini A, Dokmeci MR. Bioinks for 3D bioprinting: an overview. *Biomaterials Science.* 2018;6(5):915–46.
52. Tarassoli SP, Jessop ZM, Jovic T, Hawkins K, Whitaker IS. Candidate bioinks for extrusion 3d bioprinting—a systematic review of the literature. *Frontiers in Bioengineering and Biotechnology.* 2021;9: 616753. Published 2021 Oct 13. DOI:10.3389/fbioe.2021.616753.
53. Szychlinska MA, Bucchieri F, Fucarino A, Ronca A, D'Amora U. Three-dimensional bioprinting for cartilage tissue engineering: insights into naturally-derived bioinks from land and marine sources. *Journal of Functional Biomaterials.* 2022;13(3):118. Published 2022 Aug 12. DOI:10.3390/jfb13030118.
54. Li M, Sun D, Zhang J, Wang Y, Wei Q, Wang Y. Application and development of 3D bioprinting in cartilage tissue engineering. *Biomaterials Science.* 2022;10(19):5430–58.
55. GhavamiNejad A, Ashammakhi N, Wu XY, Khademhosseini A. Crosslinking strategies for 3D bioprinting of polymeric hydrogels. *Small.* 2020;16(35): 2002931. DOI:10.1002/smll.202002931.
56. Lim KS, Galarraga JH, Cui X, Lindberg GCJ, Burdick JA, Woodfield TBF. Fundamentals and applications of photo-cross-linking in bioprinting. *Chemical Reviews.* 2020;120(19):10662–94.
57. Hazur J, Detsch R, Karakaya E, Kaschta J, Teßmar J, Schneidereit D, et al. Improving alginate printability for biofabrication: establishment of a universal and homogeneous pre-crosslinking technique. *Biofabrication.* 2020;12(4):045004. Published 2020 Jul 9. DOI:10.1088/1758-5090/ab98e5.
58. Fu Z, Ouyang L, Xu R, Yang Y, Sun W. Responsive biomaterials for 3D bioprinting: a review. *Materials Today.* 2022;52:112–32.
59. Persaud A, Maus A, Strait L, Zhu D. 3D bioprinting with live cells. *Engineered Regeneration.* 2022;3(3):292–309.

60. Hawksworth GM. Advantages and disadvantages of using human cells for pharmacological and toxicological studies. *Human & Experimental Toxicology.* 2016;13(8):568–73.
61. Leberfinger AN, Ravnic DJ, Dhawan A, Ozbolat IT. Concise review: bioprinting of stem cells for transplantable tissue fabrication. *Stem Cells Translational Medicine.* 2017;6(10):1940–8.
62. Pittenger MF, Discher DE, Péault BM, Phinney DG, Hare JM, Caplan AI. Mesenchymal stem cell perspective: cell biology to clinical progress. *NPJ Regenerative Medicine.* 2019;4:22. Published 2019 Dec 2. DOI:10.1038/s41536-019-0083-6.
63. Halevy T, Urbach A. Comparing ESC and iPSC—based models for human genetic disorders. *Journal of Clinical Medicine.* 2014;3(4):1146–62.
64. Dufaud M, Solé L, Maumus M, Simon M, Perrier-Groult E, Subra G, et al. 3D bioprinting of articular cartilage: recent advances and perspectives. *Bioprinting.* 2022;28: e00253. ISSN 2405-8866. DOI:10.1016/j.bprint.2022.e00253.
65. Lafuente-Merchan M, Ruiz-Alonso S, García-Villén F, Gallego I, Gálvez-Martín P, Saenz-del-Burgo L, et al. Progress in 3D bioprinting technology for osteochondral regeneration. *Pharmaceutics.* 2022;14(8):1578. Published 2022 Jul 29. DOI:10.3390/pharmaceutics14081578.
66. Pan RL, Martyniak K, Karimzadeh M, Gelikman DG, DeVries J, Sutter K, et al. Systematic review on the application of 3D-bioprinting technology in orthoregeneration: current achievements and open challenges. *Journal of Experimental Orthopaedics.* 2022;9(1):95. Published 2022 Sep 19. DOI:10.1186/s40634-022-00518-3.
67. Armiento AR, Stoddart MJ, Alini M, Eglin D. Biomaterials for articular cartilage tissue engineering: learning from biology. *Acta Biomaterialia.* 2018;65:1–20.
68. Abdollahiyan P, Oroojalian F, Mokhtarzadeh A, Guardia M. Hydrogel-based 3D bioprinting for bone and cartilage tissue engineering. *Biotechnology Journal.* 2020;15(12): e2000095. DOI:10.1002/biot.202000095.
69. Wu Y, Kennedy P, Bonazza N, Yu Y, Dhawan A, Ozbolat I. Three-dimensional bioprinting of articular cartilage: a systematic review. *Cartilage.* 2018;12(1):76–92.
70. Koo Y, Choi E-J, Lee J, Kim H-J, Kim G, Do SH. 3D printed cell-laden collagen and hybrid scaffolds for in vivo articular cartilage tissue regeneration. *Journal of Industrial and Engineering Chemistry.* 2018;66:343–55.
71. Yang X, Lu Z, Wu H, Li W, Zheng L, Zhao J. Collagen-alginate as bioink for three-dimensional (3D) cell printing based cartilage tissue engineering. *Materials Science and Engineering: C.* 2018;83:195–201.
72. Łabowska MB, Cierluk K, Jankowska AM, Kulbacka J, Detyna J, Michalak I. A review on the adaption of alginate-gelatin hydrogels for 3D cultures and bioprinting. *Materials.* 2021;14(4):858. Published 2021 Feb 10. DOI:10.3390/ma14040858.
73. Schipani R, Scheurer S, Florentin R, Critchley SE, Kelly DJ. Reinforcing interpenetrating network hydrogels with 3D printed polymer networks to engineer cartilage mimetic composites. *Biofabrication.* 2020;12(3):035011. Published 2020 May 12. DOI:10.1088/1758-5090/ab8708.
74. Costantini M, Idaszek J, Szöke K, Jaroszewicz J, Dentini M, Barbetta A, et al. 3D bioprinting of BM-MSCs-loaded ECM biomimetic hydrogels for in vitro neo-cartilage formation. Biofabrication. 2016;8(3):035002. Published 2016 Jul 19. DOI:10.1088/1758-5090/8/3/035002.
75. Ding Y-W, Zhang X-W, Mi C-H, Qi X-Y, Zhou J, Wei D-X. Recent advances in hyaluronic acid-based hydrogels for 3D bioprinting in tissue engineering applications. *Smart Materials in Medicine.* 2023;4:59–68.
76. Galarraga JH, Kwon MY, Burdick JA. 3D bioprinting via an in situ crosslinking technique towards engineering cartilage tissue. *Scientific Reports.* 2019;9(1):1–12.

77. Antich C, de Vicente J, Jiménez G, Chocarro C, Carrillo E, Montañez E, et al. Bio-inspired hydrogel composed of hyaluronic acid and alginate as a potential bioink for 3D bioprinting of articular cartilage engineering constructs. *Acta Biomaterialia*. 2020;106:114–23.
78. Nedunchezian S, Banerjee P, Lee C-Y, Lee S-S, Lin C-W, Wu C-W, et al. Generating adipose stem cell-laden hyaluronic acid-based scaffolds using 3D bioprinting via the double crosslinked strategy for chondrogenesis. *Materials Science and Engineering: C*. 2021;124:112072.
79. Sahranavard M, Sarkari S, Safavi S, Ghorbani F. Three-dimensional bio-printing of decellularized extracellular matrix-based bio-inks for cartilage regeneration: a systematic review. *Biomaterials Translational*. 2022;3(2):105.
80. Behan K, Dufour A, Garcia O, Kelly D. Methacrylated cartilage ECM-based hydrogels as injectables and bioinks for cartilage tissue engineering. *Biomolecules*. 2022;12(2):216.
81. Zhang X, Liu Y, Luo C, Zhai C, Li Z, Zhang Y, et al. Crosslinker-free silk/decellularized extracellular matrix porous bioink for 3D bioprinting-based cartilage tissue engineering. *Materials Science and Engineering: C*. 2021;118:111388.
82. Wang X, Wang Q, Xu C. Nanocellulose-based inks for 3D bioprinting: key aspects in research development and challenging perspectives in applications—a mini review. *Bioengineering*. 2020;7(2):40.
83. Nguyen D, Hägg DA, Forsman A, Ekholm J, Nimkingratana P, Brantsing C, et al. Cartilage tissue engineering by the 3D bioprinting of iPS cells in a nanocellulose/alginate bioink. *Scientific Reports*. 2017;7(1). DOI:10.1038/s41598-017-00690-y.
84. Gatenholm B, Lindahl C, Brittberg M, Simonsson S. Collagen 2A Type B induction after 3D bioprinting chondrocytes in situ into osteoarthritic chondral tibial lesion. *Cartilage*. 2020;13(2_suppl):1755S–69S.
85. Bandyopadhyay A, Mandal BB, Bhardwaj N. 3D bioprinting of photo-crosslinkable silk methacrylate (SilMA)-polyethylene glycol diacrylate (PEGDA) bioink for cartilage tissue engineering. *Journal of Biomedical Materials Research Part A*. 2021;110(4):884–98.
86. Chakraborty J, Majumder N, Sharma A, Prasad S, Ghosh S. 3D bioprinted silk-reinforced Alginate-Gellan Gum constructs for cartilage regeneration. *Bioprinting*. 2022;28:e00232.
87. Critchley S, Sheehy EJ, Cunniffe G, Diaz-Payno P, Carroll SF, Jeon O, et al. 3D printing of fibre-reinforced cartilaginous templates for the regeneration of osteochondral defects. *Acta Biomaterialia*. 2020;113:130–43.
88. Mouser VHM, Levato R, Mensinga A, Dhert WJA, Gawlitta D, Malda J. Bio-ink development for three-dimensional bioprinting of hetero-cellular cartilage constructs. *Connective Tissue Research*. 2018;61(2):137–51.
89. Di Bella C, Duchi S, O'Connell CD, Blanchard R, Augustine C, Yue Z, et al. In situ handheld three-dimensional bioprinting for cartilage regeneration. *Journal of Tissue Engineering and Regenerative Medicine*. 2017;12(3):611–21.
90. Liu Y, Peng L, Li L, Huang C, Shi K, Meng X, et al. 3D-bioprinted BMSC-laden biomimetic multiphasic scaffolds for efficient repair of osteochondral defects in an osteoarthritic rat model. *Biomaterials*. 2021;279:121216.
91. Shim J-H, Jang K-M, Hahn SK, Park JY, Jung H, Oh K, et al. Three-dimensional bioprinting of multilayered constructs containing human mesenchymal stromal cells for osteochondral tissue regeneration in the rabbit knee joint. *Biofabrication*. 2016;8(1):014102.
92. Ren X, Wang F, Chen C, Gong X, Yin L, Yang L. Engineering zonal cartilage through bioprinting collagen type II hydrogel constructs with biomimetic chondrocyte density gradient. *BMC Musculoskeletal Disorders*. 2016;17:301. Published 2016 Jul 20. DOI:10.1186/s12891-016-1130-8.

93. Levato R, Webb WR, Otto IA, Mensinga A, Zhang Y, van Rijen M, et al. The bio in the ink: cartilage regeneration with bioprintable hydrogels and articular cartilage-derived progenitor cells. *Acta Biomaterialia.* 2017;61:41–53.
94. Lim KS, Levato R, Costa PF, Castilho MD, Alcala-Orozco CR, van Dorenmalen KMA, et al. Bio-resin for high resolution lithography-based biofabrication of complex cell-laden constructs. *Biofabrication.* 2018;10(3):034101. Published 2018 May 11. DOI:10.1088/1758-5090/aac00c.
95. Kessel B, Lee M, Bonato A, Tinguely Y, Tosoratti E, Zenobi-Wong M. 3D bioprinting of macroporous materials based on entangled hydrogel microstrands. *Advanced Science.* 2020;7(18):2001419. Published 2020 Jul 19. DOI:10.1002/advs.202001419.
96. Rathan S, Dejob L, Schipani R, Haffner B, Möbius ME, Kelly DJ. Fiber reinforced cartilage ECM functionalized bioinks for functional cartilage tissue engineering. *Advanced Healthcare Materials.* 2019;8(7):e1801501. DOI:10.1002/adhm.201801501.
97. Chawla S, Kumar A, Admane P, Bandyopadhyay A, Ghosh S. Elucidating role of silk-gelatin bioink to recapitulate articular cartilage differentiation in 3D bioprinted constructs. *Bioprinting.* 2017;7:1–13.
98. Guo T, Noshin M, Baker HB, Taskoy E, Meredith SJ, Tang Q, et al. 3D printed bio-functionalized scaffolds for microfracture repair of cartilage defects. *Biomaterials.* 2018;185:219–31.

Index

For Product Safety Concerns and Information please contact our EU representative GPSR@taylorandfrancis.com
Taylor & Francis Verlag GmbH, Kaufingerstraße 24, 80331 München, Germany

www.ingramcontent.com/pod-product-compliance
Lightning Source LLC
Chambersburg PA
CBHW060814220326
41598CB00022B/2616

* 9 7 8 1 0 3 2 2 2 8 6 7 9 *